Physical Illness and Drugs of Abuse

of Abuse

A Review of the Evidence

Physical Illness and Drugs of Abuse
A Review of the Evidence

Adam J. Gordon
University of Pittsburgh, Pittsburgh, PA, USA

Contributing authors

Joanne M. Gordon
Missouri State University, Springfield, MO, USA

Kevin Carl
University of Pittsburgh, Pittsburgh, PA, USA

Michael T. Hilton
University of Pittsburgh, Pittsburgh, PA, USA

Joan M. Striebel
University of California, Los Angeles, CA, USA

Michael Maher
Georgetown University, Washington, DC, USA

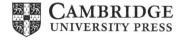
CAMBRIDGE
UNIVERSITY PRESS

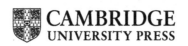

Shaftesbury Road, Cambridge CB2 8EA, United Kingdom

One Liberty Plaza, 20th Floor, New York, NY 10006, USA

477 Williamstown Road, Port Melbourne, VIC 3207, Australia

314–321, 3rd Floor, Plot 3, Splendor Forum, Jasola District Centre, New Delhi – 110025, India

103 Penang Road, #05–06/07, Visioncrest Commercial, Singapore 238467

Cambridge University Press is part of Cambridge University Press & Assessment, a department of the University of Cambridge.

We share the University's mission to contribute to society through the pursuit of education, learning and research at the highest international levels of excellence.

www.cambridge.org
Information on this title: www.cambridge.org/9780521133470

First published 2010

A catalogue record for this publication is available from the British Library

Library of Congress Cataloging-in-Publication data
Physical illness and drugs of abuse : a review of the evidence /
    Adam J. Gordon . . . [et al.].
        p. ; cm.
    Includes bibliographical references and index.
    ISBN 978-0-521-13347-0 (paperback)
    1. Substance abuse.   2. Drug abuse.   3. Comorbidity.
    4. Dual diagnosis.   I. Gordon, Adam J.
    [DNLM: 1. Substance-Related Disorders.
    2. Behavior, Addictive–complications.   3. Comorbidity.
    4. Diagnosis, Dual (Psychiatry)   5. Disease. WM 270 P5775 2010]
    RC564.68.P49 2010
    362.29–dc22   2009046278

ISBN   978-0-521-13347-0   Paperback

....

Every effort has been made in preparing this book to provide accurate and up-to-date information which is in accord with accepted standards and practice at the time of publication. Although case histories are drawn from actual cases, every effort has been made to disguise the identities of the individuals involved. Nevertheless, the authors, editors and publishers can make no warranties that the information contained herein is totally free from error, not least because clinical standards are constantly changing through research and regulation. The authors, editors and publishers therefore disclaim all liability for direct or consequential damages resulting from the use of material contained in this book. Readers are strongly advised to pay careful attention to information provided by the manufacturer of any drugs or equipment that they plan to use.

This book is dedicated to patients with
drug addictions: seek and demand the best
treatments for all your medical disorders

Contents

Foreword 1

Neglect of the high comorbidity of mental and physical illness is common despite its devastating consequences. Comorbidity worsens the prognosis of both comorbid illnesses, makes treatment less effective, and worsens the quality of life of the patient.

That comorbidity is not recognized in people who do not have contact with health services would be understandable, but that people with a physical and a mental illness who receive inpatient care get treatment for only one of them (for the physical illness in the non-psychiatric hospitals and for the mental illness in the mental hospital or ward) borders on punishable neglect, on a *vitium artis*. The situation is even worse for people who suffer from comorbid conditions and do not have access to the necessary examinations and care. Quantifying the amount of damage done by this neglect is difficult, but there are some indications showing that it is vast. For example, the life expectancy of people with schizophrenia (not in itself a disease with a fatal outcome) is about 20 years shorter than that of people without schizophrenia. This loss of years is probably mainly a result of the disease rather than to other causes of death (e.g., suicide or homicide). Similar reductions of life expectancy have been reported for other mental disorders (Angst *et al.* 2003) and for psychosocial problems such as those related to the use of alcohol and drugs.

In spite of findings of studies that show the frequency and type of comorbidity, little is done in response. Many mental hospitals have no laboratories that would help to promote the physical health of those who are admitted for treatment of their mental illness, and psychiatrists rarely make physical examinations. In Europe, 40% of the psychiatrists in private practice declare that they are examining the physical condition of their patients, but there is doubt about the quality and frequency of these examinations. Non-psychiatric institutions and healthcare workers identify only the most serious forms of mental disorders, and when they do, they usually refer patients to psychiatrists for treatment rather than undertaking it themselves.

The lack of awareness of the problem of comorbidity and the absence of service arrangements that could deal with it is not uncommon in developed countries; the situation is even worse in the developing world. Mental health programs have low priority, and there are rarely budgetary provisions for the treatment of physical illnesses in mentally ill people. Ignorance, scarcity of resources, and prejudice also prevent mental healthcare in the general health service system. Consequently, a major public health problem – providing adequate care to people with both mental and physical disorders – receives extremely little attention, even less than the treatment of mental disorders.

These were among the reasons that the Association for the Improvement of Mental Health Programmes (AIMHP), a not-for-profit non-governmental organization in Geneva, undertook to stimulate the production of a series of authoritative reviews bringing together the evidence for the comorbidity of mental and physical disorders. The goals of this initiative were to raise awareness of the problem and create an easily accessible knowledge base for programs that would address it. The project has been developed in collaboration with the World Health Organization and, in its course, the AIMHP has worked hand in hand with other organizations and associations.

The first book in the series dealt with the comorbidity of schizophrenia and physical illness (Leucht *et al.* 2007), and four others – of which the volume produced by Dr. Adam Gordon and his colleagues is one – will follow. The topics addressed in the other volumes in preparation are physical illnesses in people with intellectual disability, somatic illnesses in people with dementia, and physical illnesses in people with depressive disorders. The last will be produced in collaboration with the World Psychiatric Association, which recognized the impact of comorbidity, and in its work plan for the years 2008–2011 (Maj 2008) has undertaken to produce three volumes addressing depression comorbid with diabetes, cardiovascular disorders, and cancer.

It gives me great pleasure to see the volume produced by Dr. Gordon and his colleagues in print for three reasons. First, the problem of physical illness in people using drugs and alcohol is vast and it is important to make access to knowledge as easy as possible for decision makers and practitioners. Second, this book is produced with the encouragement and support of the US National Institute of Drug Abuse, which imparts additional credibility and contributes to the goal of the AIMHP to involve both governmental and non-governmental organizations in this endeavor. Third, Dr. Gordon's book presents a comprehensive review of knowledge in a clear and objective form, allowing its use in policy making and education.

The true reward for the tremendous amount of work that Dr. Gordon and his colleagues have undertaken will be the wide use of the knowledge that they have assembled and presented. I hope, therefore, that the readers of this book will use it in efforts to raise awareness about the nature and magnitude of the problem of comorbidity, in its prevention, and in the treatment of patients who suffer from it.

Professor Norman Sartorius, MD, PhD
President, Association for the Improvement of Mental Health Programmes
Geneva, Switzerland
May 2009

Foreword 2

Despite tantalizing evidence that drug use and drug use disorders may be related to a number of medical conditions, little work has been done to summarize this literature for the medical community. Dr. Gordon, as the editor, and the authors of this volume have addressed this gap by summarizing evidence from the world's literature over the past 20 years relating illicit substance abuse to medical conditions. This work is an essential step in integrating addiction medicine within the broader medical community. The background provided by Dr. Gordon and colleagues will serve as a base to embed addiction within a general medical framework.

According to a World Health Organization Report in 2002, illicit drug abuse (i.e., excluding alcohol and tobacco use) is among the 10 leading preventable risk factors for years of healthy life lost and disability in developed countries. The economic cost of illicit drug abuse in the USA was estimated at almost $181 billion in 2002 (Office of National Drug Control Policy 2004). While the majority of the cost of drug abuse is related to crime and the resulting costs of the criminal justice system, an increasing proportion is being spent on medical care. This is especially true as the human immunodeficiency virus and hepatitis C virus continue to spread through injection drug abuse.

The editor and writers of this text have performed a systematic review of studies detailing the epidemiological relationship of drugs of abuse and their routes of administration with the development of medical conditions, focusing mainly on the last 20 years. Yet, this text is much more than a compendium of epidemiological studies. The authors have combined their clinical experience and epidemiological knowledge to provide the context that will aid the reader in understanding how drug abuse plays a role in the etiology of a wide variety of medical conditions. This makes this text valuable as not only a clinical textbook but also as a clinical epidemiological guide that highlights the strengths and weaknesses of the wide variety of studies presented. The text is organized first by listing the specific drugs and then by highlighting a complete list of organ systems affected. We know of no other published source that provides this comprehensive and thorough a review of the current literature of physical illnesses and drugs of abuse.

Conventional wisdom would state that drug abuse is responsible for a wide variety of medical disorders. For example, one study of 747 drug-abusing patients from a large health maintenance organization were compared with 3690 demographically matched controls from the same organization (Mertens *et al.* 2003). This study found that approximately one-third of the medical conditions examined were more common among drug-abusing patients than among the matched controls, and several of the conditions were found to be the most costly. Nevertheless, conclusive associations between physical conditions and drug abuse are often not apparent. In this careful and thorough review, Dr. Gordon and the authors show that the epidemiological association between drugs of abuse and medical disorders is not always clear, partly because of the relative dearth of studies in this area, with the notable exception of infectious diseases related to injection administration. This is not surprising since addiction medicine is a relatively new specialty and the body of literature is still being developed. In addition, the physical health effects of drug abuse vary greatly. The wide spectrum of physical disorders involves virtually all of the physiological systems of the body, further confusing and complicating the association between medical conditions and drug abuse. Dr. Gordon and the authors confirm that evidence is lacking in many areas of interest, but by establishing the evidence base in a comprehensive way this text helps to point the way for future areas of investigation.

Richard A. Denisco MD, MPH
Wilson M. Compton MD, MPE
Division of Epidemiology, Services, and Prevention Research
National Institute on Drug Abuse
Bethesda, MD, USA
May, 2009

Preface

This is the one of a series of volumes addressing an issue that is emerging as a priority in the mental health field: the timely and proper recognition of physical health problems in people with severe mental disorders. It is well documented that there is a higher prevalence of severe physical diseases and a higher mortality from natural causes among people with severe mental disorders than in the general population. It is also understood that medical and psychiatric illnesses often coexist – and that an appreciation of integrating care for comorbid illness enhances patients' health and well-being. Alcohol and substance use disorders are severe mental disorders that impact patients' health and welfare.

In treatment settings, patients with substance use disorders need attention to not only their substance use but also their mental and physical health comorbidities. By screening, assessing, and treating their comorbid mental and physical health conditions, providers can improve patient-, provider-, and system-level outcomes.

Patients want and demand this type of care. As an internist and director of medical clinics in drug and alcohol treatment settings and director of a substance abuse assessment team in a large tertiary care hospital system, I have witnessed first-hand the need to provide concurrent medical care alongside well-established substance use and mental healthcare for patients with drug use disorders. Patients who use illicit substances have medical conditions such as hypertension, diabetes, and hypercholesterolemia, and they deserve attention to these disorders. As internists often consult mental health providers for psychiatric and behavioral health problems of patients who use illicit substances, so too must mental health providers who care for these patients seek consultation with physical health providers for comorbid medical disease assessment and management. As internists are more comfortable treating uncomplicated depression, so too should mental health providers care for uncomplicated physical ailments – such as those encountered in patients with substance use disorders.

Comorbidity is more than a substance use disorder and mental illness; it can also be substance use disorder and a physical health illness. This book attempts to describe the latest peer-reviewed evidence of the associations between substance use and physical health conditions. Hopefully, this knowledge will assist all clinicians to screen, assess, and treat – or refer to treatment – medical illnesses in their patients with substance use problems. Our patients deserve this awareness and integrative healthcare practice.

Adam J. Gordon, MD, MPH, FACP, FASAM
Pittsburgh, PA, USA
May 2009

Acknowledgements

Cover art

"Nebula" (1989) by Andrew S. Gordon.

Acknowledgements

The authors are indebted to the following people, centers, and programs that assisted in the development and preparation of this work. This material is based upon work supported by infrastructure support and/or funding by the National Institute on Drug Abuse; National Institutes of Health and the Department of Veterans Affairs; Veterans Health Administration; VISN 4 Mental Illness Research, Education, and Clinical Center (MIRECC); Health Services Research and Development Service Center for Health Equity Research and Promotion (CHERP); VA Pittsburgh Healthcare System; the University of Pittsburgh School of Medicine; and the Division of General Internal Medicine at the University of Pittsburgh Medical Center.

The authors wish to thank Drs. Compton Wilson, Richard Denisco, and Norman Sartorius for proposing and initiating this project in the winter of 2007. The authors also thank Drs. Darius Rastegar and Joshua Blum, other members of the Substance Abuse Interest Group of the Society of General Internal Medicine for review of portions of this manuscript. A special thank you goes to Margaret Krumm, BA, for conducting the original literature searches and editing portions of this manuscript.

Dr. Joanne M. Gordon would like to thank her husband Albert and sons Adam and Andrew for their support during this project, and also her professional colleagues and students who helped to make the classroom, clinical, and research laboratories creative and exciting learning environments.

Dr. Adam J. Gordon wishes to thank his professional and research mentors, Drs. Joseph Conigliaro, Kevin Kraemer, Thomas O'Toole, Paul Freyder, and David Macpherson – thank you for your professional stewardship and your ability to model professionalism and excitement for providing the best, evidence-based healthcare for medically underserved populations. Dr. Gordon also wishes to thank Drs. Wishwa Kapoor at the University of Pittsburgh Division of General Internal Medicine, Michael J. Fine at CHERP, and Gretchen Haas at MIRECC for ongoing professional guidance and infrastructure support. Finally, he wishes to thank his wife Molly Conroy, MD, MPH, daughter Lillian, and his parents, Albert and Joanne, for their love, patience, and support.

Abbreviations

5-HT	5-hydroxytryptamine
ADAM	Arrestee Drug Abuse Monitoring program
AIDS	acquired immunodeficiency syndrome
AIN	acute interstitial nephritis
AMI	acute myocardial infarction
ANCA	anti-neutrophilic cytoplasmic antibodies (c, cytoplasmic; p, periplasmic)
ANS	autonomic nervous system
AOR	adjusted odds ratio
ARF	acute renal failure
ASI	Addiction Severity Index
AST	aspartate aminotransferase
AUDIT	Alcohol Use Disorders Identification Test
BA	Brodmann areas
BMI	body mass index
BOLD	blood oxygen level dependent
BP	blood pressure
BRAC	Basic Rest–Activity Cycle
CAD	coronary artery disease
CAL	combined periodontal attachment loss
CARDIA	Coronary Artery Risk Development in Young Adults study
CART	cocaine-and-amphetamine-regulated transcript
CB1 and CB2	cannabinoid receptors
CHF	congestive heart failure
CI	confidence interval
CIDUS	Collaborative Injection Drug User Study
CIMDL	cocaine-induced midline destructive lesions
CIP	cocaine-induced psychosis
CK	creatine kinase
CNS	central nervous system
CRF	corticotropin-releasing factor
CT	computed tomography
CVA	cerebrovascular accidents
DAWN	US Federal Drug Abuse Warning Network
DKA	diabetic ketoacidosis
DMIOS	Determinants of Myocardial Infarction Onset Study
DSC-MRI	dynamic susceptibility contrast magnetic resonance imaging
DSM-III	*Diagnostic and Statistical Manual of Mental Disorders*, 3rd edition (DSMIII-R, 3rd edition revised)

DSM-IV	*Diagnostic and Statistical Manual of Mental Disorders*, 4th edition
DTI	diffusion tensor imaging
EC	endocannabinoids
ECG	electrocardiogram
ECHO	echoencephalography
EEG	electroencephalogram
ESRD	end-stage renal disease
FA	fractional anisotropy
FEV_1	forced expiratory volume in 1 second
fMRI	functional MRI
FVC	forced vital capacity
GABA	gamma-aminobutyric acid
GBM	glomerular basement membrane
GUD	genital ulcer disease
HAV	hepatitis A virus
HBV	hepatitis B virus
HBRA	hypnotic benzodiazepine receptor agonists
HCV	hepatitis C virus
HIV	human immunodeficiency virus
HNE	human neutrophil elastase
HPPD	hallucinogen persisting perception disorder
HSV	herpes simplex virus
IDU	injection drug users
IOM	Institute of Medicine
IQ	intelligence quotient
IUGR	intrauterine growth retardation
LBW	low birthweight
LSD	D-lysergic acid diethylamide
MDMA	3,4-methylenedioxymethamphetamine (ecstasy)
MI	myocardial infarction
MRI	magnetic resonance imaging
MRS	magnetic resonance spectroscopy
MRSA	methicillin-resistant *Staphylococcus aureus*
NAS	neonatal abstinence syndrome
NHL	non-Hodgkin's lymphoma
OR	odds ratio
PAH	pulmonary arterial hypertension
PCR	polymerase chain reaction
PET	positron emission tomography
PID	pelvic inflammatory disease
PRISM	Program of Research to Integrate Substance Use Issues into Mainstream Healthcare
RBMT	Rivermead Behavioral Memory Test
RR	relative risk
SAH	subarachnoid hemorrhage
SD	standard deviation
SEM	standard error of mean

STD	sexually transmitted disease
TB	tuberculosis
TCBC	transitional cell bladder cancer
THC	Δ^9-tetrahydrocannabinol
VC	vital capacity
WG	Wegener's granulomatosis
WHO	World Health Organization

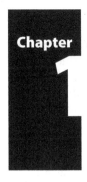

Introduction

Use of illicit substances contributes to significant morbidity and mortality worldwide. In the USA, drug use is a leading cause of preventable death and contributes to the incidence and morbidity of other mental health and physical health conditions. Healthcare providers are well aware that use of illicit substances is associated with environmental and social harms; it is not unusual for a person with an addiction to be unemployed, homeless, impoverished, or associated with illegal activities. These social morbidities also contribute to poor physical health by influencing such things as sanitation, medication compliance, and risky behaviors. Most of the current criteria to diagnose both substance abuse (four) and substance dependence (seven) disorders have little to do with the amount of substance used but rather the non-medical harm associated with its use (American Psychiatric Association 2000). Simply put, drug addiction is a complex illness that impacts mental, physical, and environmental health.

Recent advances in addiction research have indicated that a pathophysiological basis for disease exists for many illicit substances: addiction is not simply a behavior of compulsive consumption of a substance. The association of use of various illicit substances with various mental health conditions has been firmly established; however, the association between illicit substance use and physical health conditions is less known. The influence of illicit substance use on comorbid conditions is important and often under-recognized by the treatment provider. Associations of illicit substances with medical health conditions – whether epidemiological or causative in nature – play important roles in how patients interact with the healthcare system and how providers interact with patients who use illicit substances. Comorbidity among people with psychiatric conditions – including medical conditions and substance use and abuse – is recognized as a significant challenge for mental healthcare providers and even more of a challenge for generalist healthcare providers.

Nonetheless, it is becoming increasing clear that treatments that attend to patients' comorbid conditions need to be developed, and that generalist healthcare providers ought to assess and treat addiction disorders within the confines of generalist settings. In fact, recent principles of effective treatment published by the US National Institutes of Health, National Institute on Drug Abuse indicate that addictive disorders should be assessed and treated in the presence of comorbid mental health and physical health conditions (National Institute on Drug Abuse 2009).

It is challenging to encourage generalist providers to attend to addictive disorders. Perhaps generalist physician treatment of addictive disorders will be aided by the current attention to the quality of medical care. The US Preventative Services Task Force recommends routine screening for alcohol use and brief counseling interventions. In addition, a recently published report from the Institute of Medicine (IOM), *Improving the Quality of*

Health Care for Mental and Substance-Use Conditions, addresses this issue (Institute of Medicine 2005). This report was the product of an IOM consensus process in which experts in a range of disciplines impacting the broad fields of mental health and addiction medicine reviewed the literature and developed an agenda for changing the approach to the treatment and prevention of these conditions. An underlying theme of the IOM is that only by addressing substance use and mental health problems can one achieve optimal benefit for patients in medical care. Integration of mental health, physical health, and substance abuse services promotes optimal benefits to the provider and the patient (Gordon *et al.* 2007).

One of the most important recommendations of the IOM report pertains to the delivery of coordinated care by providers of primary care, mental health, and substance use treatment. The basis of this recommendation lies in the "crossing the quality chasm" rules, which endorse "shared knowledge and the free flow of information" and "cooperation among clinicians." Specifically, coordination models can be straightforward (e.g., formal agreements among providers of mental healthcare, substance use care, and primary care) or moving incrementally towards more complex arrangements (e.g., case management among systems, collocation of services, clinically integrated practices of all of these healthcare providers) (Institute of Medicine 2001). Evidence suggests that the more complex arrangements yield improved patient outcomes. Other recommendations addressed to all clinicians – including primary care physicians – included the need to screen all mental health patients for alcohol and drug use problems given the high comorbidity of these conditions and the need to maintain a patient-centered approach to the care of the patient with alcohol and drug problems.

Recent work from the Program of Research to Integrate Substance Use Issues into Mainstream Healthcare (PRISM) has revealed the impact of substance use on disparate medical conditions including diabetes mellitus, hypertension, low back pain, sleep, depression, lung cancer, chronic obstructive pulmonary disease, and osteoporosis (Howard *et al.* 2004; McFadden *et al.* 2005; Mehra *et al.* 2006; Stein *et al.* 2004; Sullivan *et al.* 2005). The increasing attention to the impact of substance use disorders on patients' medical outcomes will continue to drive efforts to engage all physicians in identifying and treating these disorders.

This book examines the epidemiological associations between physical illness and drugs of abuse. Drugs of abuse impart significant morbidity and mortality on people worldwide; in the USA, they are the ninth leading cause of preventable deaths (Mokdad *et al.* 2004). A number of reviews have examined the comorbid or co-occurring disorders of drug use and mental health disorders, but no review has systematically examined the epidemiological associations between various drugs of abuse and physical illness. Furthermore, leading textbooks in addiction medicine and internal medicine (Graham & Schultz 1998; Kasper *et al.* 2005) do not adequately review the physical morbidity associated with drugs of abuse. Recently, three textbooks have been published that highlight some physical health problems associated with alcohol and other drugs of abuse (Brick 2008; Frances *et al.* 2005; Rastegar & Fingerhood 2005). However, no systematic, comprehensive review of the recent peer-reviewed literature relating the physical diseases associated with drugs of abuse has been completed.

Therefore, the purpose of this book is to examine the relationships between drugs of abuse and physical illness. Secondary purposes are to critically review the current literature regarding these associations and to suggest future research in this field. Finally, we hope to promote practitioners' awareness, identification, and engagement of physical illnesses that afflict patients who abuse drugs.

Unfortunately, the literature regarding the associations of substance use disorders with medical illness is vast and often specific to a certain illicit drug or medical disease process. The approach in this book is to examine – comprehensively and critically – the recent evidence of causal and correlative association of substance use/abuse and physical illness. This approach will thus provide a resource for clinicians, investigators, and policy makers.

The scope of this book is narrower than that of medical literature of the same topic. First, we excluded from our evaluation of the literature associations based on the route of administration. The association of illicit substance use and increased incidence of infections by hepatitis viruses, human immunodeficiency virus (HIV), and sexual transmitted disease (STD) pathogens are well known; it is less clear whether the actual drug of abuse is the linking factor to the disease process. For instance, hepatitis and HIV are associated with intravenous drug use (particularly heroin/opioid injection), but it is likely that the intravenous administration of the illicit drug is the comorbid link, not the drug itself.

Second, we examined the identified peer-reviewed literature in PubMed (www.PubMed.gov) from January 1, 1988 through December 2008. Certainly, studies prior to 1988 examined co-occurring or comorbid medical illnesses. Recent reviews (Brick 2008; Frances et al. 2005; Graham & Schultz 1998; Rastegar & Fingerhood 2005) have noted many of them. However, our intention was to examine the latest literature. In addition, the decision to examine recent literature reflected curiosity as to whether recent studies were examining associations of substance use and medical comorbidities, and a desire to assess the quality of these studies and to examine where gaps in knowledge are occurring. Finally, the decision to examine recent literature greatly reduced the number of studies the authors needed to critically examine.

Third, the scope of this book is limited by an examination of associations of medical illnesses with only a few illicit substances. Patients around the world abuse an unknown number of illicit substances. We decided to limit our examination of the literature to four broad classes of illicit substances: cocaine, marijuana, opioids, and common hallucinogens and stimulants. These substances are more likely to affect several organ systems, have been studied intensely, have known mental health comorbid associations, and are relatively common around the world.

The book is divided into chapters by drug of abuse and subsections examining the associations between the drug and each physical illness domain. The published relationships for each of the drugs are examined with respect to each physical disease (e.g., infectious, neoplastic, musculoskeletal, etc.).

The addiction literature is rife with misleading terms and inaccuracies in diagnostic and treatment terminology. Definitions should be clear, without ambiguity. One of the most important advances in addiction medicine over the last few years is to simplify and specify terms in addiction medicine. Therefore, before embarking on examination of the literature, the following definitions will be used.

Addiction: a chronic, relapsing disease characterized by compulsive drug seeking and abuse in spite of known adverse consequences, and by functional, sometimes long-lasting changes in the brain.

Comorbidity: the occurrence of two disorders or illnesses in the same person, either at the same time (co-occurring comorbid conditions) or with a time difference between the initial occurrence of one and the initial occurrence of the other (sequentially comorbid conditions).

Mental disorder: a mental condition marked primarily by sufficient disorganization of personality, mind, and emotions to seriously impair the normal psychological or behavioral functioning of the individual.

Physical health disorder: a disease, not otherwise a mental disorder, that impairs the health of an individual and is a diagnosable illness.

Substance use: use of illicit substances that are generally not intended for use and not prescribed by a healthcare provider. Substance use may or may not meet diagnostic criteria for either substance abuse or substance dependence.

Substance abuse: defined by harmful consequences of repeated use but does not include the compulsive use, tolerance, or withdrawal, which can be signs of addiction, or substance dependence. Defined by the *Diagnostic and Statistical Manual of Mental Disorders*, 4th edition (DSM-IV).

Substance dependence: defined by criteria of DSM-IV, which may include consequences of use, compulsion to use, tolerance, and withdrawal.

The need to develop treatments that take comorbidity into account is increasingly recognized. Identifying, managing, and treating comorbid medical illness among people with psychiatric conditions – including the comorbid conditions of substance use, abuse, and dependence – is a significant challenge for clinicians, researchers, and policy makers. Substance use occurs in many patients with psychiatric disorders, and comorbidity with mental health disorders is the rule rather than the exception among some people, such as the elderly, chronically ill, or homeless patients. Comorbidity impacts the course of mental health problems and leads to exacerbations of symptoms and increased healthcare utilization. Those with mental health disorders and another comorbid condition also experience barriers to treatment.

Providers should recognize that substance use and physical health conditions also co-occur. While it is difficult to disentangle the overlapping symptoms of drug use with physical health (and mental health) disorders, an awareness of co-occurrence and association of substance use with physical conditions may prompt providers to recognize and treat these conditions. While the harm of physical health conditions and substance use is not necessarily additive, the morbidity of both types of condition contributes to deleterious outcomes and treatment responses to both. Awareness is the first step in addressing substance use and physical health comorbidity.

Chapter 2 — Methods

Similar to the methods described by Leucht *et al.* (2007), we conducted a detailed search of an electronic PubMed database to identify all articles that indicated a relationship between an illicit drug of abuse and physical illnesses. The search identified key words (and words within titles and abstracts) associated with major categories of illicit drugs of abuse (1) marijuana, (2) cocaine, (3) opioids, (4) hallucinogens, stimulants, benzodiazepines, and barbiturates and combined each with major categories of physical illness. These key words included such terms as "crack" for cocaine and "heroin" for opioids.

A broad search strategy was conducted to ensure that all physical illnesses that corresponded to an illicit drug were identified. The Medical Subject Headings (MeSH) terms for each drug of abuse were combined with the approximately 23 MeSH terms for the general disease categories of physical diseases. To obtain the latest results, the search was limited to January 1, 1988 to December 1, 2008 (approximately the last 20 years). The search was limited to peer-reviewed literature regarding human studies and in the English language. It was not restricted to only population-based or controlled studies in order to identify as many potential studies as possible that indicated even limited associations between drugs of abuse and physical illness.

The MeSH terms were included for the major categories of physical illness:
1. Infectious disease (including bacterial, mycotic, parasitic, and viral infections)
2. Neoplastic disease
3. Musculoskeletal disease
4. Digestive system disease
5. Stomatognathic disease
6. Respiratory system disease
7. Otorhinolaryngological disease
8. Nervous system disease
9. Ocular disease
10. Male urological, renal, and genital disease
11. Female urological and gynecological disease, and neonatal, congenital, and pregnancy disease
12. Cardiovascular disease
13. Dermatological disease
14. Nutritional and metabolic disease
15. Endocrine system disease
16. Immune system disease

17. Environmental disease
18. Other pathological conditions (if any).

Because the focus of the search and subsequent review of the literature were on human epidemiological associations, "animal associations" associated with illicit substances of abuse were not included in the search.

The first search was made in February 2008, and an update search was completed on December 1, 2008. After the initial search strategy, all the abstracts were read. Potentially relevant articles were then reviewed for more detailed inspection. At the beginning of each section, the number of abstracts initially reviewed in each search strategy is noted for each drug of abuse. After this initial search, known review articles, books, and book chapters were also used to supplement the search findings and identify studies that were not found in the initial search strategy. In addition, references within the identified articles were examined for additional sources of associations between the drug of abuse and physical illness, but all mentioned and summarized articles were still restricted to the time frame of the primary search (1988 to 2008).

All authors contributed to the content of every chapter, but specific authors had primary responsibility for specific chapters and led the writing for that chapter. As such, there were some deviations from secondary search strategies. The drafts of all chapters were sent for external peer review for comment on completeness and narrative (see the Acknowledgements).

Each chapter summarizes the literature in the searched time frame for a specific drug of abuse or groups of drugs of abuse. Each chapter commences with a general description of the drug of abuse. Each subsequent subsection then examines associations of that drug of abuse with the major categories of physical illness. At the end of each chapter, a summary section examines research implications and a table indicates the evidence of association between drugs of abuse and each category of physical illness, and any research implications. The quality of the literature for many associations was not strong, and many associations were "case reports" or "limited subject" descriptions of evidence. A general summary at the end of each chapter considers the quality of the literature when possible and summarizes the strengths of the associations.

It is important to note that this review is not all-inclusive of the evidence of association of drugs of abuse with the major categories of physical illness because it summarizes the recent (1988 to 2008) literature. It may be that associations have been found prior to 1988; if this is a prominent association it is often indicated but the findings are not summarized as the literature was outside the search time frame. In addition, drugs of abuse are often inhaled, injected, or otherwise administered, and the administration route may be associated with physical findings and major clinical diseases. A classic example is the strong association of injected drug use with hepatitis C virus (HCV) infection. Often, it is unclear whether the association reflects the intravenous route of administration or is specifically with the hepatitis virus. Because of this quandary, we chose not to select and summarize literature regarding associations between route of administration and illness.

Results: cocaine

Introduction

Cocaine is a powerful, addictive drug that has been used as a stimulant for centuries. The drug can be smoked, snorted, and injected intravenously, subcutaneously, or intramuscularly. Abused by over six million Americans in 2006, most of the users are between the ages of 12 and 60. At the beginning of the twentieth century, cocaine was a component of throat lozenges and tonic waters, and it was frequently used as an anesthetic. The Harrison Act of 1914 outlawed the use of cocaine and opiates, and the 1970 Controlled Substance Act in the USA further restricted use. (Das 1993; Warner 1993). However, its availability and addictive properties have made cocaine a highly abused drug in the USA.

The consequences of using cocaine vary among its users. Psychoses, violent behavior, cardiovascular and nervous system events, and altered pregnancy outcomes have all been described in the literature. This chapter reviews the epidemiological research included in the PubMed database and published between 1988 and 2008 that explores the relationship between cocaine and various health conditions. Each of the following subsections provides a synopsis of the research, followed by a commentary on the research and tables highlighting the major findings. Where appropriate, suggestions are made for additional research that might strengthen or clarify the role of cocaine in adverse health outcomes. Since research may overlap several topics, articles are cross-referenced where appropriate and may be described in several subsections.

While the review of the epidemiological literature primarily addresses the effect of cocaine use that might influence or cause altered physiology in the body systems, this introductory subsection provides some background information about cocaine that might provide insight into how cocaine might influence body function.

Cocaine HCl is a white crystalline powder derived from the coca plant (*Erythroxylum coca*) that is native to the Andes Mountains. The powder can be snorted, sniffed, or dissolved in water and injected. Crack cocaine is an inexpensive alkaloid of cocaine that is smoked, and it may be found as off-white chips, chunks, or rocks.

Cocaine binds to the dopamine transporters on presynaptic neurons and interferes with the transporter's ability to reabsorb dopamine into the presynaptic neuron. This results in an accumulation of dopamine in the synapse and a prolonged dopamine effect on the target organ. Over time, with prolonged exposure, the dopamine receptors are downregulated and signal transduction is altered. This leads to a decrease in dopamine signaling, which may contribute to addiction by affecting the brain reward system, reinforcing the need for additional cocaine use.

Besides interaction with dopamine transporters, cocaine also affects the serotonergic system by inhibiting reuptake of various members of the serotonin (5-hydroxytryptamine,

5-HT) family, resulting in an increase of some 5-HT receptors. Norepinephrine reuptake is also blocked by cocaine, resulting in stimulation of the sympathetic nervous system and subsequent sympathetic nervous system responses (e.g., elevation of blood pressure, increased heart rate). Cocaine's influence includes affecting the dopaminergic, serotonergic, and adrenergic pathways throughout the body. Some recent laboratory research has shown that cocaine can inhibit sigma receptors and serotonergic and adrenergic transmitters on placental tissue. The effect of this action on fetal development is an area of ongoing study.

Other receptors may also be affected by cocaine, including sigma receptors (where cocaine is a ligand) and the glutamate N-methyl D-aspartate (NMDA) receptors. Sigma receptor stimulation can lead to increased muscle activity and tachycardia. Seizure activity may be enhanced by cocaine stimulation of sigma receptors. Cocaine may also stimulate endothelial cells to release endothelin-1, which is a strong vasoconstrictor and can cause vasospasm, thus contributing to cardiovascular effects of cocaine.

Once in the plasma, only approximately 1% of cocaine is excreted unchanged in the urine. While most of the drug is metabolized in the liver to benzoylecgonine, other urinary metabolites include ecgonine methyl ester and ecgonine. Urine metabolites can be found within hours and as long as 10 days after heavy cocaine use. Since cocaine can be detected in the hair of users, hair samples have been used in diagnostic tests for cocaine exposure.

The physiological effects of cocaine can be experienced in 10 to 30 minutes if cocaine is inhaled or injected, or in 5 to 10 minutes after smoking. The half-life of cocaine in the plasma is approximately 50 minutes.

The action of cocaine is dose dependent. In low to moderate doses, cocaine can cause vasoconstriction and an increase in heart rate and blood pressure. Cocaine use is associated with cardiac arrhythmias, which can lead to cardiac arrest or seizures and respiratory arrest. An increased risk of cerebro- and cardiovascular incidents is possible. The behavioral effects on the central nervous system (CNS) include increased arousal, increased performance on tasks of vigilance, and alertness. Cocaine can increase self-confidence, sense of well-being, energy, and euphoria. A decreased appetite may also be seen in cocaine users.

In high doses, cocaine may lead to enhanced euphoria, arousal, and restlessness. Involuntary motor activity may also occur. Paranoia and increased irritability can increase the risk of violent behavior. Seizures may also occur. In a "cocaine crash", or withdrawal, the individual may experience depression, fatigue, jumpiness, and fearfulness.

Cocaine can interact with other drugs taken concurrently, including alcohol and nicotine. Cocaine and alcohol form cocaethylene in the liver. The effects of cocaethylene are similar to the pharmacological effects of cocaine, particularly in blocking dopamine uptake, and often results in a greater euphoria than that seen with cocaine use alone. Cocaethylene appears to be less effective in blocking norepinephrine and 5-HT transporters. Nicotine increases the dopamine levels in the CNS; consequently, the combination of nicotine and cocaine can result in increased euphoria. Nicotine appears to affect dopaminergic neurons associated with motor and cognitive function, and also has a role in motivational aspects of drug abuse.

Crack use results in consequences similar to cocaine, but because it is often smoked, there is a quicker onset and more intense response than with powdered cocaine. Crack users may have a greater likelihood of psychotic responses, hyperactivity, and violence.

Use of cocaine in any form can stimulate muscle activity, resulting in increased heat production (pyrogenic effect). Because increased dopamine and norepinephrine levels will cause increased vasoconstriction, this can lead to ischemic muscle damage, which increases the risk of rhabdomyolysis and its consequences.

Cocaine withdrawal is generally mild but may result in dysphoria, depression, sleepiness, and fatigue. Bradycardia may also occur. Unlike other drugs of abuse, cocaine causes a "crash", and patients in cocaine withdrawal "sleep off" the withdrawal effects.

Besides use as a psychological/physiological stimulant, cocaine has been used as a local anesthetic, primarily in eye and ear–nose–throat surgery. Cocaine blocks nerve action potentials and inhibits local norepinephrine uptake in the central and peripheral nervous systems. It is seldom used in the USA because of the availability of safer local anesthetics. However, cocaine is still used as a local anesthetic in some areas of the world.

Short- and long-term effects of cocaine use have been described in the literature. The following sections discuss the epidemiological research that describes the role of cocaine use in a number of body functions.

Infections

In a review of epidemiological studies published between 1988 and 2008, a search of PubMed found five articles on bacterial infections, one article on mycoses, nine articles on viral disease other than HIV, and two articles on parasitic infections. These articles are described in the following subsections. Additional discussion of infections and cocaine use may be found in other relevant subsections (e.g., genital, cardiovascular, respiratory).

Bacterial infections

Gittelman *et al.* (1991) studied individuals with rhinosinusitis in order to determine the risk of toxic shock syndrome in individuals with *Staphylococcus aureus* infections. Nasal cultures were taken from 140 patients with rhinosinusitis: 35% were identified as *S. aureus* carriers; 30% of those scheduled for surgery were *S. aureus* carriers; and 40% of those tested had isolates of the toxic strain of *S. aureus*. A statistically higher incidence of *S. aureus* was found in cocaine users, as well as those using topical decongestants and steroid nasal sprays. The authors suggested that identifying those patients at risk for toxic shock syndrome associated with the toxic strain of *S. aureus* will guide practice to prevent infection complications after rhinoplastic surgery.

In a second article exploring risk of infections, Murphy *et al.* (2001) examined soft-tissue abscesses in a case–control study. The injection drug users (IDU) studied included 151 with abscesses requiring incision and drainage, and 267 IDU without abscesses or bacterial infections in the previous year. The cases and controls were matched for age, sex, and race. The major risk factor identified was subcutaneous or intramuscular injection of abused drugs (but not intravenous injection). Those who injected heroin and cocaine (speedball) may be at risk for ischemic soft-tissue injury. Alcohol cleansing of the skin was a protective measure preventing development of abscesses. Those who were seropositive for HIV or T-lymphotropic virus type II did not have an increased risk of abscess formation.

Two articles explored notification of individuals testing positive for syphilis. In a descriptive study, Gunn *et al.* (1995) reviewed case reports of individuals with primary and secondary syphilis associated with inner-city epidemics in 1990 to 1992. Thirty percent of the cases were illegal drug users. The drug users, particularly crack cocaine users, were also associated with prostitution, had 4.2 sex partners/person, and only 1.5 named sex partners/person. Only 26% of the sex partners received treatment for syphilis. The results suggested that a greater increase in screening of high-risk groups and partner identification through social networks is needed to control syphilis epidemics.

The second article (Ross *et al.* 2006) looked at notification of syphilis in individuals in a jail-based syphilis notification database and an Arrestee Drug Abuse Monitoring (ADAM) program from 1991 to 1998. The data were compared with the ADAM database and from a large county database. Three racial/ethnic groups were studied: African American, Hispanic, and non-Hispanic. The findings showed a significant association between cocaine use and syphilis in African Americans, but not in other groups. Linear regression analysis linked cocaine use and syphilis (58% of the variance). In the African American group, the association was stronger in males than females when only the ADAM and jail notification databases were considered. The researchers suggested that crack cocaine use and increased syphilis rates were related and that there was a close association between drug abuse and some STDs.

Two articles describe bacterial infections in cocaine users. The first (Oh *et al.* 2005) described an intravenous cocaine user who developed tricuspid valve endocarditis after licking needles prior to injecting the cocaine. He apparently licked the needles in order to determine the strength of the cocaine. Three anerobes were found: *Actinomyces odontolytica*, *Veillonella* species, and *Prevotella melaninogenica*, all oral anaerobes.

Another case of bacterial infection was described by Dettmeyer *et al.* (2004). A 17-year-old female died after developing mixed bacterial infections and infarctions following splenic infarct, thought to be related to cocaine use. Microabscesses were found in the heart, meninges, and kidneys. Petechial hemorrhages were also found in various organs.

A recent study by Swaminathan *et al.* (2007) looked at the benefit of two-step testing for tuberculosis (TB) infection in drug users. A two-step TB test involves tuberculin (purified protein derivative) skin testing twice, one week apart. If both tests are negative, the individual is unlikely to have the disease. If only one test is done and is negative, an asymptomatic individual may still have latent TB. By giving a second TB test, the second test, if positive, will identify those individuals whose immune systems did not respond to the antigen initially. The "booster phenomenon" occurs when the second test is positive since the first TB test stimulates "forgetful" immune recognition. The study comprised 619 drug users in a methadone treatment program. A positive tuberculin skin test was found in 174 (28%) at the first test. After the second test (booster), 24 of 445 (5%) additional drug users had a positive test. The older age of some subjects was associated with the booster phenomenon (adjusted odds ratio [AOR] 2.38/decade; 95% confidence interval [CI] 1.34–4.22). A history of using crack cocaine also increased the odds of a booster effect (AOR 2.61; 95% CI 1.10–6.18). Prior work as a home health aide was also associated with the booster phenomenon (AOR 4.23; 95% CI 1.39–12.86). The use of the two-step test for TB increased the proportion of individuals identified with latent TB from 22 to 25%. The researchers suggested using the two-step TB test for screening drug users for better identification of persons with TB.

Table 3.1 summarizes these data for bacterial infections.

Mycoses

A case report by Jaffey *et al.* (1990) found a *Conidiobolus* infection in a crack cocaine user. This fungus infection is rare in humans and rarely disseminates except in immunocompromised individuals. In the case study described, the fungal infection caused endocarditis and also infected the lungs, kidneys, skeletal muscle, and brain. Rhabdomyolysis also occurred, with a plasma creatine kinase (CK; also known as creatinine phosphokinase) of 1.2×10^6 U/L (normal 25–200 U/L). No mention was made concerning the HIV status of the individual (Table 3.2).

Table 3.1 Bacterial infections

Study	Method	Sample	Incidence	Results
Dettmeyer et al. (2004)	Case report Lethal sepsis after splenic infarct	17-year-old female cocaine user	Multiple splenic infarcts; mixed bacterial infections; infarcts of heart, meninges, kidneys; petechial lesions also found	Splenic infarcts are rare but can lead to lethal sepsis
Gittelman et al. (1991)	Descriptive study Incidence of *Staphylococcus aureus* in nasal passages at risk for toxic shock	140 patients with rhinosinusitis	*S. aureus* found in 35% Carriers tended to use cocaine, topical decongestants, nasal steroids; 40% had toxic isolates	Cocaine users with *S. aureus* nasal colonies may be at greater risk for developing toxic shock syndrome when undergoing nasal surgery
Gunn et al. (1995)	Descriptive study Identification of contacts in syphilis cases	Case reports of individuals with primary or secondary syphilis	In 30% illegal drugs users: crack cocaine associated with prostitution, 4.2 partners/person; only 1.5 named sex partners identified; 26% received treatment	Partner notification needs to be enhanced through social network contacts
Murphy et al. (2001)	Case-control study Soft-tissue abscesses requiring incision and drainage	151 IDUs with abscesses; 267 IDUs without abscesses	Major risk: subcutaneous or intramuscular injection (but not intravenous) Speedballing (heroin and cocaine) linked to soft-tissue ischemia	Alcohol wipe use had a protective effect against abscess development HIV/human T-lymphotropic virus type II not significantly associated with abscesses
Oh et al. (2005)	Case report Polymicrobial endocarditis	Tricuspid endocarditis in IV cocaine user	Bacteria identified: three oral anaerobes, *Actinomyces*, *Veillonella*, *Prevotella*	Infection related to needle licking to judge strength of IV cocaine
Ross et al. (2006)	Ecological study Notification of syphilis infection	Three racial/ethnic groups (African American, Hispanic, non-Hispanic) involved in syphilis notification program and arrestee drug abuse monitoring	Significant association between cocaine use and syphilis in African Americans (not in other two groups)	Data suggests close association between some STDs and drug abuse
Swaminathan et al. (2007)	Descriptive study Utility of booster testing for TB; two-step TB testing Interview, test for HIV, CD4 lymphocytes	619 drug users in methadone treatment program	174/619 (28%) tested positive on initial testing; 24/445 (5%) of those testing negative on first test tested positive on second test 1 week later (booster phenomenon); boostering associated with older age (AOR 2.38/decade; 95% CI 1.34–4.22); history of use of crack cocaine (AOR 2.61; 95% CI 1.10–6.18); work as home health aide (AOR 4.23; 95% CI 1.39–12.86)	Booster TB testing can increase the number of individuals testing positive for TB by 25%; consider booster testing when screening drug users for TB

AOR, adjusted odds ratio; IDU, injection drug user; IV, intravenous; HIV, human immunodeficiency virus; STD, sexually transmitted disease; TB, tuberculosis.

11

Table 3.2 Mycoses

Study	Method	Sample	Incidence	Results
Jaffey *et al.* (1990)	Case report	Crack cocaine user with *Conidiobolus* systemic infection	Developed endocarditis after spread from leg wound; infection in lungs, kidney, skeletal muscle, brain; rhabdomyolysis (creatine kinase 1.2×10^6 U/L)	Rare infection by fungus; rarely disseminates except in immunocompromised individuals

Table 3.3 Parasitic infections

Study	Method	Sample	Incidence	Results
Sorvillo *et al.* (1998)	Medical record review and interviews Trichomoniasis in HIV-positive women	212 HIV-infected women in public clinic, 1992–1995	Trichomoniasis most common STD: 37 (17.4%) in 1998 Crude incidence rate 14.1/100 person-years experience; highest in blacks (69.0/100), those trading sex for drugs or money (51.0/100), using crack or cocaine (35.5/100), 4 or more sex partners (43.0/100), born in the USA (23.3/100)	HIV-positive women not more likely to transmit infection if they used crack/ cocaine

HIV, human immunodeficiency virus; STD, sexually transmitted disease.

Parasitic infections

One article on parasitic infections in cocaine users was found in the PubMed literature review. Sorvillo *et al.* (1998) described trichomoniasis infections in HIV-infected women in a public clinic from 1992 to 1995. At the time of publication, trichomoniasis was the most common STD, found in 37 (17.4%) of 212 women (crude incidence rate of 14.1/100 person-years experience). The crude rate was highest in those who were black (69.0/100), traded sex for drugs or money (51.0/100), had four or more sex partners (43.0), used crack cocaine (35.5/100), and were born in the USA (23.3/100). The study indicated that women may be more likely to spread trichomonas if they are black with HIV infection, or unmarried, non-black women who trade sex for money or drugs (Table 3.3).

Viral infections

Nine articles were found related to cocaine and non-HIV viral infections. The majority of the articles focused on HCV, risky behavior, and seroconversion in IDU. All of the articles were published since 2000.

Thorpe *et al.* (2000) described the characteristics of 698 young adult IDU aged 18 to 30. Infection with HCV was found in 27% and was strongly associated with age and length of intravenous drug use ($p < 0.001$). Urban users were more likely to be HCV infected than suburban users. Using multivariate analysis, sexual behavior was not related to a positive HCV test. Independent drug-related risk factors included frequency of injection, heavy crack smoking, injecting in a shooting gallery, and syringe sharing. The authors suggested there is a need to identify and educate those IDUs who are at risk for HCV infection.

Santibanez et al. (2005) explored risky behavior in individuals aged 18 to 30 years in the Collaborative Injection Drug User Study (CIDUS II) database (1997–1999). Of the 2198 individuals, 329 (15%) used crack cocaine. These users injected crack cocaine in the six months prior to the study, recently injected daily, and shared equipment, including drug solution and syringes. Lifetime crack cocaine use correlated with participation in a shooting gallery, inviting others to inject drugs, and positive blood tests for both hepatitis B virus (HBV) and HCV. The authors suggested that crack cocaine use may be a marker for high-risk behavior.

Cohen et al. (2006) also looked at risky behavior and HCV infection in 183 men who had sex with men. The men were aged 22 to 54 years; 82% were white, 35% HIV positive, 11.5% HCV infected. Those infected with HCV were more likely than others to have seen blood on shared cocaine straws, and used crack cocaine in the past six months. They were also more likely to be infected with HIV and HBV, and to have a history of rectal or urethral gonorrhea. The authors concluded that individuals with HCV infection are more likely to exhibit high-risk behavior. Men who have sex with men should be targeted to prevent HCV infection and those with HCV should be targeted to reduce the risk of HIV and other STDs.

Reimer et al. (2007) used a convenience sample of patients in an opioid detoxification program to assess the prevalence of hepatitis virus infections. Of 1512 patients in this program, 58% had antibodies to hepatitis A virus (HAV), 53% to HBV, and 75% to HCV. In patients with antibodies to only one hepatitis virus (25%), most had HCV (59%) or HAV (27%); in those with two infections (32%), HAV and HCV were most common (47%), with HBV/HCV at 41.8%. Use of cocaine was associated with HAV, HBV, and HCV infections. The HBV/HCV infections were associated with older age, a long history of intravenous drug use, and a higher incidence of rehabilitation experiences. Since IDU is associated with co-infection with hepatitis viruses, the authors suggested testing current cocaine users for antibodies for HAV, HBV, and HCV and that, when possible, users should be vaccinated to prevent HAV and HBV.

A study by Roy et al. (2007) described the information collected from the SurvUDI Network to determine the relationship between injection drug use and HCV infection. The overall prevalence rate for HCV infection in 1380 participants from the network was 60.4% (95% CI 57.7–63.0). In 543 persons initially uninfected, the HCV incidence rate was 27.1/ 100 person-years (95% CI 23.4–30.9). The independent predictors of seroconversion to HCV-positive status in 359 participants were age, drug injection one year or less, injecting with used syringes, injecting cocaine, involvement with prostitution, and recruitment from an urban setting. The authors re-emphasized the need to target new IDU and educate them in the use of sterile syringes.

In a prospective screening study, Neumeister et al. (2007) studied the risk for development of HCV infection in 243 Native Americans participating in HCV screening and completing a questionnaire assessing risk factors. The participants were mostly female (151 [62%]), had a mean age of 41 years, and included members of more than 30 tribes. Anti-HCV antibodies were found in 11.5% (95% CI 7.5–15.5). HCV RNA was detected by the polymerase chain reaction (PCR) in 8.6% (95% CI 5.1–12.1). Males were more likely to be HCV positive (13.4%; 95% CI 6.0–20.8) than females (6.2%; 95% CI 2.5–9.9). The most common risk factors for HCV were intravenous drug or cocaine use ($p < 0.0001$); however, tattooing more than five years earlier ($p < 0.0001$) and having sex partners with HCV ($p = 0.0063$) were also strong risk factors in this Native American group.

Des Jarlais *et al.* (2007) studied the relationship between herpes simplex virus (HSV) type 2 and HIV in non-IDU. The 462 study participants were recruited from a drug detoxification program, were interviewed, and serum tested for HIV and HSV-2. The subjects most often used crack cocaine, intranasal heroin, and intranasal cocaine. The prevalence of HIV was 19% (95% CI 15–22), and of HSV-2 was 60% (95% CI 55–64). The AOR for the association between HSV-2 and HIV was 1.9 (95% CI 1.21–2.98). The infection rate for HSV-2 was highest in females (86%) and 23 females who were HIV positive were also HSV-2 positive. Since HSV-2 is important in sexual transmission of HIV among non-injecting cocaine and heroin users, especially in females, the researchers suggested that HSV-2 infection needs to be prevented as well as HIV.

March *et al.* (2007) reported on a cross-sectional study of self-reported HCV and HIV infection in IDUs in 10 European cities. Face-to-face questionnaires were completed for 1131 current IDUs injecting heroin and/or cocaine. Of these, 595 (52.5%) reported they were HCV positive, and 143 (12.6%) were HIV positive. Based on multivariate analysis, those who shared needles or tested positive for TB, HBV, HIV, or other STDs were at higher risk of HCV positivity. Longer duration of drug use, sharing needles, injecting while in prison, and male gender were also associated with an increased risk for HCV. Those individuals with social exclusion and poor health status had higher incidences of HCV- and HIV-positive tests.

In a longitudinal study by Maher *et al.* (2007), the incidence of HCV and possible risk factors was researched in new IDUs. The subjects were recruited from methadone clinics and outreach needle/syringe exchange programs and followed for three to six months. The subjects in the study had injected drugs in the past six months and either did not know their HCV status or were negative; 215 were negative for HCV antibodies and 204 were new IDUs, under the age of 30, who had been injecting for six years or less. During the three to six months of follow-up, 61 seroconversions occurred (45.8/100 person-years). Several independent predictors of seroconversion were identified: duration of injecting (< 1 year, incidence rate ratio [RR] 3.10; 95% CI 1.47–6.54), female gender (incidence RR 2.0; 95% CI 1.16–3.45), culturally/linguistically diverse background (incidence RR 2.03; 95% CI 1.06–3.89), and cocaine use (incidence RR 2.37; 95% CI 1.26–4.44). In new IDUs, there also was a strong association between HCV seroconversion and sharing syringes, sharing other injection equipment, and backloading (mixing several drugs in one syringe and injecting the drugs into the syringes of other users).

Table 3.4 summarizes these data on viral infections.

Comments

Four groups of infectious diseases have been reviewed, including bacterial, fungal, parasitic, and viral (non-HIV) infections. The bacterial articles included one exploring the incidence of *S. aureus* in nasal colonies and prevention of toxic shock surgery postrhinoplasty. Although cocaine users were found to be among the 40% of individuals who tested positive for the toxic strain of *S. aureus*, more studies are needed to explore the relationship of cocaine use and *S. aureus* infection. One study on TB testing focused on the importance of a two-step TB test to identify positive reactors who might test negative on a single tuberculin screening test.

Another bacterial study identified that subcutaneous and intramuscular injection (but not intravenous injection) of heroin and cocaine was associated with abscesses requiring

Table 3.4 Viral infections (excluding HIV)

Study	Method	Sample	Incidence	Results
Cohen et al. (2006)	High-risk behavior and HCV	183 men who had sex with men; 22–54 years of age, 82% white	35% HIV positive; 11.5% HCV positive (also more likely to be HIV and HBV positive); history of rectal, urethral gonorrhea; more likely to have seen blood on shared cocaine straws, used crack cocaine in past 6 months	HCV associated with high-risk behavior; 12% HCV-positive males had no history of parental drug use
Des Jarlais et al. (2007)	HSV-2 and HIV in non-injecting heroin and cocaine users Interview and serum for HIV, HSV-2	462 non-injecting drug users in drug detoxification program: smoked crack cocaine, used intranasal heroin, intranasal cocaine	HIV prevalence, 19% (95% CI 15–22%); HSV-2 prevalence, 60% (95% CI 55–64); adjusted RR for HSV-2 plus HIV, 1.9 (95% CI 1.21–2.98) Women: 86% HSV-2 positive, 23% HIV positive; all HIV positive also HSV-2 positive	HSV-2 is an important factor in sexual transmission among non-injecting cocaine, heroin users, especially females; there is a need to prevent HSV-2 as well as HIV
Maher et al. (2007)	Longitudinal study with 3–6 months of follow-up Incidence of HCV and risk factors in new IDUs	IDUs who injected drugs in past 6 months who did not know HCV status or were negative	215, anti-HCV negative; 204, new IDU (< 30 years), injecting 6 years or less); 61 seroconversions (incidence: 45.8/100 person-years) Independent predictors of seroconversion: duration of injecting <1 year (IRR 3.1; 95% CI 1.47–6.54), female sex (IRR 2.0; 95% CI 1.16–3.45), culturally diverse background (IRR 2.03; 95% CI 1.06–3.89), IV cocaine use (IRR 2.37: 95% CI 1.26–4.44)	Strong association between HCV seroconversion and sharing syringes, sharing injection equipment, backloading new IDUs
March et al. (2007)	Cross-sectional study Self-report of HCV and HIV in IDUs in 10 European countries Questionnaire	1131 injected heroin or cocaine in past year; 71.5% male; mean age 30 years	595 (52.6%) HCV positive; 143 (12.6%) HIV positive; HCV positivity associated with sharing needles, TB and HBV positive, HIV positive, existing STDs	Social isolation associated with HCV/HIV positivity
Neumeister et al. (2007)	Prospective screening study Native Americans at risk for HCV HCV screen and questionnaire for risk factors	243 Native Americans: 161 females, 30+ tribes; mean age 41 ± 1 year	AntiHCV antibodies in 11.5% (95% CI 7.5–15.5); HCV RNA by PCR, 8.6% (95% CI 5.1–12.1) Male (13.4%; 95% CI 6.0–20.8) > female (6.2%; 95% CI 2.5–9.9)	Most common risk factors for chronic HCV were IV drug or cocaine use (p < 0.0001), tattoos over 5 years previous (p < 0.0001), sex partners with HCV (p = 0.0063)

Table 3.4 *Cont.*

Study	Method	Sample	Incidence	Results
Reimer *et al.* (2007)	Convenience sample, detoxification patients Incidence of HAV infection	1512 patients in opiate detoxification program	HAV antibodies in 57.7%; HBV antibodies in 53.0%; HCV antibodies in 75%. One hepatic marker, 24.7% (58.8% HCV; 27% HAV); two markers, 31.2% (HAV/HCV 46.7%; HBV/HCV 41.8%); all three markers, 32.9%; none, 11.2% Current use of cocaine, antibodies for HAV, HBV, HCV	Vaccination important to prevent HAV and HBV in target population
Roy *et al.* (2007)	Descriptive study using data from SurvUDI Network HCV and IDUs	1380 IDUs	HCV prevalence rate, 60.4% (95% CI 57.7–63.0%); 543 initially uninfected; HCV incidence rate, 27.1/ 100 person-years (95% CI 23.4–30.9)	Independent predictors of seroconversion (359 participants): age, injecting ≤ 1 year, injecting with used syringes, injecting cocaine, involved in prostitution, reside in urban setting
Santibanez *et al.* (2005)	Cross-sectional study using CIDUS III database High-risk behavior and HCV in six cities	2198 subjects aged 18–30 years; 329 (15%) used crack cocaine	Lifetime crack cocaine use correlated with participation in shooting gallery, inviting others to inject drugs, positive blood levels for both HBV and HCV	Crack cocaine use may be a marker for high-risk behavior
Thorpe *et al.* (2000)	Descriptive study HCV status in IDUs	698 IDU aged 18–30 years	HCV in 27%, strongly associated with age and length of injection drug use (*p* < 0.001) Multivariate analysis: sexual behavior not related to positive HCV test	Independent drug-related risk factors for HCV: frequency of injection, heavy crack smoking, injecting in a shooting gallery, syringe sharing

CI, confidence interval; IDU, injection drug users; HAV, hepatitis A virus; HBV, hepatitis B virus; HCV, hepatitis C virus; HIV, human immunodeficiency virus; IDU, intravenous drug user; IRR, incidence rate ratio; IV, intravenous; RR, relative risk; STD, sexually transmitted disease.

incision and drainage. Larger studies are needed to identify the risk of skin infection or systemic bacterial infections in individuals not seen by healthcare professionals. What is the incidence of injection site inflammation and infection in those not seen in health centers? Two syphilis studies were reviewed. In both studies, there was a relationship between STDs and cocaine use. Individuals with multiple sex partners and those engaged in prostitution were also at risk for syphilis. Risky behavior practices are a common thread in these three studies. Furthermore, the studies underscore the need for safe sex and safe injection practices, such as condom use and use of alcohol wipes prior to injecting cocaine.

Only one study on fungal infections was described in the review of the literature. This case study described a systemic infection with *Conidiobolus* in a cocaine user. No information was available regarding the HIV status of the individual. This infection is rarely seen in immunocompetent individuals. According to a Web search on *Conidiobolus*, infections with this fungus are appearing more often as an opportunistic condition.

One study on trichomoniasis described the condition in HIV-infected women. Those most at risk for the parasitic infection were black women, prostitutes, those with four or more sex partners, and those who used crack cocaine. The likelihood of infecting sex partners with this common STD may reflect the risky sex behavior associated with cocaine use.

Eight of the nine studies of viral infection in cocaine users focused on HCV infection. The ninth study reported on HSV-2 infections. A common feature in these studies is the risky behavior in those studied: frequent cocaine use and sharing of injection equipment, needles, and syringes; participating in shooting galleries; and engaging in prostitution.

These studies do not provide evidence that infections in cocaine users is associated with cocaine itself but instead tend to suggest that the risky behavior associated with cocaine use may make it easier to transmit infections from one individual to another. When possible, reduction of seroconversion of HAV and HBV may be accomplished by vaccination of high-risk populations.

Many of the studies in this section involved individuals participating in drug treatment programs or needle exchange programs or who were on drug databases. More studies are needed to look at the risk of infection in those individuals in the general population who may use cocaine. Information about co-infection with HIV or other STDs would also help in interpreting the results of some of the studies in this subsection. In some studies, drug use and HIV status was based on self-report. Since self-report can be under- or over-reporting, some cases may be missed or result in bias in reporting.

Neoplastic disease

Two abstracts were reviewed regarding neoplastic disease in cocaine users (Table 3.5). The first was a case–control study by Nelson *et al.* (1997) that compared 378 individuals with non-Hodgkin's lymphoma (NHL) with age-, race-, and sex-matched controls. Use of tobacco, alcohol, and 10 recreational drugs was determined. While use of alcohol lowered the risk for NHL (trend $p = 0.03$), use of cocaine and several other abused drugs were each associated with an increased risk of NHL, especially in frequent users. Based on multivariate analyses, use of cocaine accounted for the significant increased risk of NHL in men.

The second (Duarte *et al.* 1999) studied 198 individuals with pancreatic cancer. Thirteen were under the age of 40 (range, 19 to 31 years). Five of the thirteen were cocaine users who inhaled cocaine for at least 10 years. One other patient used marijuana. Because

17

Table 3.5 Neoplastic disease

Study	Method	Sample	Incidence	Results
Duarte et al. (1999)	Chart review Pancreatic cancer in individuals under age 40	198 patients with pancreatic adenocarcinoma; 13 patients under 40 years of age (19–37)	5 patients inhaled cocaine for over 10 years; 1 patient used marijuana	More studies needed to determine whether cocaine use is associated with adenocarcinoma of the pancreas
Nelson et al. (1997)	Case–control study Risk of NHL	378 patients diagnosed with NHL (high, intermediate grade) plus controls matched for age, race, sex	Decreased risk of NHL in women who used alcohol (trend $p = 0.03$); 50% lower in those with 5 or more drinks/week. Increased risk of NHL in males using illicit drugs (trend $p = 0.005$). Use of cocaine accounted for elevated risk in men based on multivariate analyses	Risk of NHL appears higher in cocaine users than in users of amphetamines, Quaaludes, or lysergic acid diethylamide

NHL, non-Hodgkin's lymphoma.

this cancer tends to appear in older individuals, the authors suggested that chronic cocaine exposure may influence the development of pancreatic cancer in susceptible individuals.

Comments

With only two articles associating cocaine use with cancer, more studies are needed to determine the risk cocaine use has in the development of neoplasms. Longitudinal studies may provide more risk data in the drug-abusing population.

Musculoskeletal system disease

Cocaine is associated with rhabdomyolysis. This is discussed below in the renal section. No other articles were identified in this subsection.

Digestive system disease

Eight articles were found in the PubMed database of literature published between 1988 and 2008 that explored the relationship between cocaine use and digestive system disorders. Two articles included a retrospective study and a case study on ulcer disease, and six case studies reported on cocaine-related conditions of the colon and small intestine.

Kram et al. (1992) described four patients who smoked crack cocaine and subsequently developed perforated gastroduodenal ulcers. All four were admitted to hospital with acute abdominal pain. One patient had a prior experience with peptic ulcer disease; another had an elevated white blood cell count, while two had a decreased white blood cell counts. Three of the four patients had a pneumoperitoneum on radiography. During surgery, it was apparent that all four had extensive peritoneal contamination. The authors suggested that young adults who seek medical attention because of an acute abdomen after using crack cocaine may have perforated ulcer disease that warrants prompt intervention.

Sharma et al. (1997) described the results of a retrospective study carried out over a six-year period to study the relationship between crack cocaine use and duodenal ulcer perforation. Of 78 patients who were identified with peptic ulcer disease that required surgical intervention, 24 (31%) were confirmed to have smoked crack cocaine within eight hours prior to the onset of signs and symptoms of a duodenal ulcer perforation. The 78 patients were similar in gender, use of tobacco, prior experience with peptic ulcer disease, and laboratory results. However, compared with the 54 individuals with peptic ulcer disease who did not use crack cocaine, the cocaine users were younger ($p = 0.01$), had shorter hospital stays ($p = 0.01$), and were more likely to have a perforated ulcer (75% vs. 46% for the non-cocaine users; $p = 0.04$). The researchers found that crack cocaine and alcohol use were both independent predictors of duodenal ulcer perforation. Although a cause and effect relationship could not be substantiated, a temporal relationship did exist between crack cocaine use and perforation of a duodenal ulcer.

In a case report, Garfia et al. (1990) described fatal segmental intestinal ischemia in an alcohol/cocaine-related overdose. The individual had normal mesenteric vessels with no evidence of thrombosis. However, there were unusual arteriolar lesions in the hemorrhagic areas of the intestinal submucosa.

Boutros et al. (1997) reported on a 36-year-old female who used crack cocaine twice in the two days before experiencing signs and symptoms of an acute abdomen. Pathology specimens obtained after surgery showed patchy necrosis of the transverse colon and edema and congestion of the gall bladder wall. The colon and gall bladder both had small-vessel thrombi, and the colonic mucosal findings were typical of ischemic necrosis.

Two case series described mesenteric ischemia that developed shortly after using cocaine. Sudhakar et al. (1997) described two females in their thirties who developed mesenteric ischemia. Neither had a history of atherosclerosis and both had positive toxicology screens for cocaine. Hoang et al. (1998) described three patients, one male and two females, who developed mesenteric ischemia after recent cocaine use. Angiograms were performed on all three. The 45-year-old male had small intestinal ischemia with perforation and pseudomembranous enteritis. In some submucosal arterioles, intra-luminal fibrin and intimal hyperplasia were found. Both females (aged 29 and 35 years) had occlusion of the celiac axis and superior mesenteric arteries and were treated with vascular bypasses. The two vessels and their branches were totally occluded by luminal thromboses, with evidence of recanalization. Both females had a two-year history of intravenous cocaine use.

Papi et al. (1999) described a 36-year-old male who occasionally used cocaine and developed ischemic necrosis of the transverse colon one day after injecting cocaine. The transverse colon was edematous and there was evidence of subserosal hemorrhage. The pathology report on the resected specimen described focal mucosal necrosis with patchy infiltrates of both poly-morphonuclear and mononuclear cells, and edema in the submucosa. The intestinal vessels were dilated, but there were no structural abnormalities or thromboses in the vessels.

A 33-year-old male was described who developed a distal ileum infarct after using intravenous cocaine (Osorio et al. 2000). There was no history of arteriosclerosis. The gangrenous portion of the small intestine was surgically removed. Subsequently the individual developed cocaine-induced rhabdomyolysis and acute renal failure (ARF).

Table 3.6 summarizes these findings.

Comments

These eight studies describe pathology of the stomach, duodenum, ileum, and colon that was seen in individuals who had recently used cocaine (both crack and intravenous

Table 3.6 Digestive system

Study	Method	Sample	Incidence	Results
Boutros et al. (1997)	Case study Ischemic colitis and cocaine use	36-year old female who used crack cocaine in the 2 days prior to symptoms of acute abdomen	Transverse colon with patchy necrosis; gall bladder with edema, congestion; small vessel thrombi present; colonic mucosal findings of ischemic necrosis	Recent cocaine use associated with ischemic disease of the bowel
Gaffia et al. (1990)	Case study Bowel ischemia	Fatal case caused by alcohol, cocaine overdose	Segmental bowel ischemic; unusual arteriolar lesions in intestinal submucosa in hemorrhagic areas	Intestinal ischemia should be suspected in cocaine users with acute abdominal pain
Hoang et al. (1998)	Case study Mesenteric ischemia and cocaine use	3 patients: 45-year-old male; females aged 29 and 35 years	Male: recent IV cocaine use; small intestinal ischemia with perforation; intraluminal fibrin, intimal hyperplasia in rare submucosal arterioles Females: 2-year history of IV cocaine use; occlusion of celiac axis, superior mesenteric arteries, branches with luminal thromboses, recanalization; treated with vascular bypasses	Mesenteric ischemia associated with recent IV cocaine use
Kram et al. (1992)	Case study Crack cocaine and perforated ulcer disease	4 patients with acute abdominal pain after cocaine use: 1 had history of peptic ulcer disease	1 with increased WBC count; 2 with decreased WBC count; 3 with pneumoperitoneum on radiography; all had extensive peritoneal contamination	Young patients with acute abdomen and recent cocaine use may present with normal or low WBC count; may lack evidence of perforation on radiography
Osorio et al. (2000)	Case study Distal ileum infarct and cocaine use	33-year-old male; no history of atherosclerosis	Distal ileum infarct after IV cocaine use; also developed cocaine-induced rhabdomyolysis, ARF	Recent IV cocaine use associated with distal ileum infarct

Papi et al. (1999)	Case study Ischemic transverse colon and cocaine use	36-year-old male with acute abdomen: occasional cocaine user; injected IV cocaine 1 day prior to onset of acute abdomen	Focal mucosal necrosis with infiltrates of polymorphonuclear and mononuclear WBCs; submucosal edema; vessels dilated with no structural abnormalities or thrombosis	Recent IV cocaine use associated with disease of the transverse colon
Sharma et al. (1997)	Retrospective study, 6 years Crack cocaine and duodenal ulcer perforation	78 patients with perforated ulcer disease; similar gender, tobacco use, prior history of ulcer disease, laboratory tests; 24 confirmed crack use 8 h prior to onset of acute abdomen	24 (31%) used crack cocaine; crack users were younger ($p = 0.01$), had shorter hospital stay ($p = 0.01$) than non-users, more likely to perforate (75% crack users vs. 46% non-users) Crack cocaine and alcohol use both independent predictors of perforated ulcer disease	Temporal relationship found between use of cocaine and onset of acute abdomen
Sudhakar et al. (1997)	Case study Mesenteric ischemia and cocaine use	2 females, no history of atherosclerosis; positive urine toxicology test for cocaine	Both had mesenteric ischemia	Mesenteric ischemia associated with recent cocaine use

ARF, acute renal failure; IV, intravenous; WBC, white blood cell.

cocaine). These findings were seen in individuals who did not have a history of arteriosclerosis or atherosclerosis. Concurrent uses of alcohol, other illicit drugs, or tobacco were not described. Other concurring diagnoses were identified in only one case and included cocaine-induced rhabdomyolysis and ARF. In several patients, thrombi were found in vessels – both large (celiac and superior mesenteric arteries and their branches) and small (arterioles). In other patients, occlusive disease was not found. Ischemic consequences were seen in most cases that involved perforation of the luminal wall. Those with perforations did not always display elevated white blood cell counts.

Although one study involved 24 confirmed crack cocaine users, the other seven were smaller case series (one to three patients), which suggests that recent use of cocaine may be associated with perforated gastroduodenal ulcer disease and ischemic or thrombus-related disease of the small intestine and colon. These findings could be related to the vasoconstrictive and prothrombic effects of cocaine through increases in dopamine, norepinephrine, and endothelin-1.

Given the number of users of cocaine and the number of cases described in the literature, the risk for these conditions is rare. However, healthcare providers seeing young patients with acute abdominal signs and symptoms should assess the patients for recent cocaine use and be aware that cocaine use can cause both ischemic and thrombotic vascular events. However, larger studies, including prospective cohort studies, are needed to determine the risk for digestive vascular disorders in cocaine users.

Stomatognathic disease

Articles about the jaw and mouth are included in the otorhinolaryngological section.

Respiratory system disease

Seven articles were found in the review of respiratory disease and cocaine use in the PubMed literature from 1988 to 2008, including several case–control and cross-sectional studies, and one case report.

Tashkin *et al.* (1992a) described a case–control study on respiratory effects of freebasing cocaine in 177 heavy, habitual users. These had used crack cocaine a mean of 6.6 g/week for an average of 27 months. The 75 controls in this study were age-, sex-, and race-matched non-cocaine users but may have used marijuana or tobacco. Compared with the controls, the crack users had a higher incidence of acute respiratory symptoms, including a cough, black sputum, and chest pain. They also had evidence of obstructive ventilatory impairment in the large airways and a mild, but significant, impairment of diffusion at the alveolar–capillary interface. The authors suggested that crack use can cause respiratory tract injury, chronic airflow obstruction, and alveolar–capillary diffusion abnormalities.

In another case–control study, Tashkin *et al.* (1992b) reported on 202 crack users who reported no use of intravenous illicit drugs. The controls were 99 non-users. The cases and controls were similar in race (primarily African American), non-use of marijuana (68 vs. 69%), and tobacco use. Of those smoking marijuana, more controls were current smokers than the crack users. The cocaine smokers used an average of 6.5 g/week for 53 weeks, and the median for most recently smoked was 19 days (range, 1–180 days). The authors found that the crack users had a higher occurrence than non-users for acute respiratory symptoms within 12 hours of smoking crack, including cough (43.7%), hemoptysis (5.7%), and chest pain (38.5%). They were also more likely to have mildly, but significantly, impaired diffusion capacity.

A prospective cohort study by Baldwin *et al.* (2002) looked at pulmonary microscopic damage caused by crack use. The sample included 36 healthy males and females (mean age 37.5 years), 10 who were crack-only smokers, 10 tobacco-only smokers, 10 non-smokers, and 6 who used both crack and tobacco. Bronchial alveolar lavage was used to assess alveolar macrophages. Endothelin-1 was also assessed as the lung is a major source of endothelin-1, where it is primarily secreted by the respiratory smooth muscle and also by the endothelium, airway epithelium, and other cells. Endothelin-1 is a potent vasoconstrictor and is often elevated in asthma. The crack users were healthy, with no history of hemoptysis or respiratory symptoms. Spirometry tests were within normal limits. However, compared with the tobacco smokers and non-smokers, the crack users had a significantly higher percentage of alveolar macrophages (33.8 ± 8.7% [SEM]); ($p < 0.05$). The six who used crack and tobacco had a non-significant elevation of macrophages as well. Endothelin-1 levels were significantly elevated in the crack users (6.2 ± 0.8 pg/mL) compared with the non-smokers (1.2 ± 0.4 pg/mL), tobacco smokers (1.3 ± 0.2 pg/mL), and cocaine and tobacco users (2.5 ± 0.6 pg/mL). Endothelin-1 levels were correlated with the percentage of alveolar macrophages found on bronchial alveolar lavage when the crack users and the crack and tobacco users were compared ($r = 0.64$; $p = 0.0004$). The authors suggested that microvascular injury could be found in healthy crack users without respiratory symptomatology.

Three studies focused on the relationship between asthma and cocaine use. Greenberger *et al.* (1993) reviewed clinical data, contacted next-of-kin, and reviewed autopsy and clinical laboratory results of individuals 45 years of age or younger whose cause of death was asthma. From 1985 to 1992, 39 deaths were related to asthma, including those who died from or probably died from asthma (22/39; 56.4%), those listed as indeterminant (8/39; 20.5%), and those whose deaths were coincidental (9/39; 23.1%). Of the 23 patients with laboratory information, 14 of the 23 (60.8%) tested positive for cocaine and cocaine metabolites, codeine, phencyclidine, morphine, methadone, or ethanol. The authors concluded that there was a high incidence of drug use in individuals dying from asthma.

Osborn *et al.* (1997) studied cocaine-using individuals with new onset of bronchospasms or an acute recurrence of asthma symptoms. They interviewed patients in an urban emergency department who had bronchospasm or a return of asthma symptoms after an abatement of five years. Urinalysis looked for cocaine and cocaine metabolites. In this case–control study, the 53 controls were age- and sex-matched to the 59 patients with bronchospasm. Twenty-one of the 59 (35%) patients tested positive for cocaine or cocaine metabolites in the urine, even though eight had denied using illicit drugs. Thirteen smoked crack and three snorted cocaine. In the controls, 8 of 53 tested positive for cocaine or cocaine metabolites despite denying illicit drug use. In a multivariate analysis, adjusted for age and sex, those individuals who used cocaine had a three-fold higher prevalence of new-onset bronchospasm or a recurrence of asthma (odds ratio [OR] 3.28; 95% CI 1.26–8.50).

Rome *et al.* (2000) used a cross-sectional approach to explore cocaine use and asthma. They obtained informed consent from 116 persons who were seen in an emergency department over a seven-month period. Of the 116, 103 consented to have urine samples tested for cocaine and cocaine metabolites. Those participating in the study were primarily African American (89%), female (68%), had a mean age of 33 years, and 35% were cigarette smokers. Urine samples positive for cocaine were found in 13 of the 103 (13%) and opiates in 6 (5.8%). Of the 13 patients that tested positive for cocaine, five were admitted to hospital. Two required intubation and mechanical ventilation. The cocaine users also had a significantly longer length of hospitalization than non-cocaine users (5 vs. 2.5 days; $p < 0.05$).

In a case report, van der Klooster & Grootendorst (2001) described a 40-year-old long-term cocaine user (17 years) who developed bilateral bullous emphysema, with large air- and fluid-filled spaces suggestive of pulmonary abscesses. Despite vigorous treatment with antibiotics, intubation and mechanical ventilation, the individual died of respiratory failure. With α_1-antitrypsin levels normal, and a negative HIV status, the cause of the bullous emphysema was attributed to long-term cocaine use.

Table 3.7 summarizes these results.

Comments

Two fairly large case–control studies found increased respiratory signs and symptoms in cocaine users compared with controls, who may or may not have used tobacco or marijuana. The cocaine users also had some significant changes in airway function and alveolar-arteriolar diffusion capacity. A small study showed that healthy cocaine users, with no untoward respiratory signs or symptoms, had a greater number of alveolar macrophages in bronchial secretions. Endothelin-1, a potent vasoconstrictor, was also higher in cocaine users. These three studies suggest that cocaine use can diminish respiratory function and may be occurring in healthy cocaine users. However, further studies are needed to determine risk for respiratory disease in this population.

The three studies related to asthma suggest that, compared with control subjects, cocaine users may be more at risk of new-onset bronchospasm and recurrence of asthma symptoms, experience longer hospitalizations, and also have an increased risk of death with an asthma exacerbation. These studies were small (14 to 21 patients) and were carried out in cocaine users admitted to a hospital for asthma treatment. Additional studies including cocaine users not admitted for asthma symptoms might help to determine the incidence and prevalence of asthma in these drug users.

One case study described a cocaine user who died of respiratory failure after treatment for bullous emphysema. No information was available about the tobacco smoking habits of the individual. Whether this is a rare finding in cocaine users or more common, as in those with α_1-antitrypsin deficiency, could be explored in further research.

One problem identified in at least one of these studies is the issue of the accuracy of self-report of cocaine use. Although some individuals denied illicit drug use, laboratory studies confirmed the presence of cocaine or cocaine metabolites. Researchers need to consider confirming survey data and self-report with laboratory confirmation of drug use.

Otorhinolaryngological disease

Fifteen articles were found in a PubMed search of the literature from 1988 to 2008 related to effects of cocaine on the ear and upper airway.

Schwartz et al. (1989a) examined nasal symptoms in adolescents. Questionnaires on drug use were completed by 454 adolescents enrolled in outpatient treatment facilities in five geographic regions of the USA. Cocaine use was admitted by 336 (72%) of the adolescents: 203 (60%) fewer than 25 times, 107 (32%) 25–99 times, and 26 (8%) daily or more than 100 times. Those who used cocaine the most had significantly more symptoms than ones in the 25–99 times group. Those symptoms included sniffling, sinus problems, and a diminished sense of smell. The daily users were also more likely to have nasal crusts, scabs,

Table 3.7 Respiratory system disease

Study	Method	Sample	Incidence	Results
Baldwin et al. (2002)	Prospective cohort study Microscopic respiratory damage and crack use Fiberoptic bronchoscopy, bronchial alveolar lavage, ET1 assay	36 healthy males and females, mean age 37.5 years: 10 cocaine-only smokers; 10 tobacco smokers; 10 non-smokers; 6 smoking both cocaine and tobacco	Cocaine users: no hemoptysis/respiratory distress, normal spirometry; AM increased in cocaine smokers, 33.8 ± 8.7% (compared with tobacco and non-smokers [< 2%]; $p < 0.05$); elevated but not statistically significantly in users of both cocaine and tobacco ET-1: increased in cocaine users (6.2 ± 0.8 pg/mL) compared with non-smokers (1.2 ± 0.4 pg/mL); tobacco users had smaller increase (1.3 ± 0.2 pg/mL); cocaine and tobacco users, 2.5 ± 0.6 pg/mL	There is evidence of cocaine-induced microvascular injury in healthy crack users ET-1 levels correlated with percentage AM when comparing cocaine users with cocaine/tobacco users ($r = 0.64$; $p = 0.0004$) Alveolar injury occurs in healthy cocaine smokers prior to onset of signs and symptoms
Greenberger et al. (1993)	Demographic study Cases: death from asthma Review of clinical data, contact of next of kin, informants, autopsy/laboratory studies	39 asthma deaths from 1985 to 1992 in those aged ≤ 45 years Deaths: probably from asthma: 22 (56.4%); indeterminant: 8 (23.1%); coincidental: 9 (23.1%)	Laboratory information for 23: 14 (69.8%) positive for cocaine, codeine, phencyclidine, morphine, methadone, ethanol	High incidence of drug use in out-of-hospital asthma deaths
Osborn et al. (1997)	Case–control prevalence study New-onset bronchospasm; recurrence of asthma in cocaine users Interview about illicit drug use; urine for cocaine and metabolites	Inner city emergency department patients: 21/59 (36%) positive for cocaine in urine (8 had denied illicit drug use); 10 snorted crack, 3 snorted cocaine; controls, age and sex matched: 8/53 (15%) positive for cocaine	Multivariate analysis adjusted for age, sex: use of cocaine gave three-fold higher prevalence of new-onset bronchospasm, recurrence of asthma (OR 3.28; 95% CI 1.26-8.50)	Cocaine users more likely than controls to have reappearance of asthma symptoms after 5 year abatement, or new-onset bronchospasm Unreliable drug use in self-report; verify with laboratory tests
Rome et al. (2000)	Cross-sectional study Cocaine use and asthma; adherence to treatment modalities Informed consent, questionnaire, drug screen	Adults with asthma seen over 7 months in emergency department; 116 consented to participate; 103 consented to urine samples	116 patients: 68% female, mean age 33 years, 89% African American, 35% cigarette smokers, 13% (13 of 103) urine positive for cocaine, 5.8% (6 of 103) urine positive for opiates; 5/13 cocaine users hospitalized, 2 required intubation, mechanical ventilation	22% of admitted patients tested positive for cocaine; length of stay significantly longer in cocaine users than non-cocaine users: 5 vs. 2.5 days ($p < 0.05$)

Table 3.7 *Cont.*

Study	Method	Sample	Incidence	Results
Tashkin *et al.* (1992b)	Case–control study Respiratory effects in cocaine users Questionnaire for respiratory symptoms, drug use, pulmonary function tests	202 'crack habitual smokers (no IV abuse) (6.5 g/week over 53 months); 99 controls (non-users)	Crack users: 85% black, median most recent smoke 19 days (range, 1–180); 134 marijuana users (42 current, 92 former), 68 never used marijuana, 43 current tobacco users, 25 never smoked Non-users: 96% black, 30 marijuana users (18 current, 12 former), 69 never used marijuana, 26 tobacco users, 43 never used tobacco	Crack users: higher prevalence of acute respiratory symptoms within 1 to 12 h after smoking: cough and black sputum (43.7%), hemoptysis (5.7%), chest pain (38.5%); mild significant impaired diffusion capacity
Tashkin *et al.* (1992a)	Case–control study Respiratory effects of free basing cocaine	177 heavy habitual free-base cocaine smokers (mean 6.6 g/ week over 27 months) 75 age, sex, race matched non-cocaine users Both groups may have smoked marijuana or tobacco	After controlling for smoking, cocaine users: high frequency of respiratory symptoms (cough, black sputum, chest pain); obstructive abnormalities in large airways; mild, significant impaired diffusing capacity at alveolar-capillary interface	Cocaine users more likely than non-users to have respiratory symptoms, including diffusion impairment, at alveolar–capillary interface; increased respiratory symptoms and chronic airflow obstruction
van der Klooster & Grootendorst (2001)	Case report Bullous emphysema in cocaine users Chart review, chest radiography, CT	40-year-old long-term (17 years) cocaine smoker, unknown history of cigarette use	Bilateral bullous emphysema; air/fluid-filled cavities suggested abscess Intubated, mechanical ventilation, IV antibiotics, chest tube; died of respiratory failure Sputum culture: *Enterobacter*, streptococci, normal α₁-antitrypsin	Deficiency of α₁-antitrypsin major cause of bullous emphysema; cocaine smoking also a possible cause

AM, alveolar macrophages; CI, confidence interval; ET-1, endothelin-1; IV, intravenous; OR, odds ratio.

and recurrent nose bleeds. The authors recommended that healthcare providers caring for adolescents with nasal signs and symptoms assess the patients for cocaine abuse.

Meleca *et al.* (1997) reported seven patients with burns to their upper aerodigestive tract. All seven had smoked crack or freebase cocaine and two required emergency tracheotomy.

In a review of 407 cases of epiglottitis, Mayo-Smith & Spinale (1997) found four patients, aged 22 to 33 years, with thermal injury related to inhalation of heated objects. One injury occurred from the tip of a marijuana cigarette, three others when metal pieces of crack cocaine pipes were inhaled. The signs and symptoms in the individuals were similar to that of infectious epiglottitis.

Ciorba *et al.* (2009) reported a cocaine user experiencing bilateral hearing loss after an episode of acute cocaine intoxication. The individual developed sensorineural hearing loss after intravenous injection of cocaine. Cochlear lesion sites were identified by audiological testing.

Olfactory deficits were found by Bauer & Mott (1996) in a cross-sectional study of 38 drug-abusing adults, including 19 cocaine users, and 12 controls. Upon exposure to an odorous puff of air, the cocaine-dependent and alcohol-dependent subjects had decreased olfactory evoked potentials compared with the nicotine-dependent and normal controls. This study supports case reports of damage to the peripheral and central olfactory apparatus in certain drug abusers.

Underdahl & Chiou (1998) described preseptal cellulitis and orbital bone damage in a 40-year-old male who used nasal cocaine. Computed tomography (CT) and nasal biopsy showed cartilaginous and bone destruction in the nasal septum and medial wall of an orbit, along with inflammatory exudates and cellulitis. Mucoperichondrial ischemia was evident in this cocaine user, who also had diabetes mellitus.

Damage to the nasal cavity was also found by Trimarchi *et al.* (2003) who reported on 25 cocaine-using individuals who had midline destructive lesions. All 25 had septal perforation. Partial destruction of the inferior turbinates was found in 16 (68%) and hard palate reabsorption in six (24%). Two patients with hard palate reabsorption also had soft palate disease. A diagnosis of cocaine-related necrosis was made after physical examination, endoscopy, blood and urine analyses, radiography, and nasal biopsies. Serum levels for anti-neutrophilic cytoplasmic antibodies (ANCA) were analyzed, along with antibodies against two neutrophilic compounds: proteinase-3 and myeloperoxidase. Nine of the patients tested positive for perinuclear-ANCA (p-ANCA) and five were positive for cytoplasmic-ANCA (c-ANCA). Proteinase-3 antibodies were found in all five patients with c-ANCA, while four of the nine patients with p-ANCA also tested positive for proteinase-3. (The exact role of ANCA is not clear, but it is associated with vasculitis, inflammation, and focal necrosis.)

A study by Wiesner *et al.* (2004) questioned the use of ANCA and proteinase-3 to diagnose destructive cocaine-related midline lesions (CIMDL) since ANCA and proteinase-3 are often used to diagnose Wegener's granulomatosis (WG; an uncommon inflammatory disease characterized by vasculitis). In a previous study they found antibodies to human neutrophil elastase (HNE) and ANCA (HNE-ANCA) in patients with cocaine destructive lesions but not in individuals with WG. In the 2004 study, HNE-ANCA was measured in 25 patients with CIMDL and a control cohort of 604 patients (64 with WG, 14 with microscopic polyangiitis, and 526 others) and 45 healthy volunteers. The findings are summarized in Table 3.8.

The authors suggested that ANCA–proteinase-3 testing may not be able to differentiate between WG and CIMDL and that multimodal testing and testing for HNE-ANCA may be more specific for CIMDL.

Table 3.8 Use of serological tests for diagnosis of cocaine-related midline destructive lesions

Sera	HNE-ANCA response	PR3-ANCA response
Cocaine-related midline destructive lesions	Positive in 84%	Positive in 57%
Control	Positive in 1.3%	
Wegener's granulomatosis, microscopic polyangiitis	Negative	
Healthy control sera	Negative	

HNE, human neutrophil elastase; PR3, proteinase-3; ANCA, anti-neutrophilic cytoplasmic antibodies.

In 2006, Trimarchi *et al.* reported on 30 patients with CIMDL. They compared these patients with 10 healthy patients, 10 patients with nasal polyposis, and 10 patients with WG. Nasal biopsies were taken, and subjects had blood tested for caspases 3, 9, and 8, enzymes associated with apoptosis and programmed cell death. All of the biopsies of the 30 patients with CIMDL tested positive for caspase 3 and 9 but not for caspase 8. In order to determine a time–concentration effect, an in vitro study using keratinocytic epithelial cells (HaCat) was performed. There was a positive relationship between the degree of apoptosis after a one hour of exposure to cocaine and increasing concentrations of cocaine. There was also a positive relationship between the degree of apoptosis and a stable concentration of cocaine over a six-hour period. The authors suggested that in some users cocaine may stimulate apoptotic events in the nasal cavity and ultimately the development of CIMDL.

In an attempt to clarify diagnostic and treatment algorithms in patients with necrotizing midline nasal lesions confirmed with CT, Westreich & Lawson (2004) studied three patients with WG, six with sarcoidosis, eight with cocaine abuse, and one with lymphoma. All patients had similar signs and symptoms; however, some patients also had extra-nasal lesions. Only two of the six patients with sarcoid and two of the three with WG had diagnostic serological tests. Diagnosis was confirmed in only one patient with WG, one with sarcoid, and the one with lymphoma. The degree of nasal destruction was greatest in the patients with lymphoma and WG, less in the cocaine users, and least in the sarcoid patients. Oronasal or oroantral fistulas were found only in five of the eight cocaine users and the one lymphoma patient. Only the cocaine users consistently had significantly elevated erythrocyte sedimentation rates. The authors suggested that biopsies and laboratory testing are unreliable in differentiating disease in these patients. Presence of other symptoms (e.g., neo-osteogenesis in mastoid disease in WG) may help to determine diagnosis. Hard and soft palate destruction was more commonly found in cocaine users and the patient with lymphoma.

Simsek *et al.* (2006) described four cocaine users with nasal perforation and two others with perforation through the hard palate. The laboratory findings showed ANCA in all four patients (one with c-ANCA and three with p-ANCA) and all four were carriers of *S. aureus*. The authors suggested that the bacterium may facilitate the development of ANCA and the ultimate nasal damage seen in these cocaine users.

Scheenstra *et al.* (2007) described a case of a 37-year-old cocaine user with nasal septal destruction. Acute necrotic inflammation was confirmed by biopsy. The ANCA test was positive, as was proteinase-3, suggestive of WG. However, a positive HNE-ANCA suggested cocaine-induced disease. The authors suggested that available laboratory tests may not be able to differentiate between WG and other conditions, including cocaine use.

Alexandrakis *et al.* (1999) described lacrimal duct obstruction in five women and two men who were chronic intranasal cocaine users. In addition to tearing, the patients experienced periorbital pain, edema, and destruction of the nasal septum and inferior turbinates. Three patients had extensive inflammation and fibrosis of the lacrimal duct.

After being treated for many years for necrotizing ulcerative periodontitis, a patient with gingival recession and dental erosion admitted to regularly applying cocaine to his gingival tissue. This case study, by Kapila & Kashani (1997), supports the toxic effect of cocaine and illustrates the creative misuse of the drug.

Chauhan *et al.* (2004) described a fibrous tumor in a 48-year-old chronic cocaine inhaler. The tumor was extensive, involving the entire nasal cavity and was diagnosed as a solitary fibrous tumor by immunohistochemical characteristics. According to the authors, this is the first case description of a nasal tumor in a cocaine inhaler.

These results are summarized in Table 3.9.

Comments

These studies provide some information about the possible harmful effect of cocaine on the nasal pharynx. Only one study, of adolescents in outpatient treatment programs, had a large sample size ($n = 336$). That study found that daily cocaine users (or over 100/lifetime) had an increase in nasal signs and symptoms, including inflammatory changes. Seven other studies provide some support for cocaine-related mucosal burns or destruction in the upper airway and nasal cavity. However, these studies were small, with one to 30 participants. Two studies by Trimarchi and coworkers (2003, 2006) supported their hypothesis that inflammatory and apoptotic events may be associated with cocaine use. They found that ANCA, proteinase-3, myeloperoxidase, and caspase markers were found in a number of patients with midline destructive nasal lesions. However, neither of the two studies had normal controls or healthy cocaine users; all of the cocaine users in these two studies already had diagnoses of midline destructive lesions.

Some authors question the reliability of using ANCA with or without proteinase-3 to diagnose CIMDL, primarily because of overlap with other diseases including WG, lymphoma, and sarcoidosis. Use of HNE-ANCA, as described in one study, may help to provide a biological marker for CIMDL. Further study is needed to determine the incidence and prevalence of CIMDL in a large number of cocaine users, including those who snort or smoke crack compared with injection users. It would also be helpful to determine the prevalence of ANCA, HNE-ANCA, and elevated caspase 3 and 8 in cocaine users compared with non-users.

None of the studies provides statistical data that would help to support using the research recommendations to guide practice. However, several of the studies suggested that individuals presenting with nasal or upper airway signs and symptoms should be evaluated for cocaine use.

Nervous system disease

A number of epidemiological abstracts were found in the review of research studies published from 1988 to 2008 and cited in PubMed. The review of these articles is organized by subtopics into the following categories:

- cerebrovascular studies
- strokes and subarachnoid hemorrhage (SAH)

Table 3.9 Otorhinolaryngological disease

Study	Method	Sample	Incidence	Results
Alexandrakis et al. (1999)	Case report Nasolacrimal duct obstruction CT, MRI	Chronic intranasal cocaine users (mean 11 years); 5 female, 2 male	Tear duct obstruction, periorbital edema, erythema, nasal septal destruction, loss of inferior turbinates Extensive destruction on CT, MRI: bcny orbit, opacification of sinuses, 3 with inflammation and fibrosis of lacrimal duct	Chronic cocaine use should be explored in lacrimal duct obstruction
Bauer & Mott (1996)	Cross-sectional study Olfactory apparatus competency: nasal air puff of odorous stimuli and olfactory evoked potentials	50 adults: 19 cocaine users, 7 alcohol users, 10 nicotine users, 2 anosmia, 12 free of drug with olfactory disorder	Smaller evoked potentials in cocaine- and alcohol-dependent groups compared with normal and nicotine dependent	Olfactory deficit consistent with reports of decreased smell sense; suggests lesions in peripheral or central olfactory apparatus
Chauhan et al. (2004)	Case report Fibrous tumor in nasal cavity CT scan	Female 48 years, chronic cocaine use	Immunohistochemical pattern of solitary fibrous tumor in nasal cavity	First report of fibrous tumor in cocaine user
Ciorba et al. (2009)	Case report Inner ear damage and cocaine use	IV cocaine user	Sudden, bilateral sensorineural hearing loss after cocaine use	First report of hearing loss after IV cocaine intoxication
Kapila & Kashani (1997)	Case report Gingival recession	Cocaine user initially diagnosed with necrotizing ulcerative periodontitis	Rapid gingival recession, dental erosion; user admitted to applying cocaine directly to gums	Unusual application of cocaine to gingival tissue
Mayo-Smith & Spinale (1997)	Case series Thermal epiglottitis	4 illicit drug users (aged 22 to 33 years) with epiglottitis	Thermal epiglottic burns: 3 patients from metal pieces of crack cocaine pipes; 1 from tip of marijuana cigarette	Thermal epiglottic burns and infectious epiglottitis have similar signs and symptoms
Meleca et al. (1997)	Case series Mucosal injury to aerodigestive tract	7 patients with burns to upper aerodigestive tract	All smoked crack or freebase cocaine; 2 required emergency tracheotomy	Mucosal burns can occur in users of crack, freebase cocaine

Reference	Study type / methods	Subjects	Results	Conclusion
Scheenstra et al. (2007)	Case report Necrotic nasal inflammation	37-year-old male cocaine user with necrotic inflammation of nasal mucosa	Positive for ANCA antibodies and proteinase-3 (indicative of WG); positive for HNE antibodies (more indicative of cocaine use)	Cocaine-induced nasal injury with positive ANCA similar to WG
Schwartz et al. (1989a)	Survey, demographic study Nasal symptoms in adolescent cocaine users Questionnaire	464 adolescents, non-IV drug abusers in outpatient treatment programs in five geographic regions	336 (72%) stated use of cocaine: < 25 times (203/335; 60%); 25–99 times (107/336; 32%); daily, 100+ times (26/336; 8%) Daily users: statistically significant increase in respiratory symptoms compared with < 25 time users (sniffling, sinus problems, diminished olfaction); daily users (47%) more likely than 25+ users (30%) to have nasal crusts, scabs, recurrent epistaxis	Teens with nasal signs and symptoms should be evaluated for cocaine use
Simsek et al. (2006)	Case report Midline nasal lesions	3 males (29, 30, 34 years), 1 female (36 years) with nasal septal perforation, history of cocaine use, 2 had perforation of hard palate	ANCA positive in all (1/4 c-ANCA, 3/4 p-ANCA); all nasal carriers of S. aureus	Suggests that S. aureus facilitates development of ANCA; ANCA then stimulates destructive injury
Trimarchi et al. (2003)	Midline destructive nasal lesions in cocaine users Physical examination, endoscopy, blood & urine analysis, radiography, biopsy, serum for ANCA, PR3, myeloperoxidase	25 patients with CIMDL from 1991–2001	Septal perforation in all 25; 16 (68%) with partial destruction of inferior turbinate; 6 (24%) with hard palate reabsorption (2 with soft palate involvement); 14 (56% with ANCA (9 p-ANCA, 5 c-ANCA); 9 also positive for PR3 antibodies	Individuals with sinonasal inflammation, destructive lesions should be assessed for cocaine abuse
Trimarchi et al. (2006)	Case–control study Nasal apoptosis in cocaine users Caspase 3, 8, 9 assay (nasal biopsy) Time–concentration assay with epithelial cells	30 patients with CIMDL; controls: 10 healthy patients; 10 patients with nasal polyposis; 10 patients with WG	CIMDL, all had caspase 3 and 9, not 8; controls, no caspases Time–concentration-dependent effects of cocaine seen in in vitro study	Time–dose-dependent increase in injury to cocaine-treated epithelial cells; cocaine can cause apoptosis in epithelial cells, may trigger apoptosis, leading to CIMDL

Table 3.9 *Cont.*

Study	Method	Sample	Incidence	Results
Underdahl & Chiou (1998)	Case report Midline nasal lesions	40-year-old male nasal cocaine user with diabetes mellitus	Preseptal cellulitis, inflammation, exudates with neutrophilia; cartilaginous and bone destruction of nasal septum, medial wall of one orbit; mucoperichondrial ischemia	Midline lesions associated with nasal cocaine use
Westreich & Lawson (2004)	Case report Midline nasal lesions Differential diagnosis	18 patients with similar signs and symptoms: 3 with WG; 6 with sarcoid; 8 with cocaine abuse; 1 with lymphoma	Serology tests: 2/6 sarcoid patients positive for sarcoidosis; 2/3 WG patients positive for WG Biopsy confirmed disease: 1/3 sarcoid, 1/3 WG, 1/1 lymphoma ESR consistently, statistically elevated only in cocaine users Nasal destruction: WG, lymphoma > cocaine > sarcoidosis	Laboratory tests, biopsies unreliable in all diseases; hard and soft palate defects most often seen in patients with cocaine abuse, lymphoma
Wiesner et al. (2004)	Case–control study ANCA, HNE antibodies in CIMDL	25 patients with CIMDL Control cohort 604 patients: 64 WG, 14 microscopic polyangiitis, 526 others including 45 healthy volunteers	CIMDL: HNE-ANCA 84% in one assay; PR3 positive 57% in one assay Controls: HNE-ANCA 1.3% in one assay; WG/ microscopic polyangiitis, healthy controls all negative for HNE-ANCA	HNE-ANCA may be a diagnostic marker for CIMDL, since not seen in other autoimmune disorders; it may be a more accurate diagnostic tool for CIMDL than PR3 assay (which is more diagnostic for WG)

ANCA, anti-neutrophilic cytoplasmic antibodies; CIMDL, cocaine-induced midline destructive lesions; CT, computed tomography; ESR, erythrocyte sedimentation rate; HNE, human neutrophil elastase; IV, intravenous; MRI, magnetic resonance imaging; PR3, proteinase-3; WG, Wegener's granulomatosis.

- autonomic nervous system (ANS) diseases
- CNS diseases
- demyelinating diseases
- neurological manifestations
- sleep disorders.

Cerebrovascular studies

Five studies reported on research related to the effect of cocaine on vascular flow in the CNS.

Two studies reported on cocaine-induced vasoconstriction of cerebral vessels. In the first study (Kaufman *et al.* 1998a), 23 normal males with a recreational use of cocaine of 3 to 40 lifetime exposures received either 0.2 or 0.4 mg/kg cocaine or a placebo while undergoing dynamic susceptibility contrast (DSC) magnetic resonance imaging (MRI). When regional blood flow was measured, there was no change in blood flow when the placebo was administered. However, 10 minutes after the administration of either dose of cocaine, blood flow volume decreased significantly (77 ± 4% of baseline; $p < 0.002$). The authors suggested that DSC-MRI could be used as a tool to evaluate treatments to reverse cocaine's effects.

The second study (Kaufman *et al.* 1998b) was a double-blind random controlled trial designed to determine cocaine's effect on cerebral vasoconstriction using magnetic resonance angiography. Twenty-four healthy cocaine users (lifetime exposures 3 to > 40) were given 0.2 mg/kg cocaine, 0.4 mg/kg cocaine, or a placebo. The subjects had no other illicit drug use, hypertension, or cerebrovascular disease. After 20 minutes, vasoconstriction was determined in three out of nine of the subjects receiving 0.2 mg/kg, five out of eight receiving 0.4 mg/kg, and one out of seven receiving the placebo. Vasoconstriction was dose related in those receiving cocaine ($p = 0.03$). When cocaine use was stratified by dose (3 to 10 times, 11 to 40 times, > 40 times), there was a greater likelihood of vasoconstriction in those with greater use of cocaine (over 40 lifetime uses) ($p < 0.001$). The authors suggested that cerebrovascular dysfunction might be influenced by long-term use of cocaine.

Herning *et al.* (1999) studied seven cocaine users to determine blood flow velocity during and after intravenous cocaine use. The patients were given 10, 25, and 50 mg intravenous cocaine or a placebo. Transcranial Doppler sonography was used to measure continuous cerebral blood flow velocity. Blood pressure and heart rate were also measured. After all cocaine injections, all patients had significant increases in mean and systolic velocity that lasted for two minutes. After administration of the placebo, there was no change in blood flow velocity. Their findings suggested that intravenous cocaine use causes a brief, immediate vasoconstriction in large cerebral vessels that quickly dissipates.

In a double-blind randomized study of 31 male and female cocaine users, Johnson *et al.* (2005) found that low and high doses of intravenous cocaine caused global and regional hypoperfusion. Fifteen were given low-dose cocaine (0.325 mg/kg) followed by a 48-hour rest period and then given a placebo. Sixteen were given high-dose cocaine (0.650 mg/kg) then a placebo after a similar 48-hour rest period. Positron emission tomography (PET) was used to analyze cerebral perfusion. While hypoperfusion was seen with both low and high doses, greater hypoperfusion was seen with the high dose, especially in the dopamine-rich sublobar and midbrain regions. The left hemisphere, which is more dopamine rich, was most seriously affected. The maximal effect of the hypoperfusion occurred within eight minutes of intravenous cocaine administration and mostly dissipated within 32 minutes. The authors suggested that larger doses of cocaine may increase the users' risk for ischemic stroke caused by hypoperfusion.

Rao *et al.* (2007) researched the effect of in utero cocaine exposure on the cerebral vessels of adolescents in a case–control study. Perfusion functional MRI (fMRI) was used during rest to study resting cerebral blood flow in 24 adolescents who had been exposed to cocaine in utero and 25 matched non-cocaine-exposed individuals as controls. The results showed significantly decreased global cerebral blood flow in the cocaine-exposed group, especially in the posterior and inferior brain regions (occipital cortex, thalamus), but significantly increased blood flow in the anterior and superior regions of the brain (prefrontal, cingulate, insula, amygdala, superior parietal cortex). Variation in the brain anatomy did not explain any functional modulations. The researchers hypothesized that compensatory mechanisms during neural development might explain the increase in blood flow to some areas and the decrease in flow in others. They also suggested that arterial spin-labeling perfusion MRI might be helpful to study the long-term effects of in utero exposure to cocaine.

These studies are summarized in Table 3.10.

Comments

Collectively, these studies support the vasoconstrictive effect of cocaine, cocaine metabolites, and norepinephrine effects on the cerebral vasculature. Although the number of patients in these studies were relatively small (7 to 40) and the methods quite varied (PET, structural and perfusion fMRI, cerebral angiography, sonography), it is suggested that intravenous cocaine can affect cerebral vessel size quickly and that chronic use of cocaine can also have an effect on perfusion to various areas of the brain. In utero exposure to cocaine may also have an effect on the offspring of cocaine-using mothers. Further studies with larger numbers of subjects and using similar techniques would help to determine risk of cerebral vascular changes in cocaine users.

Stroke and subarachnoid hemorrhage

Thirteen studies were found that explored the risk of stroke (ischemic and hemorrhagic) in cocaine users, including three studies on autopsy samples. Five additional studies specifically addressed SAH in cocaine users, and two studies describe patients with pontine–pituitary infarcts.

Kaku & Lowenstein (1990) studied 214 individuals, ages 15 to 44, with ischemic and hemorrhagic strokes. These 214 patients were compared with 214 controls matched for age, sex, and year of hospitalization, who had diagnoses of status asthmaticus, acute appendicitis, or acute cholecystitis. Seventy-three (34%) of the patients with strokes were drug abusers, with cocaine being the major drug abused, while only 18 of the 214 controls (8%) were drug abusers. In patients with strokes, there was a temporal relationship between drug use and the onset of the stroke in 34 patients; infectious endocarditis was the presumed cause of the stroke in 13 patients. The risk for stroke in drug abusers compared with non-users was found to be 6.5 (95% CI 3.1–13.6) when controlling for risk factors. The RR increased to 49.4 (95% CI 6.4–379) in those who had signs and symptoms within six hours of drug use. In individuals 35 years of age or younger, drug abuse was the most likely factor increasing the risk for stroke (RR 11.7; 95% CI 3.2–42.5). The authors found that among young adults, use of cocaine was a risk factor for strokes.

Table 3.10 Cerebrovascular studies

Study	Method	Sample	Incidence	Results
Herning et al. (1999)	Descriptive study Effect of cocaine on blood flow velocity Transcranial Doppler sonography, BP, heart rate	7 cocaine users given 10, 25, 50 mg IV cocaine or placebo	All doses of cocaine caused significant increased mean and systolic velocity that lasted 2 min; no change in velocity with placebo	Cocaine causes a brief, immediate vasoconstriction in large cerebral arteries
Johnson et al. (2005)	Double-blind randomized study Dose-dependent time-related effect on blood flow with IV cocaine PET scan	31 male and female cocaine users: 15 low dose (0.325 mg/kg) and placebo; 16 high dose (0.650 mg/kg) and placebo; rest phase of 48 h between treatments	Both low and high doses associated with global, regional hypoperfusion; greater hypoperfusion with high dose in dopamine-rich sublobar and midbrain regions; left hemisphere most seriously affected; maximal effect at 8 min; most effect dissipated in 32 min	High doses of cocaine used recreationally may increase risk of ischemic stroke in users; cocaine effect is time dependent on pharmacology; greater in dopamine-rich areas
Kaufman et al. (1998a)	Double-blind study Cerebral blood volume and cocaine DSC-MRI	23 healthy cocaine users (3 to 40 lifetime use)	Cerebral blood flow 10 min after 0.2 or 0.4 mg/kg IV cocaine: fall of 77 ± 4% from baseline (p < 0.002); no change with placebo	DSC-MRI may be a useful tool in assessing cerebral blood volume
Kaufman et al. (1998b)	Randomized double-blind controlled trial Effect of IV cocaine or placebo on cerebral vessels Cerebral MR angiography at baseline and 20 min later	24 healthy cocaine users, mean age 29 years, median use 8 lifetime exposures (3 to > 40)	Angiographic changes rated by two reviewers blind to treatment: vasoconstrictive response in 5/8 at 0.4 mg/kg, 3/9 at 0.2 mg/kg, 1/7 with placebo Factoring lifetime exposures, statistically strong dose-related effect: p < 0.001	Vasoconstriction in cerebral vessels occurred in the absence of other risks (polydrug use, high BP, cerebrovascular disease); cocaine use may have a cumulative effect on blood vessel reactivity with long-term use
Rao et al. (2007)	Case-control study Effect of in utero cocaine exposure on cerebral vessels in adolescent offspring Functional MRI during rest	24 adolescents exposed to cocaine in utero; 25 matched non-cocaine-exposed controls	Cocaine-exposed adolescents: significant decrease in global cerebral blood flow in posterior, inferior brain regions (occipital cortex, thalamus); significant increase in blood flow in anterior, superior regions (prefrontal, cingulate, insular, amygdala, superior parietal cortex)	Functional modulation cannot be accounted for by variation in brain anatomy; compensatory mechanisms during cerebral development may account for differences in blood flow

BP, blood pressure; DSC, dynamic susceptibility contrast; IV, intravenous; MRI, magnetic resonance imaging; PET, positron emission tomography.

Levine *et al.* (1990) studied the cerebrovascular effects of crack cocaine in 28 patients who had used crack cocaine within 72 hours of the onset of their strokes: 18 (64%) displayed neurological signs and symptoms within one hour of use and 15 (45%) had occlusive or hemorrhagic strokes associated with a severe headache. In these 28 patients, 18 had infarcts (two hemorrhagic/one fatal), five had SAH, four had intraparenchymal hemorrhage, and one had a primary intraventricular hemorrhage. Of the 18 with infarcts, the vessels involved included the middle cerebral artery (10), anterior cerebral artery (three), posterior cerebral artery (one), and vertebrobasilar artery (four). Twenty-eight patients had another risk factor for stroke, including mild mitral valve prolapse (four), hypertension (four), cigarette use (eight), and alcohol use (six). The authors suggested that there is a strong temporal relationship between crack cocaine use and stroke, particularly at a young age (23–49 years), and that young individuals with strokes should be screened for cocaine use and other illicit drugs.

Daras *et al.* (1991) described 18 patients (15 males, 3 females; 21 to 47 years) who had cerebral infarcts after using cocaine. Thirteen had hemispheric infarcts; two had brainstem strokes, two anterior spinal artery infarcts and one both a hemispheric and a cerebellar infarct. Nine smoked crack; four snorted cocaine; three injected cocaine, and two used an unknown route. Two of the patients died. Only six of the patients had traditional risk factors for cerebral vascular disease. The authors suggested that the strokes might have been caused by vasospasm, a sudden increase in blood pressure, a myocardial infarction (MI) with cardiac arrhythmias, increased platelet aggregation, or vasculitis – all outcomes reported with cocaine use.

In order to determine the proportion of strokes associated with drug abuse, Sloan *et al.* (1991) studied 167 (94%) of 178 patients with stroke who had provided information about their use of drugs. For 51 (31%), there were incomplete data. However, 11 of the remaining 116 (9.5%) acknowledged use of illicit drugs, including five (4.3%) who used cocaine. The average age of the 116 patients was 41 years (range, 25 to 56 years). The distribution of those who used illicit drugs among those with stroke was as follows: four had cerebral infarcts, two had intracerebral hemorrhages, and five had SAHs. Besides cocaine, abused drugs included over-the-counter sympathomimetics, phencyclidine, and heroin.

Kibayashi *et al.* (1995) looked at autopsy specimens from 26 individuals with cocaine-induced intracerebral hemorrhage compared with 26 with cocaine-induced cerebral aneurysm ruptures. They found that hypertensive cardiovascular disease was more prevalent in the patients with intracerebral hemorrhage and concluded that high blood pressure predisposes persons to cocaine-induced intracranial hemorrhage. An alteration in the autoregulation of blood flow caused by cocaine use was hypothesized as the cause of the hemorrhage.

Konzen *et al.* (1995) presented three cases of crack users with cerebral infarcts. In all three patients, the internal carotid artery was affected; two had large filling defects and one had vasospastic dysfunction. None had cardiac or hematological causes for their strokes. They concluded that in some cases of brain infarcts, crack cocaine can cause vasospasm of the large arteries and vascular thromboses.

Aggarwal *et al.* (1996) studied autopsy specimens from 14 individuals with intracranial hemorrhage. Intracerebral hemorrhage or SAH was found in 12 specimens. Since there were no intracranial arteriolar abnormalities or only non-specific changes, the authors suggested that the hemorrhage occurring in cocaine users occurs without any detectable vascular abnormalities.

An autopsy study by Nolte *et al.* (1996) suggested that non-traumatic fatal intracranial hemorrhage associated with cocaine use results from the pharmacological effects of cocaine rather than pathological vessel findings. In 10 of the 17 individuals studied (59%), there were positive cocaine toxicology tests. Of these, seven had parenchymal hemorrhage and three had SAHs from berry aneurysms. There was no evidence of vasculitis or other abnormalities. The authors suggested that cocaine users were at increased risk for intra-cranial hemorrhage.

In a retrospective case–control study, Qureshi *et al.* (1997) found that crack use at any time or acute crack use was not significantly associated with stroke or cerebral infarct. Comparing 66 crack users with 99 non-cocaine-using controls, the OR for stroke was 0.7 (95% CI 0.4–1.8) and the OR for cerebral infarct was 0.5 (95% CI 0.2–1.2). In acute use of cocaine (within 48 hours of incident), the OR for stroke was 1.9 (95% CI 0.7–5.1) and for cerebral infarct was 1.2 (95% CI 0.4–3.8). In this population aged 29–39 years, crack use was not significantly associated with stroke or infarct.

However, a study by Petitti *et al.* (1998) found that the use of cocaine and amphet-amines was a strong risk factor for strokes. Face-to-face interviews were carried out with 347 women experiencing strokes (aged 15 to 44 years) and 1021 randomly selected age-matched controls. Using univariate analyses, the OR for stroke in women using cocaine or amphetamines was 8.5 (95% CI 3.6–20.0). After adjusting for confounders, the OR was 7.0 (95% CI 2.8–17.9). This study was carried out with an insured urban population, in contrast to many other studies using cases from uninsured, poor, or minority populations.

A second article by Daras *et al.* (1994b) described 55 cases of cerebrovascular disease in cocaine users: 26 smoking crack, 10 snorting cocaine, and 12 injecting cocaine. Of the 55 patients, 25 had ischemic strokes and 30 had hemorrhagic strokes (one had both). Fifteen had other risk factors for stroke. Fifteen experienced their infarcts within three hours of cocaine use, and 17 had hemorrhagic strokes within three hours of use. Ten infarcts occurred after an overnight binge. Sixteen of the hemorrhagic strokes were intracerebral, nine were subarachnoid, and five were intraventricular. Angiography found four aneurysms and three arterial–venous malformations. Computed tomography identified the infarct in 15 patients, but was normal in seven patients with pure motor hemiparesis and in three patients with anterior spinal infarcts. Daras and others again suggested that cocaine-related physiological effects could have caused these strokes.

In a retrospective review, Nanda *et al.* (2006) studied 42 cocaine-using individuals experiencing strokes, 15 with bleeding aneurysms (SAH) and 27 with strokes. The mean age was 38 years, and males outnumbered females by 20 to 7. Fifteen had hypertension, and 15 tested positive for cocaine or cocaine metabolites in the urine; heroin and marijuana were found in seven others. Nine of the patients with intracranial or SAHs died. Cocaine intoxication correlated with a fatal cerebrovascular accident (CVA) ($p < 0.001$) and a poor Glasgow Outcome Score ($p < 0.001$). The authors suggested that cocaine use was associated with fatal strokes and poor outcomes.

Westover *et al.* (2007) studied young adults abusing amphetamines or cocaine and their risk for stoke. In a cross-sectional design using a quality indicators database of over three million patients discharged from 2000 to 2003, separate logistic regression models were developed for 2003 only. The 937 individuals with hemorrhagic stroke were compared with 998 individuals with ischemic strokes occurring in 2003. In both conditions, the age range for the stroke patients was 18 to 44 years. The OR for hemorrhagic stroke associated with amphetamine use was 4.95 (95% CI 3.24–7.55). The risk for ischemic stroke in amphetamine users was not significant. The OR for hemorrhagic stroke associated with cocaine use was 2.33 (95% CI 1.74–3.11), and for ischemic stroke was 2.03 (95% CI 1.48–2.79). Amphetamine users were at a higher risk for death from hemorrhagic stroke than were cocaine users. The authors suggested that, as stimulant drug abuse increases, the risk for hospital admissions for stroke and stroke-related mortality will also increase.

Three articles were specific to SAH in cocaine users. A case–control study by Fessler *et al.* (1997) reported on 33 patients with positive drug screens for cocaine and compared them with 44 patients with SAH with no evidence of cocaine use. There were 16 patients with SAH, 12 with four-vessel angiograms showing 14 aneurysms; six patients had intra-cerebral hemorrhage, and seven patients had ischemic strokes. They found that cocaine users tended to have SAH at an earlier age if incidental neurovascular anomalies were present. The average age of cocaine users with SAH was 32.8 years (with 4.9 mm diameter aneurysms), while the non-cocaine users were an average age of 52.2 years, with 11.0 mm diameter aneurysms. Eighteen (54%) indicated that their stroke occurred while using cocaine. Overall, 87.9% had their onset of stroke within the first six hours of using cocaine.

A retrospective study by Simpson *et al.* (1990) indicated that patients using cocaine had significantly poorer outcomes for SAH than patients with no known exposure to the drug.

Conway & Tamargo (2001) reported on 440 patients with aneurysmal SAH admitted over a seven-year period. Twenty-seven tested positive for cocaine in the urine or by history of cocaine use ($n = 7$). Cocaine users were more likely to have delayed clinical deficit (anywhere from 3 to 16 days after the aneurysmal SAH). After hypervolemic and hyper-tension treatment, the OR for angiographic vessel narrowing compared with the controls was 3.90 (95% CI 1.77–8.62; $p = 0.001$). The cocaine users were younger than the controls (mean age 36 vs. 52 years; $p < 0.0001$), and more likely to have an aneurysm of the anterior circulation (OR 6.89; 95% CI 1.18–47.47; $p = 0.029$). However, Glasgow Outcome Scores were no different. Recent cocaine use was independently associated with vasospasm (OR 6.41; 95% CI 2.14–19.23; $p = 0.0009$). The authors suggested that cocaine users were more likely to have increased vasospasm after an aneurysmal SAH, but that there were no differences in the neurological outcomes compared with controls.

Pituitary and pontine infarcts have also been reported in the literature. Insel & Dhanjal (2004) reported a case of a 55-year-old woman (intranasal user) with destructive nasal and paranasal lesions that involved the base of the anterior skull. Computed tomography suggested cocaine-induced ischemic necrosis involving the pituitary gland. An MRI dis-closed a decreased pituitary volume. Several pituitary hormone levels were decreased, including adrenocorticotropic hormone, luteinizing hormone, and follicle-stimulating hormone. She also had diabetes insipidus related to decreased antidiuretic hormone. In another case report, Zandio *et al.* (2008) described a 56-year-old female with hypertension and cocaine use who initially was seen with a pontine paramedian infarct related to destructive midline structural lesions. Nine months later she had a pontomesencephalic infarct. The authors suggested that older cocaine users are also at risk for cocaine-related strokes.

Table 3.11 summarizes these studies.

Comments
The varied terminology contributes to the difficulty in analyzing this particular subsection. The terms stroke, infarct, ischemic stroke, hemorrhagic stroke, SAH, intracranial hemor-rhage, and intracerebral hemorrhage may have different meanings or interpretations for the

Table 3.11 Stroke and subarachnoid hemorrhage

Study	Method	Sample	Incidence	Results
Aggarwal et al. (1996)	Autopsy findings Intracranial hemorrhage	14 patients	Intracerebral/SAH in 12; intracranial arterioles normal or non-specific changes found	Suggests hemorrhage occurred without detectable vascular abnormality
Boco & Macdonald (2004)	Retrospective study of SAH Vasoconstriction after cocaine-associated SAH Angiogram	13 cocaine users and 26 matched controls	No difference between users and controls in vessel characteristics	No evidence of narrowing of large arteries, distal narrowing, vasculitis in cocaine users
Conway & Tamargo (2001)	Retrospective study Vasospasm with cocaine use	440 patients with aneurysmal SAH; 27 (6.1%) cocaine positive in urine (within 72 h of aneurysmal SAH) or by history	Compared with controls, cocaine users younger (36 vs. 52 years; $p < 0.0001$), more likely to have anterior circulation aneurysm (97% vs. 84%; OR 6.89; 95% CI 1.18–47.47) 63% cocaine users and 30% controls had delayed clinical deficits (3–16 days), response to hypervolemic, high BP treatment or angiogram confirmed narrowing of vessels (OR 3.90; 95% CI 1.77–8.62; $p = 0.001$). Recent cocaine use independently associated with vasospasm (OR 6.41; 95% CI 2.14–19.23; $p = 0.0001$), and thick blood clot on admission CT (OR 7.46; 95% CI 2.14–19.23; $p = 0.0009$). No Glasgow Outcome Score differences	Cocaine users more likely to have delayed clinical deficits (3 to 16 days later); increased vasospasm after SAH more likely in cocaine users
Daras et al. (1991)	Case series CNS infarction with cocaine use	18 using cocaine: 15 male, 3 female; 21–47 years of age, 2 died Cocaine use: 9 smoked crack, 4 snorted cocaine, 3 injected IV, 2 unknown Traditional risk factors in 6	Types of infarcts: 13 hemispheric infarcts, 2 brainstem strokes, 2 anterior spinal artery infarcts, 1 both hemispheric and cerebellar infarct	Infarcts likely related to vasospasm, sudden high BP, AMI with cardiovascular arrhythmia, increased platelet aggregation, vasculitis

39

Table 3.11 Cont.

Study	Method	Sample	Incidence	Results
Daras et al. (1994b)	Case series Stroke and cocaine use CT	55 strokes in 54 patients Cocaine use: 26 smoked crack, 10 snorted cocaine, 12 injected cocaine Risk factors for stroke in 15; 10 infarcts after overnight binge	Strokes: 25 ischemic, 30 hemorrhagic Strokes occurred within 3 h of use in 15 with infarcts, in 17 with hemorrhagic stroke Hemorrhagic stroke: 9 subarachnoid, 16 intracerebral (8 basal ganglia, 7 hemispheric, 1 brainstem), 5 intraventricular Angiography: 4 aneurysms, 3 AVMs CT: infarcts in 15, 7 normal with pure motor hemiparesis, 3 with anterior spinal infarcts	Hemorrhage likely related to sudden increase in BP, especially in those with pre-existing aneurysm or AVM; infarcts likely caused by vasospasm, arteritis, AMI with arrhythmia, increased platelet aggregation
Fessler et al. (1997)	Case–control study SAH and cocaine Arteriogram	33 patients with SAH, association with cocaine use confirmed by drug screen (87.9% onset of stroke 6 h after cocaine use); 44 patients with SAH, no cocaine exposure	16 patients with SAH (cocaine users, mean 32.8 years; non-users, mean 52.2 years; $p < 0.05$) 12 patients had four vessel angiogram, with 14 aneurysms; 6 intracerebral hemorrhage; 7 ischemic stroke Cocaine mortality 27.3% (77.8% in patients with SAH)	Chronic cocaine use predisposes patients to have SAH at an earlier age than non-users if they have pre-existing neurovascular anomalies
Howington et al. (2003)	Retrospective study Prediction of outcome of aneurysmal SAH	108 with aneurysmal SAH, 36 (33.3%) used cocaine within 24 h of onset	Cocaine users vs. non-users more likely to: score 4 or 5 on Hunt–Hess scale (20/36 [55.6%] vs. 8/72 [11.1%]; $p < 0.0001$); experience vasospasm (28/36 [77.8%] vs. 20/72 [27.8%]; $p < 0.0001$); score between 1 and 3 on Glasgow Outcome Scale (33/36 [91.7%] vs. 20/72 [27.8%]; $p < 0.001$) Cocaine users: 3.3 times increased risk of poor outcome (95% CI 2.24–4.85)	Use of cocaine negatively affects aneurysmal SAH outcomes
Insel & Dhanjal (2004)	Case report Pituitary infarct CT, MRI	55-year-old woman with long-term nasal cocaine use	CT: destruction of paranasal sinuses into base of skull; MRI, decreased pituitary volume; laboratory tests, decreased ACTH, LH, FSH, ADH	Cocaine-induced ischemic necrosis of midline nasal structures leading to pituitary infarct

Study	Type / Focus	Sample / Details	Findings	Conclusions
Kaku & Lowenstein (1990)	Case–control study; Cocaine risk for stroke	214 with ischemic, hemorrhagic stroke; 15–44 years; 34% drug abusers (cocaine primary drug abused) 214 matched controls, (status asthmaticus, acute appendicitis, acute cholecystitis)	73 (34%) with stroke were drug abusers; 18 (8%) of controls used drugs Strokes: 34 temporal relationship with drug use; infectious endocarditis other cause in 13 Risk for stroke in drug abusers, 6.5 (95% CI 3.1–13.6); risk for stroke if signs/symptoms occurred within 6 h of drug use, 49.4 (95% CI 6.4–379); most likely factor increasing risk for stroke, drug abuse (RR 11.7; 95% CI 3.2–42.5)	In young adults, cocaine use was an increasing risk for strokes
Kibayashi et al. (1995)	Autopsy findings; Predisposition for hemorrhagic stroke	26 with cocaine-induced intracerebral hemorrhage; 26 with cocaine-induced cerebral aneurysm rupture	High BP; cardiovascular disease greater in intracerebral hemorrhage than in aneurysm	High BP predisposes to cocaine-induced hemorrhage, secondary to alteration in cerebral autoregulation of blood flow
Konzen et al. (1995)	Case series; Vasospasm and thrombus formation in strokes	3 crack users with stroke; no cardiac, hematological cause of stroke	Internal carotid involved in all patients: 2 large filling defects, 1 vasospasm	Some brain infarcts related to crack use: vasospasms of large arteries and IV thrombosis
Levine et al. (1990)	Cross-sectional study; Cardiovascualr complications with crack use	28 crack users with stroke; crack use 72 h prior to onset; 18 (64%) signs/symptoms within 1 h of use; mean age 34 years (range, 23–49); mild risk factors (mitral valve prolapse 4; hypertension 4; cigarette use 8; alcohol use 6)	5 SAH, 4 intraparenchymal hemorrhage, 1 primary intraventricular hemorrhage Types of stroke: 15 (45%) occlusive or hemorrhagic with severe headache, 18 (64%) infarcts (2 hemorrhagic; 1 fatal); vessel affected: middle cerebral (10), anterior cerebral (3), posterior cerebral (1), vertebrobasilar (4)	Strong temporal relationship between crack cocaine use and stroke, especially in young age group (23–49 years); young stroke victims should be screened for drug use
Nanda et al. (2006)	Retrospective review; Stroke and cocaine use	42 cocaine abusers with stroke; some also used marijuana and heroin; mean age 38 years; male to female ratio 20:7; 15 with high BP; 15 positive for cocaine/ metabolites in urine	15 aneurysms, 27 strokes, 9 intracerebral hematoma, 6 SAH, 1 transverse myelopathy, 4 TIA, 2 carotid occlusion, 1 slow flow vertebral system, 9 intracranial hemorrhage; 1 with SAH died	Cocaine intoxication correlated with fatal CVA ($p < 0.001$), poor Glasgow Outcome Score ($p < 0.001$)
Nolte et al. (1996)	Autopsy findings, prospective evaluation; Intracranial hemorrhage and cocaine	17 with non-traumatic fatal intracranial hemorrhage; 10/17 positive toxicology for cocaine	7/10, parenchymal hemorrhage, 3/10 subarachnoid bleed (berry aneurysm); no vasculitis or other abnormalities	Risk for fatal brain hemorrhage without pathological findings likely a result of pharmacological effects of cocaine

Table 3.11 Cont.

Study	Method	Sample	Incidence	Results
Petitti et al. (1998)	Case–control study Strokes and cocaine or amphetamine use Face to face interview	357 women aged 15–44 years with stroke; 1021 controls randomly selected, matched for age	Univariate matched OR for stroke in women using cocaine and/or amphetamines 8.5 (95% CI 3.6–20.0); adjusting for confounders, OR 7.0 (95% CI 2.8–17.9)	Use of cocaine, amphetamines increases the risk for stroke in women
Qureshi et al. (1997)	Retrospective case–control study Crack use and cocaine	Patients aged 20–39 years diagnosed with stroke; 66/144 stroke diagnosis related to crack use; 99/147 controls, stroke non-cocaine-related	Crack use at any time: OR with stroke 0.7 (95% CI 0.4–1.8), OR with infarct 0.5 (95% CI 0.2–1.2) Acute use (within 48 h): OR for stroke 1.9 (95% CI 0.7–5.1), OR for cerebral infarct 1.2 (95% CI 0.4–3.8)	Crack use at any time or acute crack use not significantly associated with stroke or cerebral infarct
Simpson et al. (1990)	Retrospective study SAH and cocaine	Cocaine users with SAH		Patients using cocaine had significantly poorer outcomes than those with no known exposure to cocaine
Sloan et al. (1991)	Descriptive study Strokes and abuse of drugs	167 patients diagnosed with stroke: 11/116 (9.5%) drug users; mean age of drug users 41 years (range, 25–56)	5/11 drug users used cocaine (45%); Types of strokes in drug users: 4/62 (6%) cerebral infarcts, 2/28 (7%) intracerebral hemorrhage, 5/26 (19%) SAH (data not significant)	Besides cocaine, other drugs abused included over-the-counter sympathomimetics, phencyclidine, heroin
Westover et al. (2007)	Cross-sectional study Amphetamine and cocaine use in stroke	Amphetamine and cocaine users aged 18–77 years: 937 hemorrhagic stroke, 998, ischemic stroke	Amphetamine users: adjusted OR for hemorrhagic stroke 4.95 (95% CI 3.24–7.55); higher risk for death; nc risk for ischemic stroke Cocaine users: OR for hemorrhagic stroke 2.33 (95% CI 1.74–3.11); OR for ischemic stroke 2.03 (95% CI 1.48–2.79)	As stimulant drug use increases, risk of hospital admissions for stroke and stroke-related mortality will increase
Zandio et al. (2008)	Case study Pontomesencephalic infarct	56-year-old female cocaine abuser with high BP	Pontine paramedian infarct with destructive midline lesions; 9 months later, pontomesencephalic infarct	

ACTH, adrenocorticotropic hormone; ADH, antidiuretic hormone; AMI, acute myocardial infarction; AVM, arterial-venous malformation; BP, blood pressure; CI, confidence interval; CVA, cerebrovascular accident; OR, odds ratio; CT, computed tomography; FSH, follicle-stimulating hormone; IV, intravenous; LH, luteinizing hormone; MRI, magnetic resonance imaging; RR, relative risk; SAH, subarachnoid hemorrhage; TIA, transient ischemic attack.

authors of these studies. Ischemic strokes typically refer to those strokes causing hypoxia to the brain tissue and caused by thrombi, emboli, systemic hypoperfusion, or venous thrombosis. Hemorrhagic strokes could refer to intracranial or intracerebral strokes. If the term intracranial hemorrhage is used, this could be interpreted as bleeding anywhere within the cranial vault. Intra-axial would apply to bleeding in the parenchyma (brain tissue; intraparenchymal), while extra-axial would refer to epidural, subdural, or subarachnoid hemorrhage. Intracerebral would refer to bleeding within the parenchyma of the brain

Despite the varied terminology, some generalizations can be made about these studies. While some structural lesions were found, many of the patients had few of the traditional risks for stroke (ischemic or hemorrhagic). Many of the studies suggest that the physiological and pharmacological effects of cocaine precipitate strokes in vulnerable populations. Several studies found that younger cocaine users with pre-existing berry aneurysms or arterial-venous malformations were at risk for hemorrhage, presumably related to the sudden vasoconstriction and intense hypertension seen within minutes of using cocaine. Several studies point out that young male users were more at risk; however, a few case studies found that older women were also vulnerable to developing cerebral infarcts.

The five studies on SAH suggest that cocaine users predisposed to cerebral aneurysm rupture are more likely to have a SAH at a younger age than their non-cocaine-using counterparts, that they are more likely to have delayed clinical deficits after the bleed, and that their residual neurological deficits were more likely to be mild compared with their non-using peers.

Although one study pointed out that crack use was not associated with stroke or infarction, and several found that neurological deficits were less common in cocaine users, most studies found that there is a strong risk for cerebrovascular disease in cocaine users and that cocaine use was associated with increased fatality.

Further studies are needed with larger sample sizes, with users of various ages and gender, and with new and chronic users to further identify the risk of cerebrovascular events in cocaine users.

Autonomic nervous system diseases

Four epidemiological studies were found that specifically researched the effects of cocaine on the ANS. All four studies involved neonates or infants. Some studies in the pregnancy complications section of this chapter also researched ANS symptoms in cocaine-exposed fetuses, neonates, and infants. Those studies are not included in the discussion here.

Bada et al. (2002a) studied 11 811 maternal–infant dyads to identify risk of ANS and CNS alterations in infants exposed to cocaine in utero. Of these, 1185 were drug exposed (717 cocaine only, 100 opiates, 92 both cocaine and opiates); 276 were unable to be confirmed by meconium testing or maternal self-report. Controls were 7442 dyads confirmed by meconium sampling; 3184 were not confirmed. After controlling for confounders, there was an increased risk for a cluster of ANS/CNS outcomes. Infants exposed to both cocaine and opioids were more likely to experience the most adverse ANS/CNS outcomes; infants only exposed to cocaine experienced the least. There was a significant increased risk of adverse effects in the cocaine exposed infants (OR 1.7; 95% CI 1.2–2.2). The OR independent of opioids was 2.8 (95% CI 2.1–3.7), and the OR for opioids and cocaine was 4.8 (95% CI 2.9–7.9). Cigarette smoking also increased the risk of ANS/CNS adverse effects: OR 1.3 (95% CI 1.04–1.55) for less than half a pack a day and 1.4 (95% CI 1.2–1.6) for half a pack or more per day. This study showed that infants exposed to cocaine or opiates in utero were at risk of having adverse ANS/CNS effects.

Table 3.12 Nervous system associations between cocaine exposure and neonatal outcomes

Signs and symptoms	Adjusted odds ratio	99% confidence interval
Jitteriness, tremors	2.17	1.44–3.29
High pitched cry	2.44	1.06–5.66
Irritability	1.81	1.18–2.80
Excessive suck	3.58	1.63–7.88
Hyperalertness	7.78	1.72–35.06
Autonomic instability	2.64	1.17–5.95

In a 2005 study, Bauer *et al.* examined the associations between cocaine exposure and neonatal outcomes. The case–control study included 171 cocaine-exposed infants and 7442 infants not exposed to cocaine. Table 3.12 illustrates the significant ANS/CNS signs and symptoms and their AOR values. Additional significant findings in the cocaine-exposed group compared with the unexposed infants included prematurity (1.2 weeks), decreased weight (536 g), decreased length (2.6 cm), and decreased head circumference (1.5 cm), all significant at $p < 0.001$. Although there were no organ defects identified by ultrasound, the cocaine-exposed infants were also more likely to have infections (OR 3.09), including hepatitis (OR 13.46), syphilis (OR 8.84), and HIV exposure (OR 12.37). They also were less likely to be breastfed, often were not discharged to the biological mother, and were involved with child protective services.

John *et al.* (2007) studied 21 neonates exposed to intrauterine cocaine and 23 control infants to assess their reaction to orthostatic stress, particularly heart rate and heart rate variability, within 120 hours of birth. During one hour of quiet sleep, electrocardiogram (ECG) records were made, followed by monitoring during 30 minutes in a supine position and then 30 minutes in an inclined position. Compared with the controls, cocaine-exposed infants had tachycardia before ($p = 0.091$) and after ($p = 0.015$) tilting. There was a clear interaction between cocaine exposure and orthostatic stress ($p = 0.049$) and heart rate variability ($p = 0.049$). The reaction of the cocaine-exposed infants to stress was delayed and prolonged. The control infants had an instantaneous increase in heart rate variability that quickly returned to normal, while the hearts of the cocaine-exposed infants had a gradual increase that did not return to normal quickly. The authors suggested that intrauterine exposure to cocaine can affect the sympathetic and parasympathetic nervous systems and alter cardiovascular function.

Schuetze *et al.* (2007) studied the effect of prenatal exposure to cocaine in 154 infants at seven months of age: 79 cocaine exposed and 75 non-exposed. In a positive affective task, the cocaine-exposed infants had a significantly higher increase in heart rate than the non-exposed infants. The non-exposed infants had a greater decrease in respiratory sinus arrhythmia when subjected to the negative affective task than the cocaine-exposed infants. The study supports other studies indicating an association between intrauterine exposure to cocaine and dysregulation of the ANS up to seven months after birth.

Table 3.13 summarizes these findings.

Comments

These studies support the risk of ANS dysfunction in infants exposed to cocaine in utero. Two of the studies were large (717 and 1185 cocaine-exposed infants) and found

Table 3.13 Autonomic nervous system

Study	Method	Sample	Incidence	Results
Bada et al. (2002a)	Cross-sectional study Drug exposure and ANS/CNS signs	11 811 maternal-infant dyads: 1185 drug exposed (717 cocaine, 100 opiates, 92 both, 276 unconfirmed drug use); 7442 controls (3184 unconfirmed drug use)	Cocaine exposure: increased OR for CNS/ANS outcomes 1.7 (95% CI 1.2–2.2); OR independent of opioid effect 2.8 (95% CI 2.1–3.7); OR opioid and cocaine additive effect 4.8 (95% CI 2.9–7.9) Smoking also increased risk:1/2 pack or less/day, OR 1.3 (95% CI 1.04–1.55), 1/2 pack or more/day, OR 1.4 (95% CI 1.2–1.6)	Cocaine and opioid use increases risk for ANS/CNS adverse outcomes; smoking also increased risk
Bauer et al. (2005)	Multisite, prospective, randomized study Neonatal effect of cocaine exposure and medical outcomes	717 cocaine-exposed infants; 7442 infants without cocaine exposure	Physical effects of cocaine at birth: 1.2 weeks younger, 536 g lighter, 2.6 cm shorter, 1.5 cm less head circumference; ANS/CNS signs, symptoms: jitteriness, tremors (AOR 2.17, 99% CI 1.44–3.29); high pitch cry (AOR 2.44, 99% CI 1.06–5.66); irritability (AOR 1.81, 99% CI 1.18–2.80); excessive suck (AOR 3.58, 99% CI 1.63–7.88); hyperalertness (AOR 7.78, 99% CI 1.72–36.06); autonomic instability (AOR 2.64, 99% CI 1.17–5.95)	ANS/CNS signs more frequent in exposed infants, but signs transient; no difference in organ function by ultrasound Cocaine-exposed infants had more infections, were less often breastfed, had more child welfare referrals, and were more likely to not be living with biological mother
John et al. (2007)	Descriptive, experimental design ANS alteration after orthostatic stress ECG: quiet sleep 1 h, supine 30 min, inclined 30 min	21 cocaine-exposed infants; 23 controls	Cocaine-exposed infants compared with controls 120 h after birth: tachycardia before ($p = 0.091$) and after ($p = 0.015$) tilting; interaction between orthostatic stress and cocaine use ($p = 0.049$) Cocaine-exposed infants: gradual increase in heart rate, slower to return to baseline than controls ($p = 0.049$)	Exposure to cocaine may alter development of sympathetic and parasympathetic nervous systems, leading to cardiovascular dysfunction after birth
Schuetze et al. (2007)	Case–control study Cocaine effect on ANS 7 months after birth Tasks eliciting positive, negative affective response; heart rate, respiratory sinus arrhythmia	79 cocaine exposed and 75 control infants	Cocaine-exposed infants compared with controls: higher heart rate with exposure to positive affective task; less suppression of heart rate to negative affective tasks	Prenatal cocaine exposure may affect cardiovascular function as long as 7 months after exposure

AOR, adjusted odds ratio; ANS, autonomic nervous system; CNS, central nervous system; CI, confidence interval; ECG, electrocardiogram; OR, odds ratio.

significant risks of cocaine exposure and ANS alterations. The study of Bada *et al.* (2002a) also showed that concurrent use of opiates increased the risk for ANS dysfunction and confirmed studies that indicated cigarette smoking also increased the risk. The study of Bauer *et al.* (2005) also confirmed the physical effects of cocaine exposure that are described in some studies in the section of this chapter on pregnancy and congenital outcomes.

One experimental study on reactions to orthostatic stress involved a small number of infants exposed to cocaine in utero. Compared with the controls, there was evidence of heart rate variability and slow responsiveness to change, suggesting ANS dysfunction in newborns. The last study looked at infants seven months after birth and found the infants' cardiovascular response to positive and negative affective tasks was exaggerated or blunted compared with the control infants; this study also had a small sample size. Support for outcomes of both of these studies would be enhanced by further studies with a larger number of infants.

Questions can also be raised whether confounders such as polydrug use, alcohol use, and demographic or socioeconomic factors affected the risk analysis in these studies. Furthermore, in the study of seven-month-old infants, determining exposure to cocaine during those seven months may help to interpret the outcome.

Central nervous system disease

A variety of studies were found in a review of the PubMed literature from 1988 to 2008 related to CNS disease and cocaine. This subsection reviews studies on cerebral atrophy, seizures, and "crack dancing."

Cerebral atrophy was described by Pascual-Leone *et al.* (1991) in a CT study of 35 habitual cocaine users, 16 self-reported first-time cocaine users, and 54 patients with head-aches, who served as controls. The subjects were between 20 and 40 years of age, did not use other illicit drugs or alcohol, were not positive for HIV, had no history of neurological disease, and had normal serum albumin levels. There were similar age and sex ratios in each of the three groups. The habitual cocaine users had significant cerebral atrophy compared with either the first-time users or controls. Moreover, there was a strong correlation between the duration of cocaine use and the degree of atrophy in the habitual users.

Four studies were found that associated cocaine use to seizure activity. Choy-Kwong & Lipton (1989) studied the incidence of seizures in 283 hospital-admitted cocaine users. They found eight patients (2.8%) who experienced seizures; four (1.4%) were focal or generalized and associated with recent cocaine use. They suggested that seizures in cocaine users are rare but seizures may appear in various forms and with various methods of cocaine use.

Pascual-Leone *et al.* (1990) reported on 474 patients with acute cocaine intoxication, 403 with no prior history of seizures and 71 with prior seizures that, by history, were not related to cocaine use. Thirty-two (7.9%) experienced seizures within 90 minutes of cocaine use. Most of the seizures were single and generalized, occurred after use of either intravenous cocaine or crack, and had no lasting neurological effects. Those individuals with seizures that were focal or multiple were more likely to use intranasal cocaine, have acute intra-cerebral complications, and be polydrug users. In the 71 who had had prior seizures that, by history, were not related to cocaine use, 12 (16.9%) had cocaine-induced multiple seizures that were the same as their previous history of seizures and induced by nasal cocaine as well as smoked or injected forms. Forty-four who had cocaine-induced seizures were habitual users and had diffuse brain atrophy on CT scan and diffuse slowing on electroencephalography (EEG) studies.

Dhuna *et al.* (1991) studied 98 of 945 cocaine-intoxicated patients experiencing seizures within 90 minutes of cocaine use. More females experienced seizures than males (18.4% vs. 6.2%). In most cases, the seizures were single, generalized convulsions. Cranial and EEG studies were normal. Those individuals with new-onset focal seizures all had cocaine-related cerebral strokes or hemorrhages. Those with a history of cocaine-unrelated seizures had convulsions precipitated by recreational use of cocaine. Four patients developed status epilepticus after massive doses of cocaine. Their seizures were refractory to medical treatment and resulted in significant mortality and morbidity. The authors found four conditions that increased the risk of cocaine-related seizures: (1) massive doses of cocaine (2 to 8 g); (2) a history of seizures (where cocaine might lower the threshold for new seizures); (3) gender (where more females are at risk than males); and (4) chronic use (where cocaine might act as "chemical" kindling, when subthreshold levels ultimately lead to stimulation and seizure activity).

Koppel *et al.* (1996) carried out a chart review of 1900 cocaine-related emergency department visits, 58 (3%) involving seizures and epilepsy. Seizure activity included idiopathic epilepsy, localization-related epilepsy, cerebrovascular disease and cocaine-use-only related seizures. In 12 of the 58 (21%), cocaine was the only explanation for seizure activity. This number was less significant than seizures associated with alcohol or head trauma. The authors suggested that cocaine-related seizures in persons with underlying epilepsy might be caused by a reduced seizure threshold associated with the toxic effect of cocaine, medication non-compliance, poor diet, or poor sleep habits.

Two case reports describe the condition "crack dancing" experienced by some cocaine users. Daras *et al.* (1994a) described seven patients with choreoathetosis, akathesia, and Parkinson-like tremors. The seven were among 701 visitors to the emergency room seen with cocaine complications over a two-year period.

Kamath & Bajaj (2007) described an adult intravenous cocaine user who developed choreiform movements after taking a large dose of cocaine; these persisted for one week after hospitalization and the movements were recorded on videotape. According to the authors, a variety of abnormal movements are associated with cocaine use, including dystonia, Tourette's syndrome exacerbation, multifocal tics, opsoclonus-myoclonus, and choreiform movements.

These studies are summarized in Table 3.14.

Comments

Cerebral atrophy was found in a small study involving habitual cocaine users. Compared with first-time users and controls with headache as the major symptom, these habitual users had significant atrophy that was correlated with the duration of cocaine use. Additional studies with larger numbers of cocaine users and users with a variety of exposure to the drug might be able to validate the risks for atrophy in cocaine users.

The risk of seizures was also discussed in this section. As Dhuna *et al.* (1991) pointed out, four conditions appear to increase the risk of seizures in cocaine users. Large doses of cocaine (2 to 8 g/use) can trigger seizures in patients with new-onset seizures and habitual users. A second risk factor is a history of a previous seizure, where cocaine may lower the seizure threshold. In their 1991 study, Dhuna *et al.* found females to be at higher risk than males; other studies in this section did not provide gender data. The fourth risk factor was chronic use, brought on by "chemical" kindling. In this phenomenon, chronic use of CNS stimulants may cause pathological changes in neurons through subthreshold stimulation.

Table 3.14 Central nervous system

	Method	Sample	Incidence	Results
Choy-Kwong & Lipton (1989)	Descriptive study Seizures in hospitalized cocaine users	283 cocaine patients admitted, 8 (2.8%) with seizures	4 seizures focal or generalized, associated with cocaine use	Seizures rare but may occur irregardless of route of entry or type of cocaine used
Daras et al. (1994a)	Case series Crack dancing	7 cocaine users	Crack dancing: chorecathetosis, akathesia, parkinsonism with tremor	Likely reflects dopamine dysfunction leading to euphoria, addiction, abnormal movements
Dhuna et al. (1991)	Descriptive study Epileptogenic properties of cocaine	98 of 945 patients (10.3%) with cocaine toxicity experiencing seizures 90 min after use	Females > males (18.4 vs. 6.2%); seizure: single, generalized convulsion; cranial CT/EEG normal New-onset seizure: focal, associated with cerebral strokes or hemorrhage Patients with cocaine-unrelated seizure history, seizure with recreacticnal use of cocaine 4 had status epilepticus after massive dose of cocaine; resistant to treatment, significant mortality, morbidity	Cocaine-related risks for seizures: massive dose of cocaine (2 to 8 g), history of seizure (related to low seizure threshold), female sex, chronic use (chemical kindling)
Kamath & Bajaj (2007)	Case series Crack dancing	Cocaine user videotaped crack dancing 4 days after using IV cocaine	Transient choreiform movements (lasted 7 days)	Cocaine abuse associated with dystonia, exacerbated Tourette's symptoms, multifocal tics, opsoclonus–myoclonus, choreiform movements
Koppel et al. (1996)	Chart review Cocaine use and seizures, epilepsy	1900 cocaine-related ER visits: 58 (3%) involved seizures, epilepsy	Seizures: idiopathic epilepsy, localization-related epilepsy, cerebrovascular disease, cocaine-use-only related seizures Cocaine likely cause in 21% (12 of 58 patients)	Seizures associated with cocaine use less significant number than seen in alcohol use or head trauma; cocaine can reduce seizure threshold in existing epileptics Other potential causes of seizures: toxic effect, drug non-compliance, poor diet, poor sleep habits

Pascual-Leone et al. (1990)	Retrospective study Cocaine and seizures	474 patients with acute cocaine toxicity: 403, no seizures; 32 (7.9%) seizure within 90 min of cocaine use; 71, seizure history not related to cocaine use; 44, cocaine-induced seizure in habitual user	Seizure soon after use: focal, multiple; mostly after intranasal administration; concurrent use of other drugs Seizures after cocaine use in individuals with prior, non-cocaine-related seizures: 12/71 had cocaine-induced seizure; seizure multiple, similar to prior seizures Cocaine-induced seizures in habitual users: CT showed diffuse brain atrophy, slowing of EEG	Cocaine use (variety of forms, administration) associated with seizures; habitual users more likely to have brain atrophy
Pascual-Leone et al. (1991)	Cross-sectional study Cerebral atrophy and cocaine use CT	35 habitual cocaine users; 16 self-report first-time users; 54 with headache Participants similar in age (20–40 years) and sex; no polydrug use, alcohol use; HIV, neurological disease; normal albumin level	Habitual cocaine users compared with first-time cocaine users and headache patients: significant cerebral atrophy; there was a positive correlation between cerebral atrophy and duration of drug use	Cerebral atrophy can be found in chronic cocaine users and is correlated with length of drug use

CT, computed tomography; EEG, electroencephalography; ER, emergency room; HIV, human immunodeficiency virus; IV, intravenous.

Ultimately, threshold levels may be reached, leading to generalized motor seizures. The studies in this section support most of these conditions. Most of the seizures described were focal, generalized, and single. Multiple seizures appeared more often in polydrug abusers. In most studies, there were no lasting neurological sequelae and cranial studies and EEGs were normal. The incidence of seizures in the cocaine user seen in healthcare settings was relatively low: 2.8–10% of cocaine users. As one author pointed out, this is significantly less than the incidence of seizures seen in alcohol users and those with head trauma.

Two case reports of "crack dancing" suggest that this cocaine-induced neuromuscular activity is more common than reported in the professional literature. As suggested by one group of authors, the condition is likely related to alteration in dopamine activity caused by cocaine use.

Demyelinating disorders

Three research studies were found in the epidemiological review of the PubMed database related to demyelinating disorders, brain volume, and cocaine use.

In the first study, Moeller et al. (2007) investigated the effect of cocaine on myelin function in 13 cocaine users and 18 healthy controls. Using diffusion tensor eigenvalues (comparing diffusion along fiber tracts with that perpendicular to fiber tracts), they found that altered myelin in the corpus callosum was more common in cocaine users than in non-users. This study supported other similar studies that found cocaine-associated alterations or damage to myelin that increased diffusion perpendicular to the tracts. Neuronal loss and/or damage to axonal tracts are possible explanations for these findings.

The second study, involving 32 cocaine users, 32 opiate users, and 32 age- and sex-matched controls (Lyoo et al. (2004), found that white matter hyperintensities were more common in cocaine users than opiate users. Brain MRI was performed on all subjects. The severity of white matter hyperintensities in the deep (and insular) and periventricular areas of white matter was graded using the Fazekas and Coffey rating scales. Cocaine users had a greater severity of white matter hyperintensities than the opioid users (OR 2.54), and the opioid users had more severe white matter hyperintensities than the controls (OR 2.90). Although there was no difference in the periventricular white matter, the deep (OR 3.25) and insular (OR 4.38) regions were more severely affected in cocaine users than in either the opioid users or normal controls. The authors suggest that since cocaine has more vasoconstrictive effects than opioids, the hyperintensities may reflect the ischemia produced by this effect. Although not statistically significant, women tended to have less severe white matter changes than males in the study; this may be explained by an estrogen effect.

Sim et al. (2007) researched gray and white matter volume in a case–control study of 40 cocaine-dependent users (27 males, average age 41.4 years) and 41 healthy age/sex-matched controls (average age 38.7 years). Voxel-based morphometry MRI was used to analyze brain mass. Compared with the control group, there were statistically significant findings in the cocaine users. In the gray matter, there was a 16.6% decrease in mass in the bilateral premotor cortex (Brodmann areas [BA] 6, 8), a 15.1% decrease in the right orbitofrontal cortex (BA 10), a 15.9% decrease in the bilateral temporal cortex (BA 20, 38), a 12.6% decrease in the left thalamus, and a 13.4% decrease in the bilateral cerebellum. There was also a 10% decrease in white matter volume in the right cerebellar lobe. These findings were significant at $p < 0.05$. There was a correlation between duration of cocaine use and cerebellar gray matter volume on the right ($r = 0.31$) and left ($r = 0.39$). When various executive function and motor function tests were performed, there was also a correlation with the duration of cocaine use and the ability to carry out these tests. These researchers suggested that, along with changes in the cerebrum, the cerebellum may also be vulnerable to changes in brain volume in chronic cocaine users.

Table 3.15 summarizes these studies.

Comments

These three small studies provide some evidence that white and gray matter changes occur in cocaine users. Additional studies with larger numbers of subjects and subjects with varying levels of cocaine use might provide further insight into the effect of cocaine on cerebral white and gray matter. The relationship between cerebral tissue changes and clinical symptoms could also be explored in more depth.

Neurological manifestations

A number of epidemiological studies related to neurological changes and cocaine use were found in a review of the PubMed literature from 1988 to 2008. The majority of studies describe cognitive manifestations and executive function. Some studies originally designated for this section are discussed in other more appropriate subsections, including those on otorhinolaryngological disorders, CNS disorders, and ocular disease.

Five articles described cognitive and executive function in cocaine users. In a case–control study, O'Malley *et al.* (1992) studied neuropsychological impairment in 20 chronic cocaine users and 20 age- and education-matched controls. Using the Neuropsychological Screening Examination, 50% (10) scored poorly on the summary index compared with 15% of the controls. The cocaine users also scored more poorly on four other tests: Halstead Category, Symbol Digit Modalities, the Wechsler Adult Intelligence Scale Revised Arithmetic, and a test of verbal memory (forgetting). Cocaine users' performance on the tests was directly related to the amount and recent use of cocaine. The authors suggested that cocaine use has a direct effect on cognitive function.

In a 1999 case–control study, van Gorp *et al.* examined declarative and procedural memory function in cocaine users during a 45-day period of abstinence. The subjects included 37 cocaine users and 27 control subjects. The following tests were administered within 72 hours of admission, and 10, 21, and 45 days following admission: CA Verbal Learning Test, recall of Rey-Osterrieth Complex Figure Test, Pursuit Rotor Task, and Profile of Mood States. Table 3.16 illustrates the findings. The findings suggested that, following a 45-day period of abstinence, non-verbal declarative memory task was negatively affected by the use of cocaine but that motor learning was improved compared with controls during this time.

Simon *et al.* (2002) studied 40 methamphetamine users, 40 cocaine users, and 80 controls matched for age, education, ethnicity, and gender. The controls were evenly paired with either the methamphetamine or cocaine group because of significant differences in age and ethnicity. The cocaine group was older and mostly African American, while the methamphetamine group was mostly white. Cognitive tests were given and information on medical history and drug use was obtained through a questionnaire. The findings showed that both the cocaine and methamphetamine groups were impaired compared with controls, but the drug users differed on type and degree of impairments.

Verdejo-Garcia *et al.* (2005) studied executive functioning in a variety of drug abusers. Subjects were users of MDMA (methylenedioxymethamphetamine [ecstasy]), cocaine, or marijuana. The 38 subjects carried out tests for executive subprocessing tasks of working

Table 3.15 Demyelinating studies

Study	Method	Sample	Incidence	Results
Lyoo et al. (2004)	Cross-sectional study Brain WMH in drug users Brain MRI; structured clinical interview for DSM-IV	32 cocaine users; 32 opiate users; 32 age-, sex-matched controls	Cocaine users greater WMH than opioid users (OR 2.54); more lesion severity in deep and insular white matter than periventricular white matter Opiate users greater WMH than controls (OR 2.90) No difference in periventricular WMH among groups; WMH changes in females less severe than in males	Cocaine-associated WMH likely caused by vasoconstriction-related ischemia
Moeller et al. (2007)	Case-control study Myelin changes with cocaine use DTI study	13 cocaine users; 18 controls	Cocaine users: altered myelin in corpus callosum	Cocaine use may cause neuronal loss, axonal tract damage
Sim et al. (2007)	Case-control study Gray vs. white matter volume Voxel-based morphometry, MRI, neuropsychological function tests	40 cocaine users (27 males, mean age 41.4 years); 41 healthy age-, sex-matched controls (26 males, mean age 38.7 years)	Cocaine-dependent group compared with controls: decreased gray matter volume 16.6% bilateral premotor cortex (BA, 6, 8); 15.1% right orbitofrontal cortex (BA. 10); 15.9% bilateral temporal cortex (BA, 20, 38); 12.6% left thalamus; 13.4% bilateral cerebellum (all p < 0.05) Decreased right cerebellar white matter volume (10%) (p < 0.05) Duration of use correlated with right (r = 0.37) and left (r = 0.39) cerebellar gray matter deficits	Executive function and motor function defects correlated with brain volume changes; cerebellum may be vulnerable to cocaine-associated brain volume changes

DTI, diffusion tensor imaging; WMH, white matter hyperintensives.

Table 3.16 Memory function in cocaine users during a 45-day period of abstinence

Test	Result at 45 days
CA Verbal Learning Test	Cocaine users and controls improved over time
Pursuit Rotor Task	Cocaine group improved at a faster rate than controls at day 10 and 45; controls showed plateau in learning rate
Rey–Osterrieth Complex Figure Test	Both improved recall; controls better than cocaine users in recalling information

memory, response inhibition, cognitive flexibility, and abstract reasoning. The results showed use of the three abused drugs affected different tests: MDMA affected working memory and abstract reasoning; cocaine affected inhibitory control; and marijuana affected cognitive flexibility. The authors hypothesized that metabolic reorganization of monoamine pathways in the frontosubcortical regions may be affected by drug use and lead to impaired executive function.

In a later study, Verdejo-Garcia & Perez-Garcia (2007) studied the performance of abstaining polysubstance abusers and controls on a variety of executive function tests. The tests measured fluency, working memory, reasoning, inhibitory control, flexibility, and decision making. The drugs abusers were divided into two groups based on drug preference: cocaine or heroin. The four components of executive function assessed were updating, inhibition, shifting, and decision making. The abstaining polysubstance abusers were cognitively impaired on all four functions (effect size from 0.5 to 2.2). Cocaine users were more impaired than heroin users and controls on inhibition and shifting functions. Regardless of choice of drug, the more drugs used, the greater the impairment. This study suggests that different drugs affect different executive functions.

Table 3.17 summarizes these results.

Comments

These studies suggest that various abused drugs seem to affect cognitive functioning in users even after a period of abstinence as long as 45 days. A limitation of most of the studies is that the numbers of subjects are relatively small, the drugs compared varied, the amount and length of use is unknown in most cases, and the tests used to assess cognition varied. Two studies involved polydrug abusers, but it is unclear whether these subjects used one or more drugs. If each subject was a polydrug user, the results of each individual's test could be influenced by the multiplicity of drugs used. Long-term studies might provide some insight whether cognition can improve over a period of time greater than 45 days. Studies using the same cognitive tests might also be helpful in determining which cognitive functions are impaired. Another problem is that these studies cannot establish a cause and effect relationship because persons with poorer cognitive and executive function may be more likely to use drugs. One would need to do longitudinal studies and look at these factors over time.

Sleep disorders

Four studies and two reviews were found in a PubMed search of sleep conditions and cocaine use published between 1988 and 2008.

Weddington *et al.* (1990) described changes in mood, craving, and sleep during cocaine abstinence in 12 male cocaine addicts and 10 non-addict controls. The two differences

Table 3.17 Neurological manifestations

Study	Method	Sample	Incidence	Results
O'Malley et al. (1992)	Case–control study Neuropsychological impairment and cocaine Neuropsychological Screening Examination	20 chronic cocaine users; 20 age-, education-matched controls	50% of cocaine users scored poorly on summary index compared with 15% of controls; cocaine users also scored less well on four other tests	Cocaine has a direct effect on cognitive function
Simon et al. (2002)	Case–control study Cognitive performance and cocaine Cognitive function tests	40 cocaine users; 40 methamphetamine users; 80 controls, matched for age, education, ethnicity, gender	Both cocaine and methamphetamine users were impaired on cognitive tests compared with controls; type and degree of impairment differed	
van Gorp et al. (1999)	Case–control study Declarative and procedural memory function and cocaine use Tested on day 1, 10, 21, 45	37 cocaine users, 27 control subjects	After 45 days abstinence, both groups improved in recall function (controls more than cocaine users), both groups improved in verbal learning, cocaine group improved faster than controls in Rotor Task Test	Following 45-day abstinence, non-verbal declarative memory tasks negatively affected by cocaine use
Verdejo-Garcia et al. (2005)	Cross-sectional study Executive function in polydrug users Executive function tests	38 polysubstance abusers: MDMA, cocaine, marijuana	MDMA: poorer function on working memory, abstract reasoning tests Cocaine: poorer function on inhibitory control Marijuana: poorer function on cognitive flexibility tests	Impaired executive function may be related to metabolic reorganization of monoamine pathways in cerebral cortex
Verdejo-Garcia & Perez-Garcia (2007)	Cross-sectional study Executive function in polydrug users Executive function tests	Cocaine users, heroin users	Both groups cognitively impaired on four functions; cocaine users more impaired than heroin users and controls on inhibition and shifting functions	Different drugs affect different executive functions

MDMA, 3,4-methylenedioxymethamphetamine.

between the addicts and controls were diagnoses of psychoactive substance abuse and antisocial personality. During short-term abstinence (28 days), the cocaine users demonstrated greater mood distress and depression, which decreased over time. No sleep difficulties were identified except falling to sleep and having a clear head upon rising.

A case–control study involving three cocaine-dependent men was published by Johanson et al. (1999). Subjects had an abstinence phase of 8 to 10 days, followed by five days of intranasal cocaine before bedtime, and then a second abstinence phase of 14 to 16 days. During the cocaine-administration phase, typical cocaine-related changes in mood and blood pressure occurred and sleep was severely disrupted. During the second abstinence phase, daytime sleepiness increased, but there were no differences in mood from the cocaine-administration phase. Two weeks after the study was completed, sleep patterns as assessed by polysomnograms remained different from age-matched controls.

The effect of cocaine binge–abstinence cycles was reported by Pace-Schott et al. (2005). Five chronic cocaine users had a three-day abstinence cycle, followed by a three-day binge cycle, which was then followed by a 15-day abstinence cycle. Polysomnography and Nightcap ambulatory monitor were used to record physiological sleep, and a questionnaire was used to assess subjective sleep. After binging and 15-day abstinence period, sleep quality progressively worsened based on changes in sleep duration, efficiency, and latency. However, self-reported subjective sleep did not change over this period. The study found that sleep deteriorated over the binge–abstinence period although the perception of sleep quality did not change. The researchers suggested that the sleep homeostat was disrupted by cocaine use and this resulted in a difference between the subjective and objective determination of sleep quality.

Morgan et al. (2006) carried out a randomized controlled trial with 12 subjects to study occult insomnia and the effect on procedural learning. The 12 subjects received either cocaine on days 4 through 6 and then a placebo on days 18 through 20 (for a 12 day abstinence), or a placebo on days 4 through 6 and then cocaine on days 18 through 20 (for an 18-day abstinence). Simple and vigilance reaction times were tested and a motor sequence test of procedural learning was given during the study. Sleep was measured by polysomnography, a Nightcap sleep monitor, and a sleep self-report. There was no correlation between the reported quality of sleep and the physiological sleep results. For example, total sleep time and latency were worse on days 14 through 17 even though the subjects reported a better quality of sleep. Procedural learning ability did correlate with total sleep time and was impaired at 17 days of abstinence compared with two or three days of abstinence. Slow-wave sleep was lowest on days 4 through 9 of abstinence and highest during cocaine use and days 10 through 17 of abstinence. Although cocaine users reported better sleep during sustained abstinence, they slept less and vigilance and procedural learning was impaired. The authors suggested that homeostatic sleep drive function was impaired by cocaine and the patterns displayed were similar to those seen in chronic insomnia.

Sleep patterns during cocaine abstinence were reported in a review article by Morgan & Malison (2007). They found that profound sleep disturbances occurred during the first three weeks of drug abstinence. Although subjects reported no sleep difficulties, there was no indication that recovery of normal sleep patterns occurred after continuing abstinence. The review discussed sleep pathways and the relationship between cocaine and sleep.

Another review (Valladares & Irwin 2007) described the usefulness of using polysomnography as a tool to evaluate sleep patterns in cocaine users. The goal of the review was to encourage more studies on sleep alteration in cocaine users in order to decrease morbidity related to disturbed sleep patterns.

The results are summarized in Table 3.18.

Comments

The four studies on sleep are similar; they all looked at sleep patterns in cocaine-using subjects enrolled in inpatient settings, involved comparing affective behaviors and sleep cycles during periods of abstinence and cocaine use, involved chronic cocaine users, were carried out in 38 days or less, and involved 12 patients or less. Only one of the studies used a control group; three of the studies used polysomnography as the physiological tool to measure sleep. Some of the studies used cognitive function tests during the course of the study. While some of these features are positive, some limit the generalizability of the study.

It is difficult to compare the findings of the studies since they used different protocols for periods of abstinence and cocaine use. There is a suggestion that normal sleep patterns may not reappear for a longer period of time than the 38 days of abstinence in one of the studies. One wonders when "normal sleep patterns" became "abnormal." Studies looking at sleep patterns in first-time users, occasional users, and long-term users might be helpful in determining the onset of altered sleep patterns and the conditions under which this change occurs.

A central theme in these studies is that there is a difference in the perception of sleep quality and the physiological findings on the polysomnogram. There is a suggestion that altered function of the sleep homeostat may be related to this discrepancy. Studies including plasma levels of hormones or neurotransmitters associated with sleep might provide some hint to the cause of the changes in sleep patterns seen in chronic cocaine users. One group of researchers suggested that the altered sleep in cocaine users is similar to chronic insomnia.

Measurement of plasma corticotropin-releasing factor (CRF) might be helpful to correlate sleep patterns with increases or decreases of CRF. A review by Roth *et al.* (2007) suggested that CRF is elevated in primary insomnia and also in major depressive disorder. The authors suggested that an increase in CRF is involved in the hyperarousal seen in insomnia. Arzt & Holsboer (2006) described the role of CRF in adaptation to stress and suggested that, if adaptation fails, an increase in CRF can be neurostimulatory through stimulation of CRF-1 receptors and lead to affective mood disorders, anxiety and altered cognition, appetite, and sleep. In a laboratory study, Orozco-Cabal *et al.* (2008) demonstrated that the normal synergistic role of dopamine and CRF in stimulation of dopamine receptors leads to synaptic depression. In chronic cocaine use, dopamine and CRF become stimulatory and can stimulate the basal amygdala and prefrontal cortex, leading to glutamatergic transmission. They suggested that functional and receptor changes can occur in dopamine and CRF with cocaine use and ultimately may affect normal nervous system pathways, cognitive functioning, and drug craving.

Ocular disease

Eleven articles were found in a PubMed search for publications on cocaine use and ocular disorders, 10 being case reports. Five articles describe incidents of corneal ulceration or infection; one describes iritis in a cocaine user, and another describes retinal damage associated with cocaine use. Two articles discuss color vision changes and two report on the development of acute glaucoma related to cocaine exposure.

Table 3.18 Sleep

Study	Method	Sample	Incidence	Results
Johanson et al. (1999)	Case–control study Effect of cocaine on mood and sleep (abstinence 8 days, intranasal cocaine 5 days, abstinence 14–16 days) Polysomnography	3 abstaining cocaine users, 3 age-matched controls	During cocaine phase, typical mood and blood pressure changes; sleep severely disrupted Second abstinence phase: increased daytime sleepiness, no difference in mood from cocaine phase	Sleep patterns remained different from controls (on polysomnography)
Morgan & Malison (2007)	Literature review Sleep patterns during cocaine abstinence			Profound dysregulation of sleep during first 3 weeks of abstinence; no indication of recovery; subjective reports do not correlate with physiological sleep patterns
Morgan et al. (2006)	Randomized control trial Cocaine effect on occult insomnia and procedural learning Polysomnography, Nightcap sleep monitor, self-report of sleep	12 cocaine users received either cocaine on days 4–6 and placebo on days 18–20 or placebo on days 4–6 and cocaine on days 18–20	No correlation between quality of sleep and physiological measurements (e.g., measured sleep worse while quality reported better) Slow wave sleep lowest day 4–9 of abstinence, highest during cocaine use and day 10–17 of abstinence During sustained abstinence: decreased sleep, impaired vigilance, impaired procedural learning, but reported better sleep	Sleep study suggestive of chronic insomnia; altered homeostatic sleep drive function
Pace-Schott et al. (2005)	Descriptive study Effect of cocaine binge–abstinence on sleep Polysomnography, Nightcap ambulatory monitor; sleep questionnaire	5 cocaine users; binge–abstinence 3 days abstinence, 3 days binge, 3 days binge, then 15 days abstinence	Poor quality sleep progressively occurred based on polysomnography (sleep duration, efficiency, latency); self-report of subjective sleep did not change; sleep deteriorated over binge–abstinence cycle but perception of sleep quality did not change	Sleep homeostat likely disrupted by cocaine use, causing difference in subjective and objective sleep quality
Valladares & Irwin (2007)	Literature review Evaluation of sleep patterns in cocaine users Polysomnography			More studies could use polysomnography, with goal of decreasing morbidity associated with sleep disturbances in cocaine users
Weddington et al. (1990)	Case–control study Mood, craving, and sleep in cocaine users	12 male cocaine users, 10 male non-users	During 28-day abstinence, cocaine users demonstrated greater mood-distress and depression, which decreased over time; no sleep difficulties were identified except for difficulty falling to sleep and lack of clear head upon rising	

57

Sachs *et al.* (1993) described 10 cases of infectious keratitis and four cases of sterile epithelial defects seen in crack cocaine users. The sterile defects were associated with vigorous eye rubbing after using crack. Although no visual complications occurred after treatment, the authors suggested that certain subsets of young crack users may be pre-disposed to corneal complications.

Colatrella & Daniel (1999) reported a case of corneal inflammation and infection after vigorously eye rubbing following exposure to and use of cocaine. The individual was treated with antibiotics and had no reported negative outcomes. The authors suggested that use of cocaine should be investigated as a cause of keratitis if no other risk factors are identified.

Pilon & Scheiffle (2006) reported a 42-year-old female who was admitted to a drug treatment program. Her left eye had a purulent discharge and a deep stromal ulcer of the cornea, which subsequently grew *Candida albicans*. Besides testing positive for cocaine, she also had a positive heroin toxicology screen.

Ghosheh *et al.* (2007) described four cases of corneal ulcers seen in crack users. Three of the patients had streptococcal infections; the fourth had *Capnocytophaga* sp. and *Brevibacterium casei*. Although all four patients responded to antibiotic therapy, two required a tarsorrhaphy, where the eyelids were partially sewn together to protect the cornea.

Pachigolla *et al.* (2007) reviewed the records of 131 patients with keratitis. Corneal scrapings were taken and organisms were found in 73 of 139 samples (52.5%). The most common organism found was *Pseudomonas* spp. and *S. aureus* was the next most common. Four risk factors for keratitis were identified: pre-existing ocular disease, contact lens use, trauma, and cocaine use. Cocaine use was reported by 5% of the patients. Complications were rare in the uninfected group and, after healing, visual acuity improved in the uninfected group as well. More severe complications were reported in the patients with infectious keratitis ($p = 0.041$).

Rofsky *et al.* (1995) described microtalc retinopathy and glaucoma-like retinal nerve fiber layer defects in 60 cocaine users. These findings were only found in users of freebase cocaine. According to Maloney (2002), the fillers used in drugs such as cocaine may include magnesium silicate, which cannot be broken down once in the body. After absorption into the bloodstream, small particles may reach the eye and become trapped in the retinal capillaries as microemboli. The macula of the eye is particularly vulnerable because of a dual blood supply by the retinal and choroidal vessels. Rofsky and others speculated that the talc particles may cause microvascular changes in other parts of the body in addition to the eyes.

Talc retinopathy was also described in a case report of a patient with a 20-year history of cocaine and heroin use (Tran & Ilsen 2007). The individual had no systemic diseases such as diabetes mellitus, sarcoidosis, or sickle cell anemia that might have explained the neovascularization seen in the retinal vessels of both eyes. A variety of vascular changes were seen on fundoscopic examination including pinpoint deposits on both maculas, engorged vessels, intraretinal hemorrhage, exudates, and preretinal hemorrhage. The peripheral neovascularization was treated by panretinal photocoagulation.

In addition to corneal and retinal disease, cocaine was found to be associated with a case of iritis in a 31-year-old male (Wang 1991). The individual had a previous episode of iritis; both events were associated with casual cocaine use.

Desai *et al.* (1997) carried out a case–control study to evaluate color vision loss in cocaine users. Thirty-one cocaine users undergoing withdrawal were compared with 31 matched controls on their performance on two color vision tests. On the Farnsworth–Munsell 100-hue test, 23 of the 31 cocaine users experienced blue–yellow color loss, compared with 3 of 31 of the controls ($p < 0.001$). Blue–yellow color loss was also detected by the Lanthony desaturated D-15 color test in 15 of the 31 cocaine users, compared with 2 of 31 controls ($p < 0.001$). Since dopamine has a role in normal color vision signaling in the retina, color vision distortion was not unexpected in this study.

Two cases of acute-angle-closure glaucoma in cocaine users have been described in the literature. Mitchell & Schwartz (1996) described a 55-year-old male who developed acute-angle-closure glaucoma in his right eye after intranasal cocaine use. Cocaine is known to cause mydriasis, which can precipitate angle closure in predisposed individuals with a shallow anterior chamber. Hari et al. (1999) described the development of acute-angle-closure glaucoma in a 46-year-old female who received 2% cocaine paste to her nasal mucosa during an antral washout under general anesthesia. Postoperatively, she developed pain and loss of vision.

Table 3.19 summarizes these studies.

Comments

These 11 articles provide cases of corneal, retinal, and iris conditions associated with cocaine use. Although these are all case reports, healthcare providers should consider cocaine use in individuals presenting with inflammatory eye disorders. Prompt culturing and appropriate antibiotic therapy could help to prevent chronic eye damage.

Microtalc emboli, discussed in two case reports, may provide some insight into the cause of retinal damage and could further explain ischemic and inflammatory changes seen elsewhere in the body. Further study of the mechanisms of cell pathology is needed.

Changes in color vision may be induced by cocaine-related alterations in dopamine signaling in the retina. One group of researchers suggested color vision may be useful to study in cocaine users. Further study to assess the risk of vision distortion would be helpful.

Based on the two patients described, the risk for acute-angle-closure glaucoma in susceptible individuals with shallow anterior chambers could be increased in cocaine users and in non-users undergoing procedures where cocaine-containing anesthetics are used.

Male urological disease

A number of epidemiological studies were found in a review of PubMed published on genitourinary problems and cocaine use for the period of 1988 to 2008. This review is divided into three subsections: male genitalia, renal dysfunction, and miscellaneous renal disorders.

Male genitalia

One article by Cocores et al. (1988) described the influence of alcohol and cocaine on sexual dysfunction. In a population of 80 male patients addicted to both drugs and who resided in a drug treatment center, 50 (62%) indicated that they had sexual dysfunction. No articles were found that reported on sexual dysfunction in only cocaine users. Some evidence from laboratory studies indicates that erectile dysfunction may occur with cocaine use; two reports related to this topic were found in the literature.

Two articles have been published since 1999 describing six cases of priapism occurring in males with no predisposition for the condition. In a report, Altman et al. (1999) described three males who used cocaine in the previous 24 hours and tested positive on toxicology tests. Because of the delay in seeking medical care, intracavernosal aspiration and

Table 3.19 Ocular disease

Study	Method	Sample	Incidence	Results
Ghosheh et al. (2007)	Case series Corneal ulcers	4 crack users	3 streptococcal infections; 1 with Capnocytophaga and Brevibacterium; 2 required tarsorrhaphy	Aerosolized crack can lead to corneal ulcers
Pachigolla et al. (2007)	Review of keratitis over 5 year period Corneal scrapings	131 patients (139 eye scrapings)	Organisms found in 73 (52.5%); Pseudomonas predominant; also S. aureus; 114 (87.1%) had one or more risk factors: pre-existing ocular disease, contact lens use, trauma, cocaine use (5%)	Complications uncommon in sterile group; vision more acute in sterile group after treatment
Rofsky et al. (1995)	Review of cases of retinal damage	60 with microtalc and retinal nerve fiber layer defects	Glaucoma-like findings	Findings only seen in users of freebase cocaine
Sachs et al. (1993)	Case series Corneal complications	Crack users: 10 infectious keratitis, 4 sterile epithelial defects	Those with sterile epithelial defects had rubbed their eyes vigorously after cocaine use	A subset of young crack users may be predisposed to corneal complications after use.
Wang (1991)	Case report	31-year-old male with iritis associated with intranasal cocaine use	Two separate incidences of iritis	
Pilon & Scheiffle (2006)	Case report	42-year-old female, tested positive for cocaine and heroin use	Deep, paracentral stromal ulcer on left cornea; culture, Candida albicans	Without other risk factors, cocaine use should be considered with corneal ulceration
Colatrella & Daniel (1999)	Case report	40-year-old male	Corneal infiltrate, epithelial defect; vigorously rubbed eyes after cocaine use; no adverse effects after treatment	Prompt recognition and treatment important in successful outcome

Desai et al. (1997)	Case–control study Color vision change during cocaine withdrawal	31 cocaine-withdrawing cocaine users, 31 matched controls	More blue–yellow color loss in cocaine users: Farnsworth–Munsell 100-hue test positive in 231 cocaine users, 3 controls ($p < 0.001$); Lanthony desaturated D-15 Color Vision Test positive in 15 cocaine users, 2 controls ($p < 0.001$)	Color vision testing might be useful in identification of cocaine users
Hari et al. (1999)	Case report Glaucoma and cocaine	46-year-old female received 2% cocaine paste for nasal surgery	Developed painful acute-angle-closure glaucoma 24 h after cocaine application	Cocaine, sympathetic nervous system stimulation causes mydriasis and can lead to acute-angle closure in individuals with shallow anterior chambers
Mitchell & Schwartz (1996)	Case report Glaucoma and cocaine use	55-year-old male, intranasal cocaine user	Developed acute-angle-closure glaucoma in one eye; treated with laser peripheral iridotomy	Cocaine use can cause mydriasis and angle-closure-glaucoma in susceptible individuals
Tran & Ilsen (2007)	Case report Talc retinopathy	Chronic cocaine, heroin user with no systemic disease (diabetes, sarcoidosis, sickle cell)	Bilateral peripheral retinal neovascularization in peripheral retina secondary to cocaine use; retinal vascular emboli from talc deposits	Impurities in cocaine mix can lead to talc retinopathy

irrigation were unsuccessful. Cavernous spongiosal shunting also failed in two patients. A partial penectomy for infected, gangrenous distal penile tissue was ultimately performed on one patient. Early diagnosis of cocaine use may help to prevent a recurrence of priapism in the drug user.

Munarriz *et al.* (2003) described three cases of priapism induced by cocaine or ephedrine-containing non-prescription drugs for weight loss. They also carried out a laboratory study on rabbit cavernosal penile tissue by electrically stimulating the tissue after either cocaine or ephedrine application. Both drugs caused sustained contraction for several hours. The researchers hypothesized that long-term use of cocaine or ephedrine could deplete nor-epinephrine from nerve endings in the sympathetic nervous system, resulting in sustained contraction.

Four studies looked at the prevalence of genital ulcer disease (GUD) in cocaine users. Most cases of GUD are associated with STDs, although there may be other causes.

Chirgwin *et al.* (1991) studied 194 patients with STDs who were tested for HIV. More women than men participated in the study. The OR determined for crack use and GUD was 15.15 (95% CI 3.27–inexact), and the OR for crack use and multiple simultaneous STDs was 13.87 (95% CI 4.62–inexact). Presence of HIV antibodies was associated with a history of crack cocaine use: OR 2.98 (95% CI inexact–9.61). Infection with HIV was independently associated with GUD and crack cocaine use. The researchers indicated the association between cocaine use and GUD, STDs, and HIV was a result of the high-risk behavior characteristic of this population, including drug-related prostitution.

A review of the literature by Martin & DiCarlo (1994) supported the hypothesis that drug-related prostitution was part of cocaine users' risky behavior. The presence of *Haemophilus ducreyi*, the cause of chanchroid, in males was strongly associated with crack cocaine use but was also strongly related to sexual exposure to cocaine-using women. The authors suggested that the syphilis and chancroid epidemics in the USA were related to crack use, since drug use was associated with sexual activity with cocaine-using women.

Bauwens *et al.* (2002) studied 47 patients with GUD in an effort to determine the source of GUD in HIV, syphilis, and GUD outbreaks. Patients were tested for syphilis, HIV, HSV-2, and *Chlamydia*. Cultures were obtained from GUD lesions; lymph node aspirates were also obtained. Almost half tested positive for HIV ($n = 20$ [43%]), but other findings included confirmed lymphogranuloma venereum ($n = 8$), and possible lymphogranuloma venereum ($n = 9$), but also GUD in seven others without lymphogranuloma venereum. Inguinal lymphadenopathy (bubo) was found in 15 of the 17 patients with confirmed or possible lymphogranuloma venereum. Genital herpes was detected in 13, chancroid in 7, and syphilis in 4 patients. The authors suggested that lymphogranuloma disease is often transmitted with other STDs.

Gomez *et al.* (2002) conducted a retrospective case–control study to study the inter-relationship between crack use and GUD and HIV infections. During 1985 to 1990, cocaine use in Bahamian patients with STDs was associated with GUD (OR 3.3; 95% CI 2.1–5.1), with secondary syphilis (OR 5.5; 95% CI 2.4–12.6), and HIV (OR 8.1; 95% CI 4.3–15.2). Their findings showed a temporal trend in epidemics in the area: cocaine use initially increased, then GUD, followed by HIV infections.

A case of recurring Stevens–Johnson syndrome was described by Hofbauer *et al.* (2000) in a 26-year-old male cocaine snorter with genital skin erosion. He also had erosion of the oral mucosa. A diagnosis of Stevens–Johnson syndrome was based on histological findings during the patient's second episode of skin lesions. Stevens–Johnson syndrome is a systemic allergic reaction that often manifests with a rash and lesions of the skin and mucous membranes. After treatment with systemic steroids, the patient's symptoms cleared. He was advised to avoid a particular cocaine street mix he had used prior to the two earlier episodes.

Table 3.20 summarizes these results.

Renal dysfunction

A number of studies were found that described acute and chronic renal failure in cocaine users, some of whom also had hypertension, rhabdomyositis, or rhabdomyolysis.

One longitudinal study by Vupputuri *et al.* (2004) reported on the association of illicit drug use with declining renal function. Interviews were carried out with 640 patients in a Veteran's Association (VA) hypertension clinic regarding drug use from 1977 to 1999 and the patients were followed for seven years thereafter. The endpoint was an increase in serum creatinine levels of ≥ 0.6 mg/dL (≥ 53.0 μmol/L). The drugs used included marijuana (22.7%), cocaine (6.7%), amphetamines (9.3%), psychedelics (3.1%), and heroin (4.3%). After adjusting for a number of confounders, the RR for mild kidney function decline associated with any drug use was 2.3 (95% CI 1.0–5.1) and with cocaine use was 3.0 (95% CI 1.1–8.0). The only other drugs with an increased RR for declining renal function were psychedelics.

Brecklin *et al.* (1998) reported on a study designed to determine the prevalence of chronic hypertension in chronic cocaine users. They studied 301 black males with normal renal function in an addiction treatment program for cocaine use. Despite positive cocaine toxicology tests, 62% were normotensive. During a two-week observational period, 20% had acutely elevated blood pressures that returned to normal levels in one day, and 18% had chronically elevated blood pressure above 140/90 mmHg. Cocaine users with elevated blood pressures did not have microalbuminuria. The authors concluded that hypertension in cocaine users is predominantly an acute situation, and not chronic.

Fine *et al.* (2007) reported on an 11-year review of kidney biopsy results in 193 HIV-infected patients. Excluding those with hypertension and diabetes, of the 53 remaining patients, 29 (55%) had hypertensive renal changes on biopsy (arterial internal fibrosis and arteriolosclerosis). Sixteen (55%) of the patients with hypertensive renal changes were also cocaine abusers and 6 of the 24 patients without hypertension renal changes also used cocaine. The OR for developing hypertensive renal changes in cocaine users was 3.7 (95% CI 1.2–11.7). Cocaine use was significantly associated with hypertension and renal changes in an adjusted analysis (OR 3.55; 95% CI 1.04–12.14). These authors suggested that the risk of hypertensive renal changes is high in HIV-positive cocaine users even though hypertension was not evident.

Ruttenber *et al.* (1999) reviewed 150 cases of rhabdomyolysis reported in the medical literature and identified 58 individuals in an autopsy registry with fatal excited delirium. One hundred and twenty-five individuals dying from fatal acute cocaine toxicity were also identified. Comparing the three groups, those with rhabdomyolysis and excited delirium were very similar in age, gender, route of cocaine use, and symptoms of excitement, delirium, hyperthermia, and lack of seizure activity. Those individuals with acute cocaine toxicity were very different from the other two groups. The authors suggested that rhabdomyolysis and excited delirium are different stages of the same syndrome in cocaine users. In both cases, the probable cause is a change in dopamine processing that occurs with chronic, intense use of cocaine, and not toxic effects of the drug.

A case of cocaine-induced ARF mimicking thrombotic thrombocytopenia purpura was described by Volcy *et al.* (2000). A 38-year-old female inhaled crack cocaine and developed

63

Table 3.20 Male genitalia and genital ulcer disease

Study	Method	Sample	Incidence	Results
Altman et al. (1999)	Case series. Priapism and cocaine	Priapism in 3 males using cocaine in previous 24 h	Treatment failures: intracavernosal aspiration, irrigations; cavernous spongiosal shunting, 1 required partial penectomy (infected, gangrenous distal penile tissue)	Urine toxicology screen may help earlier diagnosis and treatment and could help to prevent recurrence of priapism in cocaine users
Bauwens et al. (2002)	Descriptive study. Source of GUD in HIV, syphilis, GUD outbreaks. Tested for syphilis, HIV, HSV-2, chlamydia, LGV; cultures of GUD, lymph node aspirates	47 with GUD	20 (43%) HIV positive; 17 (36%) LGV or possible LGV (15/17 had inguinal lymphadenopathy); 7/30 patients without LGV had adenopathy); 13 (28%) genital herpes; 7 (15%) chancroid; 4 (9%) syphilis	LGV also a possible STD transmitted through unprotected sex; associated with cocaine outbreaks
Chirgwin et al. (1991)	Descriptive study GUD in urban heterosexuals	194 patients with STD, also tested for HIV	Crack use and GUD, OR 15.15 (95% CI 3.27–inexact); crack use and multiple simultaneous STDs, OR 13.87 (95% CI 4.62–inexact); HIV antibodies associated with history of crack cocaine, OR 2.98 (95% CI inexact–9.61)	GUD associated with high-risk sexual behavior, including drug-related prostitution
Cocores et al. (1988)	Descriptive study. Sexual dysfunction in dual alcohol and cocaine users	Individuals in treatment center	50 (62% of those providing a sexual history) self-reported sexual dysfunction	
Gomez et al. (2002)	Retrospective case–control study. Review of inter-relatedness among crack use, GUD, HIV infection	Bahamians with STDs	Cocaine use in patients with STDs (1985–1990): associated with GUD (OR 3.3; 95% CI 2.1–5.1), associated with syphilis (OR 5.5; 95% CI 2.4–12.6), associated with HIV (OR 8.1; 95% CI 4.3–15.2)	A temporal relation exists in epidemics: cocaine use > GUD > HIV
Hofbauer et al. (2000)	Case report. Stevens–Johnson syndrome (first case reported)	24-year-old cocaine snorter	2 incidences of oral, genital erosive skin changes after snorting coke; diagnosed as recurring Stevens–Johnson syndrome; signs and symptoms cleared 4 days after treatment	Recommendation: avoid a particular street mix of cocaine
Martin & DiCarlo (1994)	Literature review		Haemophilus ducreyi in males strongly associated with crack cocaine, but more important risk of sexual exposure to cocaine-using women	Crack use is associated with syphilis, chancroid epidemics in the USA
Munarriz et al. (2003)	Case series. Priapism and ephedrine and cocaine users	3 cocaine or ephedrine users	Laboratory study of rabbit penile tissue with cocaine or ephedrine application: sustained contraction for several hours	Alpha-adrenergic function normal; long-term use of drugs may deplete sympathetic nervous system norepinephrine stores, leading to priapism

CI, confidence interval; GUD, genital ulcer disease; HIV, human immunodeficiency virus; HSV-2, herpes simplex virus type 2; LGV, lymphogranuloma venereum; OR, odds ratio; STD, sexually transmitted disease thrombocytopenia and ARF requiring hemodialysis. However, she did not develop the hemolytic anemia typically found in thrombotic thrombocytopenia purpura. Her renal biopsy did show thrombotic microangiopathy and glomerular ischemia. She continued to have renal insufficiency after the acute phase of her illness; one month later, after using cocaine again, her condition worsened and she experienced ARF, anemia, and thrombocytopenia. The authors hypothesized that the renal biopsy findings could be caused by endothelial injury, vasoconstriction or impaired vasodilation capabilities, procoagulant activity, or antiplatelet activity.

Perneger et al. (2001) carried out a case–control study to determine the association between illicit drug use and end-stage renal disease (ESRD) using 716 patients with ESRD selected from a registry and 361 controls randomly selected by phone. Statistical analyses showed that the risk factors for ESRD included lifetime use of heroin, cocaine, or other addictive drugs. Adjusting for age, sex, race, socioeconomic status, diabetes, and high blood pressure, there was an association between ESRD and cocaine, crack, or psychedelic drug use (AOR 19.1; 95% CI 1.7–208.7), but not a separate association with heroin use.

Norris et al. (2001) carried out a cross-sectional study of 201 African American patients in two outpatient hemodialysis units in order to study the association between cocaine use and patients requiring hemodialysis with and without a diagnosis of hypertension-related ESRD. The subjects included 106 males and 87 females, with a mean age of 49.28 years and 55 (28%) used cocaine prior to initiating hemodialysis. Among the 55 cocaine users, 49 (89.1%) had hypertensive ESRD while 64/138 (46%) of the non-users did not: an OR of 9.44 (95% CI 3.79–23.49; $p < 0.0005$). Compared with those who did not use cocaine, cocaine users with hypertensive ESRD were younger (40.7 vs. 53.8 years) and had a shorter duration of hypertension (5.3 vs. 12.7 years) (both $p < 0.0005$ adjusted for age and sex). The authors concluded that in the hemodialysis population, there is a strong association with a history of cocaine use and earlier onset of ESRD. They hypothesized that cocaine could be the cause of ESRD in cocaine users without other identifiable cause.

In a case study, de Mendoza et al. (2004) looked at four patients with renal insufficiency. Two had malignant hypertension, one had rhabdomyolysis associated with cocaine use, and one was a cocaine user with severe ischemic neurological lesions. The authors concluded that differentiating the cause of ARF is difficult.

Fernandez et al. (2005) carried out a chart review to look for predictors of ARF and the need for hemodialysis in patients with rhabdomyolysis. Charts were reviewed over a four-year period, and they identified 93 males and 4 females with a diagnosis of rhabdomyolysis and a CK level > 1000 U/L. The mean age of the patients was 35.7 years. The three major causes of rhabdomyolysis were cocaine use (30 patients), exercise (29 patients), and immobilization (18 patients). In 17 of the 97 patients (17.5%) ARF developed; eight (8.25%) required hemodialysis. The authors found that only the initial serum creatine and blood urea nitrogen levels could predict the need for hemodialysis.

A case study by Rivero et al. (2006) described a young African American cocaine user who developed ARF but who did not have rhabdomyolysis. The patient recovered with supportive therapy. The researchers hypothesized that the intense vasoconstriction might have led to the ARF.

Gu & Herrera (2007) described two cases of malignant hypertension associated with cocaine use. Renal biopsies showed morphological features of thrombotic microangiopathy. Fibrinoid necrosis of the arteries and glomerular tufts were also pathological features seen.

Table 3.21 summarizes these studies.

Table 3.21 Renal dysfunction

Study	Method	Sample	Incidence	Results
Brecklin et al. (1998)	Descriptive study Chronic high BP in chronic cocaine users Urine toxicology tests	Black males enrolled in addiction treatment program for cocaine use; 301 with normal renal function tests and no microalbuminuria	62% normotensive regardless of toxicology screen status; 20% acutely elevated BP, normalized in 1 day; 18% chronic elevation of BP (> 140/90 mmHg); no significant difference in BP with age	Hypertension in cocaine users likely to be acute, not chronic; cocaine use not associated with microalbuminuria
de Mendoza et al. (2004)	Case series Acute renal insufficiency and cocaine	4 cocaine users: 2 with malignant high BP, 1 with severe ischemic neurological lesions, 1 with rhabdomyolysis		Variety of causes of acute renal insufficiency in cocaine users
Fernandez et al. (2005)	Chart review, retrospective study Prediction of ARF and HD in patients with rhabdomyolysis Creatinine > 1000 U/L	93 males, 4 females; mean age 35.7 years	Causes: cocaine in 30, exercise in 29, immobilization in 18; 17 (17.5%) developed ARF; 8 (8.25%) required HD	Only initial CK and blood urea nitrogen level predicted need for HD
Fine et al. (2007)	Descriptive study Cocaine use and chronic renal disease in HIV-positive patients 11 year review of kidney biopsies	193 HIV-positive patients, 53 with no history of high BP or diabetes; 29/53 (55%) hypertensive renal changes on biopsy; 16/29 (55%) used cocaine; 6/24 without hypertensive changes used cocaine	Use of cocaine and developing hypertensive renal changes compared with those without such changes, OR 3.7 (95% CI 1.2–11.7); adjusted analysis of cocaine use associated with hypertensive changes on renal biopsy, OR 3.55 (95% CI 1.04–12.14)	Cocaine users can develop hypertensive renal changes even without evidence of high BP
Gu & Herrera (2007)	Case series Malignant hypertension and renal failure Biopsy	2 patients with renal failure	Cocaine-induced malignant hypertension with morphological features of thrombotic macroangiopathy; biopsy showed fibrinoid necrosis of arterioles, glomerular tufts	
Norris et al. (2001)	Cross-sectional study Cocaine use in HD with and without diagnosis of hypertension-related ESRD	201 black patients from two outpatient HD units: 106 males, 87 females (193 in study); 55/193 (28.5%) used cocaine before HD	Hypertensive ESRD: 49/55 (89.1%) cocaine users, 64/138 (46%) non-users (OR 9.44; 95% CI 3.79 –23.49; p < 0.0005) 49/113 (43.4%) with hypertensive ESRD had history of cocaine abuse	Cocaine users younger (40.7 vs. 53.8 years; p < 0.0005), shorter duration of high BP (5.3 vs. 12.7 years; p < 0.0005) adjusted for age/sex; In HD, there is a strong association with history of cocaine use, earlier onset of ESRD

Study	Type/description	Population	Findings	Comments
Perneger et al. (2001)	Case–control study. Association between drug use and ESRD	716 patients treated for ESRD in 1991; 361 controls (similar age, 20–65 years), randomly selected by telephone interview	Risk factors for development of ESRD: lifetime use of heroin, cocaine, other addictive drugs; association for ESRD adjusted for age, sex, race, socioeconomic status, diabetes, high BP, crack use in cocaine users, psychedelic drugs (OR 19.1; 95% CI 1.7–208.7)	Risk for ESRD associated with cocaine and psychedelic drugs, but not separated from heroin effects
Rivero et al. (2006)	Case report. ARF without rhabdomyolysis	Young African American	No evidence of rhabdomyolysis; recovered with supportive therapy	Likely cause intense vasoconstriction
Ruttenber et al. (1999)	Case–control study. Literature review. Cocaine-associated rhabdomyolysis	150 with rhabdomyolysis in literature; 58 with FED; 125 fatalities from cocaine toxicity	Rhabdomyolysis and FED patients similar in age, gender, race, route of cocaine administration; mostly black, male, younger than cocaine toxicity victims; experienced excitement, delirium, hyperthermia, no seizures	Suggests rhabdomyolysis in cocaine users and FED are part of the same syndrome with different stages, caused by change in dopamine processing and not drug toxicity
Volcy et al. (2000)	Case report. Cocaine-induced ARF	Female 38 years old inhaled crack cocaine; after treatment, use of cocaine 1 month later caused return of ARF	Developed ARF, thrombocytopenia, requiring HD; renal biopsy indicated thrombotic microangiopathy, glomerular ischemia, not thrombotic thrombocytopenia purpura	Possible mechanisms: endothelial injury, vasoconstriction or impaired vasodilatation, procoagulant activity, antiplatelet activity
Vupputuri et al. (2004)	Longitudinal study at Veteran's Association clinic for high blood pressure. Effect of illicit drug use and kidney function. Interview for drug use	640 patients followed for 7 years (1977–1999)	Drugs used: marijuana, 22.7%; crack cocaine, 6.7%; amphetamines, 9.3%; psychedelics, 3.1%; heroin, 4.3% Mild kidney function decline: associated with any drug use (RR 2.3; 95% CI 1.0–5.1), cocaine use (RR 3.0; 95% CI 1.1–8.0)	Only other drugs with significant RR were psychedelics

ARF, acute renal failure; BP, blood pressure; ESRD, end-stage renal disease; FED, fatal excited delirium; HD, hemodialysis.

Miscellaneous renal dysfunction

Two case studies were published that describe the development of ARF in patients who also used cocaine. In the patients described, an autoimmune anti-glomerular basement membrane (GBM) disease was found in individuals who also were cocaine users. However, no relationship between anti-GBM and cocaine use was established. Peces *et al.* (1999) described a case of glomerulonephritis in a 35-year-old intranasal cocaine user who developed circulating anti-GBM antibodies and, on biopsy, had IgG and C3 (complement) deposits in the tissues, confirming a diagnosis of anti-GBM disease. He had no evidence of rhabdomyolysis or circulating myoglobin. Sirvent *et al.* (2007) described a 26-year-old female who inhaled cocaine and developed anti-GBM glomerulonephritis and pulmonary hemorrhage (characteristic of Goodpasture's syndrome). She required hemodialysis for initial treatment and also on a continual basis.

In a review of the literature, Jaffe & Kimmel (2006) described chronic nephropathy in cocaine users. They found that, although the literature supports a relationship between cocaine use and renal disease, there was no evidence that heroin and renal disease were related. In vitro cell and animal studies did support cocaine injury with renal pathology. The findings included non-specific changes in the renal glomeruli, interstitial matrix, and renal tubules.

Two case reports described individuals who had renal dysfunction after using cocaine. Decelle *et al.* (2007) described a 42-year-old male who developed acute interstitial nephritis after sniffing cocaine. Initially requiring hemodialysis, the patient fully recovered. Bemanian *et al.* (2005) described a 48-year-old male with flank pain after cocaine use. By exclusion of other possible diagnoses, a diagnosis of cocaine-induced renal infarct was made.

These results are summarized in Table 3.22.

Comments

This section includes a variety of studies covering a broad range of topics. Many are case studies of cocaine-using individuals and manifestations related to the genital–urinary–renal system. The etiologies of most of the dysfunctions in the studies are hypothetical, although some laboratory studies may support the hypotheses.

Sexual dysfunction

The one published article on sexual dysfunction in cocaine users also relates to alcohol use since the subjects in the study were dual users. There is some laboratory science that suggests that erectile dysfunction might occur with cocaine use through several mechanisms: elevated serum endothelin-1, which can be released with endothelial damage; decreased release of the vasodilator nitric oxide; and elevated tissue myeloperoxidase, found in granular leukocytes. However, few studies were found that support an association between cocaine use and sexual dysfunction.

Genital ulcer disease

Four studies showed a relationship between cocaine use and risky sexual behavior that ultimately led to GUD and transmission of STDs. The diseases most commonly described include HIV, syphilis, *Chlamydia*, HSV-2, chancroid, and lymphogranuloma. Trading sex for drugs and unprotected sex appear to be a part of the risky behavior seen in cocaine users. Some statistically significant results were found for the association of GUD with

Table 3.22 Miscellaneous renal dysfunction

Study	Method	Sample	Incidence	Results
Bemanian *et al.* (2005)	Case report Cocaine and renal infarct	48-year-old male, 4 day history of flank pain after cocaine use	Diagnosis: cocaine-induced renal infarct	
Decelle *et al.* (2007)	Case report Cocaine use and acute nephritis	42-year-old male, acute interstitial nephritis after cocaine sniffing	Required initial HD but fully recovered	
Jaffe & Kimmel (2006)	Literature review Chronic nephropathy and cocaine use		Heroin as cause of renal disease not supported by literature Cocaine use and renal disease: renal hemodynamic changes, glomerular matrix synthesis, degradation, oxidative stress, renal atherogenesis	In vitro cell and animal studies support cocaine injury to kidney; heroin cause not supported
Peces *et al.* (1999)	Case report Glomerulonephritis in cocaine user	35-year-old male, intranasal cocaine use; no rhabdomyolysis, no plasma myoglobin	Circulating anti-GBM antibodies; biopsy showed IgG, complement C3 deposits; diagnosis: anti-GBM disease	Autoimmune disease targeting GBM
Sirvent *et al.* (2007)	Case report and review of the literature Cocaine user and Goodpasture's syndome	26-year-old female, inhaled cocaine	Anti-GBM glomerulonephritis and pulmonary hemorrhage; required chronic HD; diagnosis Goodpasture's syndrome	Autoimmune disease targeting kidney and lung

HD, hemodialysis; GBM, glomerular basement membrane.

cocaine use, HIV, and other STDs. Two studies found a relationship among an increase in cocaine use, epidemics of GUD, and subsequent HIV infections.

Immunology

Allergic and autoimmune disorders are also described in several studies. Stevens–Johnson syndrome, an allergic condition, was described in one individual with genital skin erosion. The cause was attributed to a particular street mix of cocaine being used by the individual. Two articles described anti-GBM in patients with glomerulonephritis. A renal biopsy confirmed the presence of anti-GBM antibodies, IgG antibodies, and C3 (complement). Another patient had anti-GBM antibodies and pulmonary hemorrhage. Both cases suggest a diagnosis of Goodpasture's disease, a rare autoimmune disorder diagnosed in one per million population a year. These persons may also test positive for ANCA (described previously). It is possible that these patients had a susceptibility to anti-GBM disease or Goodpasture's syndrome and the use of cocaine is coincidental or a trigger for developing the disorder. Alternatively, the toxins in cocaine may be a precipitating factor in development of the disease. More studies are needed to clarify the role of cocaine in autoimmune renal disease and allergies.

Hypertension and renal disease

The combined link of cocaine, hypertension, and renal disease is strong, but questions still remain. A seven-year longitudinal study found that there is an increased risk for a mild decline in kidney function in cocaine users. Case–control longitudinal studies would strengthen the evidence for or against cocaine use and decreasing renal function. One study found hypertensive changes in kidney biopsies of HIV-positive cocaine users, even though hypertension was not seen in the users. While hypertensive renal changes occurred in HIV-positive cocaine users without hypertension, no such changes were found in other users. Another study found that although initial blood pressure was elevated in some cocaine users admitted to treatment facilities, one-fifth of the patients were normotensive within one day, suggesting that cocaine use is not a risk factor for chronic hypertension. Another one-fifth remained hypertensive but had no evidence of microalbuminuria, which would suggest renal dysfunction.

These studies provide some evidence that cocaine users are at risk for developing renal disease. However, more studies are needed to explore the dose and length of use of cocaine needed to depress renal function. Renal biopsy results might help to identify the type of renal pathology occurring in cocaine users. Most of the studies followed cocaine users only, suggesting that studies have some selection bias. Questions also have to be raised whether the renal disease occurred prior to the development of hypertension, since it is known that pre-existing renal disease can cause hypertension.

Rhabdomyolysis

The role of rhabdomyolysis in cocaine users may be associated with ischemic muscle changes induced by intense vasoconstriction, exacerbated by cocaine. As myoglobin is released in the circulation, obstructive casts may form in the renal tubules, resulting in ARF. Microvascular clots may also form. A laboratory study by Rozhinskaia et al. (1989) found myoglobin autoantibodies in serum from individuals with circulating myoglobin. The authors suggested that the autoantibodies may be a method for the body to remove serum myoglobin through the action of the reticuloendothelial system.

One study suggested that some cases of rhabdomyolysis reported in the literature may be related to excited delirium, and that both conditions are part of the same syndrome seen in some cocaine users.

Further study is needed to look at the development of rhabdomyolysis in cocaine users and to determine the mechanism(s) that cause a release of myoglobin into the circulation. Epidemiological studies are needed to determine the risk of this potentially fatal event among cocaine users.

Acute renal failure

Several articles suggested that cocaine-induced renal failure is related to elevated levels of endothelin-1, thrombotic microangiopathy, abnormal platelet function, and glomerular ischemia. These conditions could be explained by toxic effects of cocaine on the vascular bed, resulting in endothelial injury and stimulation of procoagulant and antiplatelet activity. The review of the literature by Jaffe and others suggested chronic cocaine users were likely to develop chronic renal disease associated with cocaine-induced hemodynamic changes, alteration of glomerular synthesis and degradation, oxidative stress, and renal atherosclerosis.

According to one study, acute renal insufficiency in cocaine users can be attributed to malignant hypertension, rhabdomyolysis, and severe ischemic lesions. Another paper reported ARF in a cocaine user who did not have rhabdomyolysis. A case was described of a female requiring hemodialysis because of renal failure similar to thrombotic thrombo-cytopenia purpura, although the hemolytic anemia commonly seen in this condition was not found. The renal biopsy showed similar findings to other conditions associated with renal vasoconstriction and imbalances of the procoagulant and anticoagulant regulatory system. Another study described two patients with malignant hypertension whose renal biopsies showed arterial necrosis and thrombotic macroangiopathy.

End-stage renal disease

Several studies looked at the risk for ESRD in cocaine users. There is some evidence that use of cocaine or psychedelic drugs may be associated with hypertensive ESRD. In one study of patients on hemodialysis, 89% were cocaine users; these individuals tended to be younger than other patients on hemodialysis and had an earlier onset of ESRD.

Some cases of ESRD or cases of ARF requiring hemodialysis have been described in cocaine users. In one large study, approximately one-half of all patients requiring hemo-dialysis were cocaine users who did not have hypertension but had evidence of hypertensive renal changes. These individuals were younger than other patients requiring hemodialysis. In another study, almost a third of the patients with rhabdomyolysis and renal disease were cocaine users. That study found that initial CK levels and urea nitrogen were the only predictors for those patients who required hemodialysis therapy.

More epidemiological studies are needed to determine the risk of renal disease in cocaine users, including hypertensive changes seen in renal tissue. Renal disease in indi-viduals with and without a diagnosis of chronic hypertension, and the association between duration of cocaine use and amount of use over time, needs to be explored more fully. The role of rhabdomyolysis in cocaine users also needs to be studied to identify the risk factors and quantify the risk for cocaine users in developing this condition, which can lead to acute or chronic renal failure and ESRD.

Summary

Based on the variety of case studies of cocaine users developing renal disease, particularly ARF, clinicians need to be aware of the physiological effects of cocaine use (vasocon-striction, increased norepinephrine levels, alterations in procoagulant and anticoagulant function) and consider a variety of possible pre- and intrarenal causes for ARF. These possibilities include malignant hypertension, renal macro- and microvascular occlusion, rhabdomyolysis secondary to muscle ischemia, and autoimmune renal disease, which may or may not be related to cocaine use. Monitoring renal function tests is important in those cocaine-using individuals with renal dysfunction so appropriate therapy can be initiated.

Female genital and neonatal/congenital disease

A number of articles were found in the PubMed search for epidemiological studies pub-lished between 1988 and 2008 on the female genital and reproductive system and cocaine use. This subsection includes genital, pregnancy complications, and infant studies.

Genital ulcer disease

Four studies were described in the previous section on cocaine and urology, which also relate to genital disorders in females. These studies showed a relationship between cocaine use and risky sexual behavior in females as well as males that ultimately led to GUD and transmission of STDs. The infections most commonly described include HIV, syphilis, *Chlamydia*, HSV-2, chancroid, and lymphogranuloma. Trading sex for drugs and unprotected sex appear to be two of the risky behaviors seen in cocaine users. Some statistically significant results were found for the association of GUD with cocaine use, HIV, and other STDs. Two studies found a relationship among an increase in cocaine use, epidemics of GUD, and subsequent HIV infections.

One additional study by Mertz *et al.* (1998) related to GUD in females as well as males reviewed cases of atypical genital ulcers in an STD clinic in 1994. Using PCR assays, the following causes were identified in 143 patients: 44 (31%) *Haemophilus ducreyi*; 44 (31%) HSV; and 27 (19%) *Treponema pallidum*. More than one organism was detected in 12 (8%) and 14 (10%) of the patients with GUD were seropositive for HIV. The males in this study who had chancroid were significantly more likely to report having sex with crack cocaine users, having multiple sex partners, and exchanging money or drugs for sex. The findings in this study were consistent with the findings in the studies described in the male urology section above.

Pelvic inflammatory disease

One study, by Jossens *et al.* (1996) looked at risk factors and markers for symptomatic pelvic inflammatory disease (PID) in 234 females in a metropolitan hospital compared with 122 controls in a women's clinic. The controls were similar to the cases in sociodemographic, reproductive, sexual, and medical histories. In a univariate analysis, crack cocaine was identified as one of several risk factors for PID. Multivariate analysis found that the following were significant independent risk factors for PID: parity > 0, more than one sex partner in the previous 30 days, sex during the previous menses, and lack of use of a contraceptive. Although cocaine use did not appear as a significant independent risk factor in the multivariate analysis, cocaine use has been associated with four factors that were significant. This suggests that cocaine use may be a marker for persons who engage in risky behavior, rather than a cause of this risky behavior.

Table 3.23 summarizes these studies.

Pregnancy complications and cocaine

A number of studies were found that provided information about complications and neonatal consequences in pregnant women who used cocaine. Because many of the studies combined information regarding maternal complications and fetal or neonatal consequences, some of those studies are combined in this subsection. Table 3.24 compares the findings of the pregnancy complications found in these studies. Other pregnancy complications and congenital conditions in infants exposed to cocaine are found later in this section.

Burkett *et al.* (1994) described the effect of cocaine binging and pregnancy outcomes in 905 multiethnic, multiracial, inner city pregnant women who were identified as cocaine users during their pregnancy. They were divided into three groups: group 1, 78 aggressive drug seekers who were erratic bingers (where binges lasted 26.4 to 34.4 hours); group 2, 67 daily cocaine users; and group 3, 760 women who were cyclical users (intervals of three, five, seven days, or over seven days). The researchers found that complications were proportional to the frequency of binging ($p = 0.0007$). There was a similar high prematurity rate in group 1 (35.9%) and group 2 (34.3%). Acute problems in group 1 included vaginal bleeding (21.8%), placenta abruptio (14.3%), and stillbirth (20.5%). Groups 2 and 3 were more likely to have chronic problems, including infants small for gestational age (32.8%),

Table 3.23 Female genital disorders[a]

Study	Method	Sample	Incidence	Results
Jossens et al. (1996)	Case–control study Risk factors for PID	234 women hospitalized with PID, 122 controls in a women's clinic Groups similar for demographics, medical and sexual history	Univariate analysis: risk factors for PID include crack cocaine use Multivariate analysis controlling for confounders: risk factors included parity (OR 4.44; 95% CI 2.34–8.42), > 1 sex partner in previous 30 days (OR 11.08; 95% CI 4.31–28.5), sex during previous menses (OR 5.22; 95% CI 1,88–14.48), lack of contraception (OR 7.6; 95% CI 4.10–14.09)	Unprotected sex and risky sexual behavior, as seen with cocaine use, associated with increased risk for PID
Mertz et al. (1998)	Case–control study Atypical genital ulcers	143 patients at a STD clinic	Patients with genital ulcers were more likely to be HIV seropositive than patients without genital ulcers ($p < 0.001$); men with chancroid were more likely than male patients without ulcers to report sex with crack cocaine users, exchange money for sex or drugs, and have multiple sex partners. Disease organisms identified: Haemophilus ducreyi, 56/143 (39%); herpes simplex virus, 44/143 (31%); Treponema pallidum, 27/143 (19%)	Epidemics of GUD are associated with transmission of STDs and appear to be associated with cocaine use and risky sexual behavior

GUD, genital ulcer disease; HIV, human immunodeficiency virus; PID, pelvic inflammatory disease; STD, sexually transmitted disease.
[a] See Table 3.20 for additional studies on GUD involving females.

systemic infections (31.3%), anemia (35.6%), and a low maternal weight under 100 pounds (45 kg) (32.8%). Women who tested positive for cocaine at the time of delivery were two to three times more likely to be at risk for prematurity, placenta abruptio, and vaginal bleeding than those testing negative. However, other factors were likely to be involved in the development of placenta abruptio in group 1 (the erratic bingers) since the risk did not change whether the individual tested positive or negative for cocaine.

Singer et al. (1994) carried out a case–control study comparing 100 women testing positive for cocaine during their pregnancy with 100 matched controls. They found that cocaine use was the best predictor for preterm birth and low birthweight (LBW) controlled for prematurity. After controlling for prematurity, dual use of cocaine and alcohol decreased linear growth. Cocaine use was found to increase negative birth outcomes; however, abortion history and lack of prenatal care were also associated with poor outcomes.

Table 3.24 Increased pregnancy complications and cocaine use in mothers: a comparison of outcomes (18 studies)

Study	Date	No.	Preterm labor	Placenta abruptio	Fetal death	SGA	LBW	Length (decreased)	Placenta previa	Spontaneous abortion	Heart anomalies	IUGR	Sml C	Miscellaneous[a]
Bada	2002	1072					+	+				+	+	
Bateman	1993	361	32%				31%	+					+	
Burkett	1994	905	35%	OR 2–3	20.5%	32.8%								1
Cherukuri	1988	55	50.9%									RR 3.6	+	
Dombrowski	1991	592	+	2 times		+	+							
Dusick	1993	86		18%							7%			2
Handler	1994								OR 1.4					
Hoskins	1991	314	+			+	+	+						
Kistin	1996	64	RR 4.0	RR 10.0	RR 5.3	RR 4.2	RR 5.3		RR 2.4					
Little	1989	53	+				+				+			3
Macones	1997	40							AOR 4.39					
Martinez	1996	13			18.2%	ns	ns							
Ness	1999	400								OR 1.4				
Ney	1990	14	9.9%		+									
Singer	1994	100	+				+							
Spencer	1991	63	4 times											
Sprauve	1997	483	OR 1.9	OR 3.0			AOR 1.6					AOR 1.7		
Weathers	1993	137	15%		2%									

No, women or children positive for cocaine; SGA, small for gestational age; LBW, low birthweight; IUGR, intrauterine growth retardation; Sml C, small head circumference; +, positive finding, increased incidence; RR, relative risk; OR, odds ratio; AOR, adjusted OR; ns, studied, not significant; times, increased risk.
[a]Miscellaneous: 1, increased infection, anemia, low maternal weight; 2, seizures (17%); 3, arrhythmias.

In a retrospective cohort study comparing use of cocaine with cigarette smoking, Kistin *et al.* (1996) found that cocaine users were at a higher risk for a variety of prenatal conditions, while smokers had similar outcomes but less risk than cocaine users. The study compared 64 cocaine users who did not smoke cigarettes, marijuana, or use heroin with 3209 cigarette smokers who did not use illicit drugs or alcohol, and 13 043 women who did not use cocaine, illicit drugs, or cigarettes. Significant risks for following outcomes were found in cocaine users compared with women who did not use cigarettes or drugs: LBW, RR 5.3 (95% CI 3.0–9.3); infants small for gestational age, RR 4.2 (95% CI 2.4–7.3); prematurity, RR 4.0 (95% CI 2.3–7.0); placenta abruptio, RR 10.0 (95% CI 3.5–29.0); placenta previa, RR 2.4 (95% CI 0.3–17.8); and perinatal death, RR 5.3 (95% CI 1.9–15.2). Although cigarette smokers had less increased risk, the number of infants affected was considerably larger since many more women smoke cigarettes than use cocaine.

Ness *et al.* (1999) studied the effect of cocaine use and cigarette smoking on spontaneous abortion. Cocaine use was self-reported and tested with urine or hair samples; cigarette smoking was self-reported or confirmed with urine analysis. The women were African American, of low socioeconomic status, pregnant adolescents and women seen in an inner city emergency room. Four hundred women had spontaneous abortions on admission or during follow-up to 22 weeks of gestation, and 570 carried their fetuses beyond 22 weeks. Of those who did not have a spontaneous abortion, 20.5% were adolescents and 21.8% were non-adolescents. In those with spontaneous abortions, 28.9% used cocaine and 21.8% smoked cigarettes. The presence of cocaine in the hair was independently associated with an increased risk for spontaneous abortion (OR 1.4; 95% CI 1.0–2.1; adjusted for demographic variables and drug use). However, self-report and positive urine tests for cocaine were not associated with an increase in spontaneous abortion. The presence of cotinine in the urine was independently associated with an increased risk for spontaneous abortion (OR 1.8; 95% CI 1.3–2.6). The study found a 24% increased risk for spontaneous abortion related to combined cocaine and tobacco use.

Martinez *et al.* (1996) studied pregnancy outcomes in 102 Hispanic and African American women suspected of having preterm labor. The women who tested positive for cocaine (12.7%) were older than the others (27.8 vs. 22.1 years; $p = 0.002$), and had a higher mean parity (two vs. one). More of the women with preterm labor were African American (92.3%) than Hispanic ($p = 0.0004$). The cocaine users had greater cervical dilation when first seen (3 cm vs. 1 cm; $p = 0.008$), were more likely to be admitted to the hospital (85% vs. 32%; $p = 0.0001$), and less likely to receive medicine to decrease labor contractions owing to advanced dilation or pregnancy complications (36% vs. 79%; $p = 0.0002$). There was no significant difference in gestational age or birthweight in the newborns; however, there was higher risk of fetal deaths in cocaine users (18.2% vs. 0%; $p = 0.02$). The authors concluded that recent cocaine use had a significant impact on pregnancy outcomes.

In a retrospective cohort study, Cherukuri *et al.* (1988) studied 55 women who used crack during their pregnancy; 60% of these had prenatal care. The controls were 55 women without a history of drug use and similar in age, parity, socioeconomic status, alcohol use, and prenatal care. The crack users were more likely than controls to have an early delivery (< 37 weeks) (50.9% vs. 16.4%; $p = 0.001$), had a 3.6 times greater risk of retarded intrauterine growth ($p < 0.006$), and had more infants with small head circumference for gestational age (10th percentile or less; $p < 0.007$). The crack users also had a 1.8 times greater risk for premature membrane rupture ($p = 0.03$). Few neurobehavioral symptoms were found in the children of cocaine-using mothers.

In a cohort study, Little *et al.* (1989) compared the pregnancy outcomes for 53 cocaine users with 100 women without cocaine exposure. The researchers found that cocaine users were more likely to have preterm labor ($p < 0.05$), infants with complications at birth (tachyarrhythmia, meconium presence), LBW ($p < 0.05$), and an increase in congenital heart anomalies ($p < 0.01$).

Ney *et al.* (1990) compared 141 women with preterm labor with 108 women with uncomplicated labor. Within the group with preterm labor, 24 (17%) tested positive for drugs in their urine, 14 of the 24 for cocaine. Only 3 of the 108 women with uncomplicated labor tested positive for drugs in their urine, with one of the three testing positive for cocaine. The authors encouraged practitioners to obtain toxicology urine tests on preterm women in order to guide management, including appropriate neonatal care and counseling and prenatal care for the substance-abusing women.

In a case–control study, Dombrowski *et al.* (1991) studied 592 women who reported using cocaine to decrease the length of labor; 4687 non-drug users were the controls. The cocaine users were older and had a higher parity than the controls. The researchers found that the belief that cocaine shortens labor was not supported in this study. Moreover, there was greater morbidity in the cocaine users, which included a decrease in birthweight, birth weight percentile for gestational age, and doubled increase in placenta abruptio.

Spence *et al.* (1991) studied 500 pregnant women admitted for labor and delivery. Urine screens were carried out on all patients: 15.3% tested positive for cocaine (95% CI 11.8–18.8), and the prevalence for no prenatal care among all subjects was 62% (95% CI 47.2–76.6). Those testing positive for cocaine in the urine were four times more likely to have a preterm labor and two times more likely to have a premature infant with an Apgar score at one minute of 6 or less. The use of the urine screen was found to be helpful in identifying potentially unrecognized problems with drug use.

Handler *et al.* (1994) studied the effect of cigarette or cocaine use on placenta previa, comparing 304 women with placenta previa with 2732 matched controls. The authors found a dose–response relationship between cigarette smoking and placenta previa independent of other known risks (trend $p < 0.01$). Women who smoked 20 or more cigarettes a day were two times more likely to have placenta previa than non-smokers (OR 2.3; 95% CI 1.5–3.5). Women using cocaine were 1.4 times more at risk for placenta previa than non-cocaine users (OR 1.4; 95% CI 0.8–2.4); however, the risk was not statistically significant. The study confirmed the risk for placenta previa in cigarette smokers and suggested that more research is needed to determine risk in cocaine users.

Macones *et al.* (1997) also studied the risk of placenta previa in a case–control study, comparing 40 women with placenta previa at delivery with 80 women without placenta previa. In a multilogistic regression model adjusting for other variables, maternal use of cocaine was an independent risk factor for placenta previa (AOR 4.39; 95% CI 1.17–16.4). Additional risk factors for placenta previa were prior cesarean section, prior elective abortion, and parity.

A retrospective cohort study by Sprauve *et al.* (1997) reported on adverse pregnancy outcomes in 483 cocaine users testing positive for cocaine and 3158 women who had a negative drug screen and served as the controls. They found that cocaine users and their infants were more likely than the non-drug users to have the following adverse outcomes: LBW (31.3% vs. 14.9%; OR 2.6; 95% CI 2.1–3.2), intrauterine growth retardation (IUGR; 29% vs. 13%; OR 2.7; 95% CI 2.2–3.4), preterm infant (28.2% vs. 17.1%; OR 1.9; 95% CI 1.5–2.4), placenta abruptio (3.3% vs.1.1%; OR 3.0; 95% CI 1.6–5.6), and low Apgar score at five minutes (7.9 vs. 4.5%; OR 1.8; 95% CI 1.2–2.7). Adjusting for confounders, the only two outcomes with significant risks were LBW (AOR 1.6; 95% CI 1.03–2.4) and IUGR (AOR 1.7; 95% CI 1.2–2.3). For those infants born of mothers who tested positive for cocaine one week before delivery, the Apgar score at five minutes was significantly different from that in those who did not (OR 2.4; AOR 2.0; 95% CI 1.1–3.7).

Dusick et al. (1993) conducted a prospective cohort study with mothers and their infants with very LBW (< 1499 g). Of the 232 infants, 86 (37%) were exposed to cocaine in utero; 26 of these (30%) were identified by meconium analysis only. The control group was the remaining 146 non-cocaine-exposed infants (identified by negative urine tests, history, and meconium analysis); 91 other infants were excluded because of early death (80) or missing tests (11). Based on intracranial ultrasound findings, there was no difference between the two groups in the number with intraventricular cerebral hemorrhage (36% and 35% for cocaine exposed and unexposed, respectively), grade III intraventricular hemorrhage (36% and 35%, respectively), or periventricular leukomalacia (4% and 2%, respectively). The incidence of placenta abruptio was significantly higher in the cocaine group compared with controls (18% vs. 8%; $p = 0.046$), as was surgical ligation of a patent ductus arteriosus (7% vs. 1%; $p = 0.02$), as well as evidence of seizures (17% vs. 5%, $p = 0.004$). The findings suggest that cocaine-exposed LBW infants are not at increased risk for intracranial hemorrhage but are at risk for other adverse outcomes.

In a secondary analysis, Bada et al. (2002b) studied 11 811 maternal–infant dyads. Of these, 1072 infants were exposed to cocaine in utero, 7565 tested negative for cocaine with meconium results or maternal history, and 3174 infants were excluded from the study. Growth deceleration after 32 weeks was based on the estimated birthweight, length, and head circumference. There was a significant interaction between cocaine use and gestational age. At 40 weeks, controlling for confounders, the cocaine-exposed infants had a decrease in birthweight (151 g), length (0.71 cm), and head circumference (0.43 cm). Other substances also affected some of these parameters, including smoking, which had a negative impact on all measurements; alcohol, which decreased weight and length only; and opiates, which decreased weight only.

Weathers et al. (1993) looked at weight, length, and head circumference in 137 community-based children exposed to cocaine in utero (prevalence, 1.0%); 89 tested positive on urine drug screen, and 48 mothers reported cocaine use. Twenty-one were premature (15%; 95% CI 9–21), and two died of sudden infant death syndrome. Half of the infants were followed 12 months later and percentiles for weight, length, and head circumference were obtained: weight at birth, 23rd percentile; weight at 12 months, 43rd percentile; length at birth, 29th percentile; length at 12 months, 49th percentile; head circumference at birth, 18th percentile, head circumference at 12 months, 54th percentile. These findings suggest that infants move toward the median percentiles within one year after birth.

Bateman et al. (1993) looked at birthweight and preterm delivery in 2810 inner city mothers and infants. Cocaine-exposure was identified by urine testing and maternal history for 361 infants (12.8%). Their developmental parameters were compared with 387 control infants without cocaine exposure. Cocaine-exposed infants were more likely than the controls to have LBW (< 2500 g) (31% vs. 10%) and prematurity (32% vs. 14%). Multivariate analysis found that cocaine-exposed infants had decreased mean birthweight (154 g), length (1.02 cm), and head circumference (0.69 cm) compared with the unexposed infants. The duration of gestation in the cocaine-exposed infants was 0.74 weeks shorter. Birth weight was particularly decreased in crack-exposed infants (200 g) compared with a decrease of 195 g in infants of mothers who used cocaine with other drugs.

These results are summarized in Table 3.25.

Table 3.25 Pregnancy complications

Study	Method	Sample	Incidence	Results
Bada et al. (2002b)	Secondary analysis of data (Maternal Lifestyle Study) Cocaine use and intrauterine growth	11 811 mother–infant dyads: 1072 infants exposed to cocaine; 7565 negative by maternal history, meconium results; 3174 excluded, unconfirmed exposure	Growth deceleration after 32 weeks: significant interaction between cocaine use and gestational age At 40 weeks controlling for confounders, cocaine exposure associated with decrease in birthweight (151 g), length (0.71 cm), head circumference (0.43 cm)	Besides cocaine influence, smoking cigarettes had a negative impact on all measurements; alcohol use decreased weight and length only; opiates decreased weight; intrauterine drug exposure had no effect on growth and development
Bateman et al. (1993)	Case–control study Pregnancy outcomes and cocaine exposure LBW (< 2500 g) and preterm delivery	2810 inner-city deliveries (1 year): 361 live births of cocaine-exposed infants; 387 controls, no drug exposure	LBW: cocaine 31%, controls 10%. Preterm delivery: cocaine 32%, controls 14% Multivariate analysis, controlled for demographic variables, lifestyle, gestation: in cocaine exposed, decreased birthweight (154 g), length (1.02 cm), head circumference (0.69 cm), duration of gestation (0.74 weeks)	Birthweight deficit higher in infants exposed to other drugs in addition to cocaine and crack; fetal growth retardation and decreased gestation found in this population
Burkett et al. (1994)	Cross-sectional study Cocaine binging and pregnancy outcomes	905 multiethnic, multiracial inner city cocaine-using women: group 1, 78 erratic bingers (26.4–34.4 h); group 2, 67 daily users; group 3, 760 cyclical users (intervals of 3–5, 7, 7+ days)	Pregnancy complications proportional to frequency of binging (p = 0.0007) High prematurity rate in groups 1 (35.9%) and 2 (34.3%) Acute problems: group 1, vaginal bleeding (21.8%), placenta abruptio (14.3%); stillbirth (20.5%) Chronic problems: groups 2, 3: small for age (32.8%), systemic infection (31.3%), anemia (35.6%), low maternal weight (< 100 lbs [45 kg]) (32.8%)	Prematurity, placenta abruptio, vaginal bleeding 2 to 3 times more likely if cocaine positive at time of delivery; placenta abruptio likelihood similar with cocaine use or not at time of delivery; other factors must be involved
Cherukuri et al. (1988)	Retrospective method cohort study Crack use and pregnancy outcomes	55 crack users, 55 women with no history of drug use and matched for age, parity, socioeconomic status, prenatal care, alcohol use	Crack-using women compared with controls: more likely to have early delivery (< 37 weeks) (50.9% vs. 16.4%; p = 0.001); infants with IUGR (3.6 times increase; p < 0.006); infants with small head (10th percentile) for age (p < 0.007); premature membrane rupture (1.8 times increased risk; p < 0.03)	60% crack users had no prenatal care; infants had few, mild neurobehavioral symptoms

Study	Design	Sample	Results	Conclusions
Dombrowski et al. (1991)	Case–control study. Testing myth that cocaine use shortens labor	592 cocaine-using women, 4687 controls	Cocaine users: older, higher parity, decreased birthweight, percentile, and gestational age at birth, 2 times increased risk of placenta abruptio	Labor was not statistically shortened in cocaine users, length of labor similar to controls; morbidity was increased in the cocaine group
Dusick et al. (1993)	Prospective cohort study. Infant intraventricular hemorrhage and cocaine exposure. Intracranial ultrasound	323 very VLBW infants (< 1499 g) of which 91 excluded (80 early death, 11 missed tests); 86/232 cocaine-exposed infants (by maternal history, maternal, infant urine tests, meconium assay), 146 non-cocaine-exposed	No difference in infants in intraventricular hemorrhage (36% vs. 35%), grade III and IV hemorrhage (14% vs. 14%), periventricular leukomalacia (4% vs. 2%) Adverse outcomes with cocaine exposure compared with controls: placenta abruptio (18% vs. 8%; $p = 0.046$), surgical ligation patent ductus arteriosus (7% vs. 1%; $p = 0.02$), seizures (17% vs. 5%; $p = 0.004$)	For LBW infants, no increased risk to infants exposed to cocaine and intraventricular hemorrhage Cocaine-exposed infants increased risk for other adverse outcomes
Handler et al. (1994)	Case–control study. Cigarette smokers vs. cocaine users and PP	304 women with PP, 2732 controls	Dose-response relationship between cigarette use and PP independent of other known risks (p trend < 0.01) Cigarette smokers (20 or more/day) more likely to have PP than non-smokers (OR 2.3; 95% CI 1.5–3.5); cocaine users 1.4 times more likely to have PP than non-users (95% CI 0.8–2.4)	Cigarette smoking increases risk for PP; more study needed for cocaine users
Hoskins et al. (1991)	Cross-sectional study. Umbical artery Doppler flow velocimetry (systolic/diastolic [s/d] ratio)	314 infants	31/112 (28%) delivered at or before 36 weeks, 13/112 (12%) small for gestational age; 33/112 (29%) LBW s/d ratio: normal in most women positive for cocaine; abnormal in all women with placenta abruptio; 14/64 (22%) cocaine users had preterm labor with abnormal s/d ratio	Cocaine users had a significant correlation between placental abruption and abnormal s/d ratio ($p < 0.05$) and between abnormal s/d ratio and preterm birth, small for gestational age, and low birthweight babies
Kistin et al. (1996)	Retrospective cohort study. Cocaine vs. cigarette use and pregnancy outcomes	64 cocaine users with no cigarette use, no other drugs or alcohol; 3209 smoking cigarettes only, 13 043 controls with no cocaine, other illicit drug or cigarette use	Higher risk for cocaine users: LBW (RR 5.3; 95% CI 3.0–9.3), small for age (RR 4.2; 95% CI 2.4–7.3), prematurity (RR 4.0; 95% CI 2.3–7.0), placenta abruptio (RR 10.0; 95% CI 3.5–29.0), placenta previa (RR 2.4; 95% CI 0.3–17.8), perinatal death (RR 5.3; 95% CI 1.9–15.2) Smokers: same outcomes with lesser magnitude	Though cigarette smokers had lesser magnitude of complications, more people smoke, so more infants affected

Table 3.25 Cont.

Study	Method	Sample	Incidence	Results
Little et al. (1989)	Cohort study Cocaine users and pregnancy outcomes	53 cocaine users and infants, 100 non-cocaine users and infants	Cocaine-using women and infants: increased preterm labor ($p < 0.05$), infant complications at birth (meconium, tachycardia, LBW) ($p < 0.05$), increased congenital heart anomalies ($p < 0.01$)	
Macones et al. (1997)	Case–control study Placenta previa and cocaine use	40 placenta previa, 80 normal labor cocaine use: self-reported or urine toxicology screen	Multiple logistic regression analysis, adjusted for other variables: maternal cocaine use independent risk factor for placenta previa (AOR 4.39; 95% CI 1.17–16.4)	Other risks for placenta previa: prior cesarean section, prior elective abortion, parity
Martinez et al. (1996)	Descriptive study Fetal death and preterm labor	102 mainly African American and Hispanic women suspected of having preterm labor; 13 (12.7%) tested positive for cocaine (urine test)	Positive for cocaine compared with non-users: older (27.8 vs. 22.1 years; $p = 0.002$); higher parity (2 vs. 1); black (92.3%; $p = 0.0004$); more cervical dilatation (3 cm vs. 1 cm; $p = 0.008$); more likely to be admitted (85% vs. 32%; $p = 0.0001$); less likely to receive tocolysis because of advanced labor, complications (36% vs. 79%; $p = 0.0002$); increased fetal deaths in cocaine users (18.2% vs. 0% in non-users; $p = 0.02$)	No difference in gestational age or birthweight in infants of cocaine-using mothers Recent cocaine use in some segments of urban population at significant risk for poor outcomes
Ness et al. (1999)	Descriptive study Cigarette and cocaine use and spontaneous abortion	400 women with spontaneous abortion (22 weeks or less); 570 women pregnant longer than 22 weeks	Those with spontaneous abortion 28.9% used cocaine (positive hair analysis); 34.6% smoked cigarettes (positive urine test) Maintained pregnancy > 22 weeks: 20.5% adolescents; 21.8% adult women Presence of cocaine in hair independently associated with increased risk of spontaneous abortion (OR 1.4; 95% CI 1.0–2.1; adjusted for demographic variables, drug use);	Cocaine in urine test or by self-report not associated with spontaneous abortion Urine test for cotinine in urine (smoking indicator) also independently associated with increased risk for spontaneous abortion (OR 1.8; 95% CI 1.3–2.6) Risk of spontaneous abortion was 24% for cocaine or tobacco use

Study	Design and focus	Sample	Results	Conclusions
Ney et al. (1990)	Case–control study. Cocaine use and preterm labor	141 women in preterm labor, 108 with uncomplicated labor	Preterm labor: 24/141 (17%) positive toxicology urine test; 14/24 positive for cocaine (9.9%). Uncomplicated labor: 3/108 (2.8%) positive toxicology urine test; 1/3 positive for cocaine	Preterm laboring women should be encouraged to get urine test to guide management
Singer et al. (1994)	Case–control study. Outcomes with cocaine use	100 women positive for cocaine during pregnancy, 100 matched controls	Cocaine use best predictor of preterm birth, LBW (controlled for prematurity); cocaine and alcohol used together decreased linear growth	Cocaine use has direct negative effects on pregnancy outcomes. Alcohol effect also important in negative outcomes
Spence et al. (1991)	Descriptive study. Cocaine use and pregnancy outcomes	500 women admitted for labor/delivery	15.3% tested positive for cocaine (95% CI 11.8–18.8); those without prenatal care 62% prevalence (95% CI 47.2–76.6). Cocaine users (urine test) 4 times more likely to have preterm labor; 2 times more likely to have premature infant with Apgar < 6 at 1 min	Urine screen helpful to identify potentially unrecognized cocaine users
Sprauve et al. (1997)	Retrospective cohort study. Adverse pregnancy outcomes	483 women positive for crack cocaine drug abuse, 1 week before delivery; 3158 controls, negative drug screen	Users vs. controls: LBW, 31.3% vs. 14.9% (OR 2.6; 95% CI 2.1–3.2); IUGR, 29% vs. 13% (OR 2.7; 95% CI 2.2–3.4); preterm, 28.2% vs. 17.1% (OR 1.9; 95% CI 1.5–2.4); placenta abruptio, 3.3% vs. 1.1% (OR 3.0; 95% CI 1.6–5.6); low Apgar score, 7.9% vs. 4.5% (OR 1.8; 95% CI 1.2–2.7) Adjusted for confounders: LBW, AOR 1.6 (95% CI 1.03–2.4); IUGR, AOR 1.7 (95% CI 1.2–2.3); Apgar at 5 min, OR 2.4, AOR 2.0 (95% CI 1.1–3.7) for users with positive drug screen	
Weathers et al. (1993)	Descriptive study. Cocaine use prevalence at delivery. Growth and development parameters	137 mother–infant dyads exposed to cocaine (prevalence 1.0%): 89 tested positive at urine drug screen, 48 self-report (mothers)	Prematurity (< 37 week) 21 (15%; 95% CI 9–21), 2 sudden infant death syndrome. Growth parameters (percentiles) at birth and 12 months (50% lost to follow-up): weight 23% and 43%, length 29% and 49%, head circumference 18% and 54%	Infants had lower growth parameters at or near the mean at 12 months

AOR, adjusted odds ratio; IUGR, intrauterine growth retardation; CI, confidence interval; LBW, low birthweight; OR, odds ratio; PP, placenta previa; RR, relative risk.

Table 3.26 Miscellaneous pregnancy and infant studies

Study	Method	Sample	Incidence	Results
Towers et al. (1993)	Case series Pre-eclampsia and cocaine use Laboratory tests for pre-eclampsia, drug screen for cocaine	11 third trimester pregnant women, positive cocaine drug screen, with hypertension, headache, blurred vision, abdominal pain, or seizures	Diastolic BP ≥ 90 mgHg, back to normal 45–90 min after admission; all had one or more sign/ symptom of pre-eclampsia; no positive laboratory tests for pre-eclampsia	Consider cocaine intoxication in pregnant women presenting with signs and symptoms of pre-eclampsia who rapidly improve after admission

Miscellaneous pregnancy and infant studies

Pre-eclampsia and cocaine

In a 1993 study, Towers et al. described 11 pregnant women presenting with signs and symptoms of pre-eclampsia. They all had high blood pressure, with a diastolic pressure > 90 mmHg, blurred vision, abdominal pain, or seizures during their third trimester. Within 45 to 90 minutes after admission, the signs and symptoms abated and the blood pressure was normal. Although all women tested positive on the urine drug screen, none of the laboratory tests was positive for pre-eclampsia. The authors suggest that cocaine intoxication in pregnant women can mimic pre-eclampsia, based on the rapid improvement after admission and absence of positive laboratory tests for this pregnancy complication (Table 3.26).

Umbilical artery velocimetry

Hoskins et al. (1991) conducted a cross-sectional study using umbilical artery velocimetry in 314 women divided into five groups based on the following variables: cocaine use, cocaine non-use, placenta abruptio, and preterm labor. Of these, 88 (28%) delivered at or before 36 weeks, 38 (12%) had infants small for gestational age, and 91 (29%) had babies with LBW. Almost all of the women testing positive for cocaine had normal systolic/ diastolic umbilical artery velocimetry ratios; all the women with placenta abruptio had abnormal ratios, as well as 14 of the 64 women with preterm labor and a history of cocaine use. There were no abnormal umbilical artery velocimetry ratios in women with preterm labor or in the controls. The cocaine users had a significant correlation between placenta abruptio and abnormal ratios ($p < 0.05$), and also between abnormal ratios and preterm birth, infants small for gestational age, and infants of LBW. This study is summarized below in Table 3.27.

Cardiovascular studies in fetuses and infants exposed to cocaine

Schuetze & Eiden (2006) studied heart rates and respiratory sinus arrhythmia in a case-control study comparing 77 cocaine-using mothers and their cocaine-exposed infants with 64 non-exposed mothers and infants. The infants were studied at four to eight weeks of age during a 15-minute sleep period. The researchers found a dose-dependent effect on respiratory sinus arrhythmia with cocaine exposure that could not be attributed to fetal growth or exposure to other substances. There was an association between cocaine exposure and heart rate that was mediated by birthweight. The authors suggest that in utero exposure to cocaine can have lasting effects still seen four to eight weeks later.

Frassica *et al.* (1994) studied the incidence of arrhythmias in cocaine-exposed infants by identifying the rates of cardiac consultations in children prenatally exposed to cocaine and in children with no known cocaine exposure. The study between 1988 and 1991 identified 18 cocaine-exposed infants, 13 with arrhythmias: 12 with supraventricular arrhythmias and four with low-grade ventricular ectopy. Five of the 13 developed congestive heart failure (CHF). After the neonatal period, five infants had arrhythmias, including high-grade ventricular arrhythmias and two cardiorespiratory arrests. The authors found that cocaine-exposed infants were more likely to have a higher rate of cardiac consultations than infants not exposed to cocaine. Arrhythmias in the cocaine-exposed infants tended to persist after the neonatal period and may lead to life-threatening events.

Myocardial ischemia in infants was the focus of a case–control study by Mehta *et al.* (1993), who compared 21 infants exposed to cocaine with 20 control infants similar in birthweight, gestational age, and postnatal age. The infants were monitored for ST segment and heart rate variability with a Holter monitor for 48 hours after birth. Six of the cocaine-exposed infants (29%) had transient ST segment elevation suggestive of ischemia, and one of the unexposed infants had a transient ST segment elevation (OR 7.6; 95% CI 1.14–50.64). Heart rates and arrhythmias were similar in the two groups, but the cocaine-exposed group had an increase in vagal activity. They suggested that infants of cocaine-using mothers could develop transient myocardial ischemia.

Lipshultz *et al.* (1991), in a historical cohort study, examined the incidence of cardiac anomalies in 554 infants reviewed over an 18-month period. Cocaine-positive drug screens were found in 214 out of the 554 infants; 340 infants tested negative (RR 3.7; 95% CI 1.4–9.4). Based on a comparison with the cocaine-negative group, the rate of cardiac anomalies was higher in the cocaine-exposed infants than in the general population of infants (650/1000 vs. 18/1000). Some of the infants with high-grade ventricular ectopy had cardiorespiratory arrest. The findings suggested that exposure to cocaine in utero predisposes infants to structural cardiac malformations, ECG abnormalities, and cardiopulmonary autonomic dysfunction.

Rana *et al.* (1995) examined 635 placentas at 24 weeks of gestation to determine an umbilical coiling index (number of coils/length of the cord). Three groups were compared: hypocoiled (below the 10th percentile), normal coiled (10th to 90th percentile), and hypercoiled (over the 90th percentile). Compared with infants with normal coiling indices, infants with hypocoiled cords had an increase in fetal heart rate disturbances (28.6% vs. 15.9%; $p = 0.01$) and also the need for interventional delivery (19% vs. 7.1%; $p = 0.002$). Infants with hypercoiled cords were more likely than those with normal coiling to experience premature delivery (33.3% vs. 12%; $p < 0.0001$). Hypercoiling was more frequently seen in cocaine-exposed infants than in unexposed infants (12.7% vs. 3.3%; $p = 0.0006$). The authors suggested that the degree of cord coiling could be a predictor of certain pregnancy outcomes.

A longitudinal prospective study was carried out by Shankaran *et al.* (2006), who studied intrauterine growth and risk for hypertension at age six years. Of 1388 infants, 600 (43%) were cocaine exposed in utero. They were matched by sex, gestational age, and race to 781 non-exposed infants and 69% of both groups were followed for up to six years. Of 516 full-term births, 144 (28%) were diagnosed with IUGR at birth. At age six, 93 of 516 (18%) had hypertension (95th percentile); 35/144 (24%) of the IUGR children had hypertension compared with the non-IUGR infants (58/372; $p < 0.05$). There was no significant difference in the prevalence of hypertension between the cocaine-exposed and non-exposed groups. When analyzed adjusting for confounders including cocaine use, IUGR was significantly associated with hypertension and the child's body mass index (BMI) (RR 1.8; 95% CI 1.2–2.7). The authors suggested that IUGR may be a marker for development of hypertension in adults.

Table 3.27 summarizes these studies.

Other congenital studies in fetuses and infants exposed to cocaine

Congenital syphilis

Several studies reported on the incidence of congenital syphilis in infants exposed to cocaine. An ecological study by Webber & Hauser (1993) identified 17 219 cocaine-dependent women and 2229 newborns of all races in selected residential zip code areas in NYC. The city-wide congenital syphilis rate in those areas had increased from 1.2 to 5.8/1000 live births; cocaine dependence had also increased from 23.3 to 423.5/100 000 women. City-wide, the congenital syphilis rate had increased from 1.8 to 10.6/1000 live births in newborns of African American women. Based on grouping the women into four quartiles based on rates of cocaine dependence (1 being the highest and 4 the lowest), the findings showed that congenital syphilis rates increased the most in the highest cocaine-using quartile: quartile 1, from 1.9 to 14.6; quartile 2, from 2.1 to 12.4; quartile 3, from 1.5 to 7.6, and quartile 4, from 1.6 to 2.8.

Rawstron et al. (1993) carried out a retrospective chart review and prospective analysis involving 403 pregnant women with syphilis: 75 (18%) of their newborns had congenital syphilis and of these, 35 were live births and 40 stillborn. The infants did not have typical signs or symptoms of congenital syphilis (rash, hepatosplenomegaly, or adenopathy), but they tested positive through radiography, cerebrospinal fluid analysis, Venereal Disease Research Laboratory test, conjugated bilirubin, and plasma aspartate aminotransferase (AST). Statistical analyses found that there was a significant association in three areas: lack of prenatal care, lack of treatment for syphilis, and a high rapid plasma reagin titer. However, there was no significant association with a reported history of crack or cocaine use.

A study by Sison et al. (1997) identified 1012 infants positive for drugs in meconium analyses ($n = 449$ [44.3% of the total]): 401 (39.6%) tested positive for cocaine, 71 (7%) tested positive for opiates, and 31 (3.1%) tested positive for marijuana. Slightly over 7% of the mothers had positive rapid plasma reagin and fluorescent treponemal antibody absorbed tests. Based on the US Center for Disease Control and Prevention definitions, 46 (4.5%) of the infants were diagnosed as having congenital syphilis. A positive rapid plasma reagin test and congenital syphilis diagnosis was higher in infants with positive drug screen results compared with those with a negative drug screen. Cocaine-positive mothers were significantly more likely to have infants diagnosed as having positive rapid plasma reagin test and congenital syphilis ($p < 0.01$). The researchers concluded that cocaine use was associated with an increase in congenital syphilis rates in the population tested.

A 1991 case–control study by Greenberg et al. examined a syphilis epidemic in New York City from 1987 to 1989. Their study found that cocaine use was a maternal risk for having a child with congenital syphilis (OR 3.9; 95% CI 2.8–5.3). Based on their findings, they suggested that epidemics of congenital syphilis might be related to an increase in crack and cocaine use.

Subependymal cysts

Smith et al. (2001) used cranial sonograms to evaluate subependymal cysts in a retrospective review of medical records for 122 premature infants. The sonogram findings of a

Table 3.27 Cardiovascular studies in fetuses, infants exposed to cocaine

Study	Method	Sample	Incidence	Results
Frassica et al. (1994)	Historical cohort study Rates of cardiac consultation for arrhythmias in infants exposed to cocaine	18 exposed to cocaine in utero, controls infants with no known cocaine exposure	3 infants developed fetal arrhythmias in neonatal period (2 bradycardia-related cesarean sections) 13 with arrhythmias: 12 supraventricular, 4 low-grade ventricular ectopy, 5 of 13 (38%) developed CHF After neonatal period, 5 infants with high-grade ventricular arrhythmias, 2 respiratory arrests	Cocaine-exposed infants more likely to to have cardiac consultation than non-cocaine-exposed infants
Hoskins et al. (1991)	Cross-sectional study Umbical artery Doppler flow velocimetry (systolic/diastolic [s/d] ratio)	314 infants	Infants: 31/112 (28%) delivered at or before 36 weeks, 13/112 (12%) small for gestational age, 33/112 (29%) LBW Most women positive for cocaine, normal s/d ratio All women with placenta abruptio abnormal s/d ratio; cocaine users: 14/64 (22%) preterm labor with abnormal s/d ratio	Cocaine users: significant correlation between placental abruption and abnormal s/d ratio ($p < 0.05$) and between abnormal s/d ratio and preterm birth, small for gestational age, and LBW babies
Lipshultz et al. (1991)	Historical cohort Cardiovascular abnormalities in cocaine-exposed infants	554 drug-screened neonates: 214 (39%) positive for cocaine; 340 (61%) negative for cocaine (matched controls)	Cocaine-exposed infants increased cardiac anomalies (650/1000 vs. 18/1000 in controls; RR 3.7; 95% CI 1.4–9.4) Arrhythmias: high-grade ventricular ectopy, cardiorespiratory arrest	Cocaine exposure in utero predisposes structural cardiac malformation, ECG abnormalities, autonomic dysfunction for change in posture
Mehta et al. (1993)	Prospective case–control study Myocardial ischemia in infants Cardiac Holter monitoring over 48 h	21 infants exposed to cocaine, 20 controls, similar birthweight, gestational age, postnatal age	Transient ST elevation suggestive of ischemia: 6 (29%) cocaine-exposed infants and 1 (5%) controls (OR 7.6; 95% CI 1.14–50.64)	Heart rate and arrhythmias not significantly different, but increased vagal tone in cocaine-exposed infants and greater risk of transient ischemia
Rana et al. (1995)	Placenta analysis Coiling of umbilical cord (umbilical coiling index is the number of coils/length of cord): hypocoiled < 10th percentile, normal 10–90th percentile, hypercoiled > 90th percentile	635 placentas, 24 weeks of gestation or more	Hypocoiled compared with normal: increased fetal heart rate disturbances (28.6% vs. 15.9%; $p = 0.01$), increased interventional delivery (19% vs. 7.1%; $p = 0.002$), increased premature delivery (33.3% vs. 12.0%; $p < 0.0001$), higher cocaine exposure (12.7% vs. 3.3%; $p = 0.006$)	

Table 3.27 *Cont.*

Study	Method	Sample	Incidence	Results
Schuetze & Eiden (2006)	Case–control study Physiological parameters in cocaine-exposed infants Tested between 4 and 8 weeks of age during 15 min of sleep (respiratory sinus arrhythmia; heart rate)	77 mother–infant dyads, cocaine exposure; 64 mother–infant dyads, no cocaine exposure	Respiratory sinus arrhythmia: dose-dependent effect not associated with fetal growth or exposure to other substances Heart rate: birthweight-mediated association between cocaine exposure and heart rate	In utero exposure to cocaine has lasting effects seen 4 to 8 weeks after birth
Shankaran et al. (2006)	Prospective study (longitudinal: 6 years). IUGR and risk of hypertension BP data at 6 years of age	1388 infants from 4 centers in NICHDNR network: 600 cocaine-exposed infants: 415 cocaine-exposed infants available at 6 years, 535 non-exposed infants matched for gestational age, race, sex	144/415 cocaine-exposed infants: (28%) diagnosed with IUGR at birth At age 6, 93 (18%) of 516 full-term babies had high BP (95th percentile); 35/144 (24%) had high BP compared with non-IUGR 58/372 (16%) ($p < 0.05$) IUGR significantly associated with high BP (RR 1.8; 95% CI 1.2–2.7) High BP seen in 20% cocaine-exposed 6-year olds vs. 16% of non-exposed children ($p = 0.20$, not significant)	No significant difference in high BP between cocaine- and non-cocaine-exposed groups; IUGR associated with high BP in early childhood

BP, blood pressure; CHF, congestive heart failure; CI, confidence interval; ECG, electrocardiogram; IUGR, intrauterine growth retardation; LBW, low birth weight; NICHDNR, National Institute of Child Health and Human Development Neonatal Research Network; OR, odds ratio; RR, relative risk.

cocaine-exposed group were compared with those for infants not exposed to cocaine. Sixteen (14%) had subependymal cysts. Cysts were more frequently found in cocaine-exposed infants (8/18; 44%) than non-exposed infants (8/99; 8%) ($p < 0.01$). They concluded that cocaine-exposed infants were at higher risk for subependymal cysts than non-exposed infants. According to Behnke *et al.* (1999), subendymal cysts occur in 3–5% of newborns and tend to have no significant effect on growth and development. They found that subependymal cysts, though benign, are often associated with hemorrhage, hypoxic–ischemic damage, and neurotropic infection, and the neurological consequences often are linked to the causative factors.

Urogenital defects

Chavez *et al.* (1989) studied infants born between 1968 and 1980 with urinary and genital anomalies. Data were obtained from the Atlanta Birth Defects Case–Control Study. In infants of mothers who used cocaine during the first trimester, urinary defects were found in 276 infants, and genital anomalies were found in 791. The crude OR for urinary defects in 276 cocaine-exposed infants compared with 2835 controls was 4.39 (95% CI 1.12–17.24). There was no significant difference when genital anomalies were compared in the two groups (OR 2.26; 95% CI 0.67–7.62). This study's findings were consistent with other animal and clinical studies.

Table 3.28 summarizes these studies of congenital abnormalities in fetuses and infants exposed to cocaine.

Comments

Female genital disorders

The studies discussed in the section on urology and those included here support the increased risky sexual behavior of individuals using crack and cocaine. Use of these drugs is associated with an increase in unprotected sex and sex with multiple partners, and thus the risk of transmitting STDs. The one study described in this subsection showed no specific risk associated with cocaine use for PID, but the risky sexual behavior of those using cocaine will increase the risk of PID. More studies are needed to explore whether there is a direct relationship between cocaine use and PID.

Pregnancy complications and cocaine

Eighteen studies described some of the complications seen in women who used cocaine during their pregnancy. From Table 3.24, one can appreciate the myriad of pregnancy complications seen in women using cocaine. Preterm labor and infants of LBW were frequently seen in these studies. Many of the studies had large sample sizes (100 to 1072 women–infant dyads) and significant findings for preterm labor, LBW infants, infants small for gestational age, placenta abruptio, and fetal death. Other complications included decreased infant length, placenta previa, IUGR, small head circumference, cardiac anomalies, and spontaneous abortion. What is not clear is the effect of lack of prenatal care (40–60% in some studies), and the interaction between cigarette smoking and alcohol use on fetal growth and development. Studies that might be interesting would include the comparison of lack of prenatal care in non-cocaine-using women and cocaine users for pregnancy outcomes. In one study, infants of cocaine users were not small for gestational age nor did they have LBW. This small study (13 infants) contradicted the findings of a number of other studies that showed these outcomes were risk factors in cocaine-using mothers.

Table 3.28 Other congenital studies in fetuses, infants exposed to cocaine

Study	Method	Sample	Incidence	Results
Chavez et al. (1989)	Descriptive study based on Atlanta Birth Defects Case–Control Study Urogenital anomalies	Infants exposed to cocaine in first trimester 1968–1980: 276 urinary anomalies, 791 genital anomalies Controls: 3835 infants without birth defects	Risk of urinary anomalies in cocaine exposed vs. 2835 controls: crude OR 4.39 (95% CI 1.12–17.24) Risk of genital anomalies in cocaine exposed vs. 2973 controls: OR 2.26 (95% CI 0.67–7.62) (not significant)	Increased risk of urinary but not genital anomalies in cocaine-exposed infants (consistent with other studies)
Greenberg et al. (1991)	Case–control study Congenital syphilis		Maternal risk of having an infant with congenital syphilis, odds for exposure to cocaine 3.9 times greater among patients than controls (95% CI 2.8–5.3)	Epidemics of syphilis may be related to increased cocaine, crack use
Rawstron et al. (1993)	Retrospective chart review, prospective analysis Congenital syphilis	403 pregnant women with positive serology for syphilis	73 (18%) infants with congenital syphilis: 35 live births, 40 stillborn Infant signs/symptoms: no rash, hepatosplenomegaly, or adenopathy Infant positive laboratory tests: radiography, CSF, VDRL, conjugated bilirubin, AST	Significant association with lack of prenatal care or treatment for syphilis, higher reagin titer, no association between congenital syphilis and crack or cocaine use
Sison et al. (1997)	Descriptive study Congenital syphilis	1012 infants positive for drugs (meconium analysis) 1012 mothers, positive RPR and FTA-ABS (72/1012: 7.1%)	449 infants: meconium positive for drugs: 401 (39.6%) for cocaine, 71 (7%) for opiates, 31 (3.1%) for marijuana Congenital syphilis diagnosis in 46 (4.5%) based on CDC definitions Positive RPR and congenital syphilis higher in infants with positive results compared with negative drug screen; significantly increased (p < 0.01) in infants with cocaine-positive mothers compared with negative mothers	Cocaine use is associated with increased congenital syphilis rates
Smith et al. (2001)	Retrospective review Subependymal cysts in premature infants Cranial sonograms	122 premature (< 36 weeks) infants: group 1, cocaine exposed; group 2, not exposed 16/117 (14%) with subependymal cysts	Cysts found in 8/18 (44%) cocaine-exposed infants, 8/99 (8%) non-exposed infants (p < 0.01)	Increased risk of subependymal cysts in cocaine-exposed infants; findings similar to other studies
Webber & Hauser (1993)	Ecological study Congenital syphilis	17 219 cocaine-dependent women; 2229 newborns New York City (1982–1988) 4 groups, residential zipcode	Congenital syphilis rate increased from 1.2 to 5.8/1000 live births; cocaine dependence increased from 23.3 to 423.5/1000 women of all races	Increase in cocaine dependence associated with increased rate of congenital syphilis

AST, aspartate aminotransferase; CDC, US Centers for Disease Control and Prevention; CSF, cerebrospinal fluid; FTA-ABS, fluorescent treponemal antibody absorbed test; RPR, rapid plasma reagin test; VDRL, Venereal Disease Research Laboratory test.

Many of the studies differed in how they measured "prematurity" – 37 weeks or less, or 36 weeks or less. They also used different measures to assess "exposure to cocaine." Sometimes maternal self-report was used (typically unreliable); other times meconium and hair samples for cocaine were assessed (reliable tests). Urine tests seemed to identify some cocaine-using mothers but were not as reliable as hair and meconium samples. Many of the women assessed in these studies were of low income but there were also women from health clinics and a variety of socioeconomic levels.

One study looked at debunking the myth that cocaine use can shorten the time of labor. The researchers showed that labor time was the same in cocaine users and non-users, but that cocaine users were prone to adverse fetal outcomes. Another study found no increased risk of intracranial hemorrhage in cocaine-exposed infants. In both cases, additional studies might help to clarify the role, if any, of cocaine in these outcomes. One study looked at growth parameters at birth and 12 months later. Initially, the infants were small for gestational age, had LBW, and had small head circumferences; however, by 12 months, these children were in the 40th to 60th percentiles, indicating growth retardation did not persist after the first year of life.

While these studies provide some insight into the role of cocaine and pregnancy outcomes, consideration of the pathophysiology associated with cocaine use can also provide some explanation for these outcomes. Cocaine is a vasoconstrictor that increases dopamine and norepinephrine levels. These two neurotransmitters are also powerful vasoconstrictors in high doses. Consequently, use of cocaine during pregnancy could increase the risk of vascular complications such as placenta abruptio.

Cocaine is also an appetite depressant. A decreased caloric intake in cocaine-using pregnant women could result in infant outcomes such as LBW, small for gestational age, small head circumference, and IUGR. One study did find that cocaine-using mothers' weight under 100 pounds (45 kg) was an increased risk for poor infant outcomes.

Pre-eclampsia

One study found that some cocaine-using women were likely to develop signs and symptoms of pre-eclampsia, including elevated diastolic blood pressure and seizures. However, within a few hours (presumably after the cocaine high), these women no longer had pre-eclamptic symptoms. Intense vasoconstriction and hypertension could have been brought on by the use of cocaine. More studies are needed to verify the findings of this small study of 11 patients.

Cardiovascular studies

Several studies looked at cardiovascular outcomes in infants exposed to cocaine in utero. In one study, respiratory sinus arrhythmia was found to persist for four to eight weeks after birth. Other studies point to an increase in cardiac structural anomalies and supraventricular and ventricular arrhythmias that in some cases led to fatal consequences. One study found no difference in cocaine-exposed infants regarding heart rate or arrhythmias, but found ST segment changes in 29% of the infants.

One study looked at the degree of umbilical artery coiling and infant risks. Prematurity was increased in those infants with hypercoiling compared with a control group of infants with normally coiled cords. The role of hypercoiling is unclear, and further exploration of this phenomenon is needed.

Another study looked at the risk for hypertension at age six years in children diagnosed with IUGR during the neonatal period. There was no difference in the cases and controls in this study; however, IUGR was associated with hypertension and low BMI.

More studies are needed to confirm the findings of several of these studies as some had small sample size (21 to 77 patients) and some did not appear to control for confounders. In longitudinal studies, the effect of continuing exposure to a cocaine-user's family members was not addressed. Studies are needed to determine the effect of continuing exposure to cocaine during the growth and development periods of childhood.

Congenital syphilis

The four studies describing the increase in congenital syphilis coupled this phenomenon with increased use of cocaine by pregnant women. Several studies indicated that some of the pregnant women were not treated for their diagnosed syphilis, lacked prenatal care, and that the risk of congenital syphilis was not always related to cocaine use. Cocaine use, however, was related to an increase in STDs through risky sex behavior. Not all pregnant women with syphilis had children with congenital syphilis; the incidence was 4.5% to 18%. Most of the infants in one study were asymptomatic and only diagnosed by laboratory tests.

Other congenital conditions

Two other studies described congenital anomalies found in cocaine-exposed infants. Subependymal cysts were found to be more common in cocaine-exposed infants than in controls. These cranial abnormalities are found in 3–5% of all newborns and thought to be benign but were found in 44% of cocaine-exposed infants ($n = 8$) in one study. Hypoxia and ischemia is thought to be a cause of these abnormal lesions. Given that cocaine and the catecholamines are vasoconstrictors, an increased risk of these cysts might be explained by cocaine use, but further study is needed to confirm this relationship.

Another study confirmed that urinary defects were more likely to occur in cocaine-exposed infants than in controls. However, the incidence of genital anomalies was the same in both groups. This study's findings were consistent with finding of similar studies on urogenital congenital anomalies.

Cardiovascular disease

In a review of the PubMed literature from 1988 to 2008, 35 epidemiological studies related to cocaine use and cardiovascular disease describe the risk for acute MI (AMI), arrhythmias, and cardiac arrest (16 publications), dysfunction of the coronary vessels (9), and cardiac morphology changes and vascular disease in individuals using cocaine (5). Four publications provide some evidence that platelet activation and thrombus formation may be a risk factor of cocaine use, and one other article links cocaine use with increased aortic wall lipid.

The physiological cardiovascular effects of cocaine have been described in the scientific literature and include vasoconstriction, increased heart rate and blood pressure, cardiac arrhythmias, chest pain, and risk for AMI. At a cellular level, cocaine interferes with the reabsorption of dopamine and is also a strong alpha-adrenergic stimulant. Catecholamine levels are increased after cocaine use. Recent laboratory research suggests that cocaine can upregulate endothelial cell adhesion molecules and enhance inflammatory cell activity in the blood vessels. Some of the vascular constriction effects of cocaine may be related to endothelin-1 release. Myocardial depression, sometimes seen in cocaine users, may be related to the drug's suppression of calcium influx during cardiac systole and desensitization of adrenergic receptors. Coagulation defects in cocaine users may be related to altered regulation of endothelial procoagulant and anticoagulant factors. These studies and others may help to explain some of the cardiovascular consequences seen in cocaine users.

Coronary artery reactivity

Lange *et al.* (1989) published an article on the effect of intranasal cocaine used as a nasal/laryngeal anesthetic and coronary artery constriction. The occurrence of chest pain was evaluated for 45 males and 11 females between the ages of 36 and 67 years. During angiography, intranasal cocaine (2 mg/kg body weight) was administered. A control group of 16 patients received saline intranasally. Fifteen minutes after cocaine administration, there was an increase in heart rate and arterial blood pressure. There was a decrease in coronary sinus blood flow and an 8–12% decrease in left coronary artery diameter ($p < 0.01$ for all parameters compared with controls). The group receiving cocaine did not experience chest pain or evidence of ischemia (by ECG). After administration of phentolamine, an α-adrenoceptor blocking agent, the cardiovascular parameters returned to baseline values. There was no difference in the responses of those individuals with left coronary artery cardiovascular disease ($n = 28$), and those who were disease-free ($n = 17$). Since the dose of the intranasal cocaine was similar to that found in cocaine topical anesthetics, the authors suggested that recreational drugs are likely to produce more pronounced cardiovascular symptoms.

Dressler *et al.* (1990) studied 22 necropsy specimens from cocaine addicts to evaluate the effect of cocaine and coronary artery narrowing. Blood levels of cocaine were elevated (3.2 mg/L) in 13 patients at the time of death. Nine cocaine users died from non-cocaine-related causes. The specimens were from 17 males, 19 African Americans and three white, with a mean age of 32 years. In 8 of the 22 specimens (36%), one or more of the four major coronary arteries were narrowed more than 75% with atherosclerotic plaque. When segments of four coronary vessels from the 17 individuals were analyzed, 8% of the segments were narrowed 76–100% in 12 patients who died from cocaine use, and 19% of the segments were narrowed 51–75%. In five patients who were drug addicts but died from other causes, 3% had segmental narrowing of 76–100%, and 7% had segmental narrowing of 51–75%. There was narrowing of the coronary arteries in 17 of the 22 patients. The authors found more coronary artery disease in those who had elevated cocaine levels in their blood at the time of death than those dying from others causes.

In a case–control study, Flores *et al.* (1990) examined the coronary arteries of 18 patients (15 men; ages 35 to 67 years), 12 who received intranasal cocaine (2 mg/kg body weight) and six who received saline. Compared with those receiving saline, those receiving the cocaine had a decrease in lumen size in both diseased and non-diseased segments of coronary arteries 15 minutes later, but to a greater extent in diseased segments ($p < 0.05$). They concluded that cocaine is a vasoconstrictor of both diseased and non-diseased coronary artery segments, with greater constriction in diseased vessels.

Kolodgie *et al.* (1991) reviewed 5871 autopsy records and found 495 (8.4%) with positive cocaine toxicology findings. At the time of death, six (1.2%) of the individuals positive for cocaine showed total thrombic occlusion of the left anterior descending coronary vessel. Matched by age and gender, two controls were specimens from individuals dying from cocaine overdose and those dying from sudden thrombin-caused cardiac death in non-substance abuse individuals. The researchers examined the coronary artery specimens and found significantly more mast cells in the vessels of cocaine users than in the controls. A positive relationship between the number of mast cells and vessel narrowing ($r = 0.68$) was found in the cocaine users with left anterior descending coronary vessel occlusion. Despite the young age of the patients (29 ± 2 years), there were significant

Table 3.29 Results of administration of cocaine or cigarettes on coronary arteries

	Rate–pressure product (% increase) $(n = 30)$[a]	Non-diseased artery diameter (% decrease)	Diseased artery diameter (% decrease)
Intranasal cocaine	11 ± 2 ($p < 0.001$)	7 ±1 ($p < 0.001$)	9 ± 2 ($p = 0.001$) ($n = 18$)
One cigarette	12 ± 4 ($p = 0.021$)	7 ± 1 ($p < 0.001$)	5 ± 5 ($p = 0.037$) ($n = 12$)
Intranasal cocaine and one cigarette	45 ± 5 ($p < 0.001$)	6 ± 2 ($p < 0.001$)	19 ± 4 ($p < 0.001$) ($n = 12$)

[a] Heart rate × systolic blood pressure.

atherosclerotic lesions without plaque hemorrhage in those with cocaine-associated thrombi. Five subjects had one or more vessel narrowed significantly (75% or more). The researchers hypothesized that adventitial mast cells may have a role in development of vasospasm, thrombosis, and sudden death in long-term cocaine users.

Majid *et al.* (1992) examined coronary artery narrowing in six cocaine users hospitalized for prolonged chest pain and ST and T wave changes on ECG. The patients were administered up to 32 mg of intravenous cocaine, at a level enough to produce a "high." A computer-assisted quantitative technique was used to assess coronary artery diameter. After the cocaine administration, there were no changes in coronary artery diameter, myocardial perfusion, left ventricular wall motion, or ECG, even though there was an increase in both heart rate and mean systolic arterial blood pressure. Blood flow in the coronary sinus increased, presumably from an increase in cardiac output (62%; $p < 0.007$). This study suggests that cocaine-related chest pain is not related to coronary artery vasospasm or decreased myocardial perfusion.

A study by Brogan *et al.* (1992) suggested that cocaine metabolites (benzoylecgonine and ethylmethylecgonine) could cause coronary vasoconstriction. In a randomized double-blind, controlled clinical trial, 18 patients with a history of chest pain (16 men; 37 to 65 years of age) were administered saline (8 patients) or cocaine (10 patients; 2 mg/kg body weight) while undergoing a cardiac catheterization. Cineangiographic measurements were taken on the left coronary artery at 30, 60, and 90 minutes. Cocaine and cocaine metabolite levels were measured at the same time. The eight control subjects showed no change in coronary blood flow; however, those administered cocaine had a significant decrease ($p < 0.05$) in vessel diameter at 30 minutes (at the peak blood cocaine level). The vessels returned to the baseline level at 60 minutes and narrowed again at 90 minutes ($p < 0.05$). The 90-minute interval corresponded to an increase in blood level of cocaine metabolites. The study suggests that initial vasoconstriction is related to the direct effects of cocaine, but that the metabolites also contribute to vasoconstriction occurring as long as 90 minutes after using cocaine.

In a cross-sectional study, Moliterno *et al.* (1994) administered intranasal cocaine (2 mg/kg body weight) to 42 smokers; 36 had coronary artery disease (CAD), 28 were male, and the age range was 34 to 79 years. The rate–pressure product (heart rate multiplied by systolic blood pressure) and coronary artery diameter were measured after intranasal cocaine administration (6 patients; 2 mg/kg body weight), after smoking one cigarette (12 patients), and after both intranasal cocaine administration and smoking one cigarette (24 patients). Table 3.29 illustrates the results and indicates that both cocaine and cigarette smoking increase vasoconstriction in normal and diseased coronary arteries. However, the degree of change in the rate–pressure product and diseased artery diameter was significantly increased in those administered both cocaine and smoked tobacco. The authors hypothesized that an increase in metabolic requirement for oxygen and decreased arterial diameter contributed to the findings in the cigarette and cocaine users.

Kontos *et al.* (2003) studied 90 patients with cocaine-related chest pain who had been seen in the emergency room within the previous five weeks. On angiography, 45 (50%) had significant CAD (> 50% stenosis): 29 (32%) had significant single vessel disease, and 14 (16%) had significant disease in two or three vessels. Stenosed by-pass grafts occurred in 3%. Of those individuals with an MI or increased blood troponin-I levels, 77% had significant vessel disease compared with 35% without an MI or increased troponin levels. Of the 35% with significant disease, only seven (18%) had no history of CAD. The study found that prior MI, increased troponin-I levels, and elevated cholesterol levels are predictors of significant CAD in cocaine users.

Coronary artery aneurysms were found in 0.2–5.3% of patients with atherosclerotic disease, Kawasaki's disease, and rare disorders. Satran *et al.* (2005) studied the incidence of coronary artery aneurysms in 112 cocaine users and compared their findings with a control group of 76 of similar age and risk. The mean age for the predominantly male (80%) cigarette smokers (95%) was 44 years. The control group had more atherosclerosis, diabetes mellitus, and CAD than the cocaine users. Of the cocaine users, 45% had a prior AMI, although 48% had non-obstructive CAD. Thirty-eight percent of the control group had a previous AMI. Using univariate and multivariate analyses, cocaine was a strong predictor of coronary artery aneurysms. Over 30% of the cocaine users had coronary artery aneurysms compared with 7.6% of the control group ($p < 0.001$). The findings suggest that cocaine use may predispose individuals to develop coronary artery aneurysms and lead to an AMI.

Table 3.30 summarizes these studies.

Chest pain, ischemia, electrocardiology changes, and acute myocardial infarction

Nademanee *et al.* (1989) studied the effect of cocaine withdrawal on myocardial ischemia. The study comprised 21 chronic cocaine users in a 28-day patient treatment program, 42 volunteers, and 119 patients with stable or unstable angina. The subjects' ECGs were monitored with a 24-hour ambulatory Holter monitor and exercise treadmill. Among the cocaine users, eight had frequent ST elevation in the first two weeks of withdrawal. One cocaine user had a positive treadmill test for ischemia. During the Holter monitoring, none of the volunteers or patients with stable angina had ST segment changes but 4% of those with unstable angina experienced some ST segment changes. The authors concluded that ST segment elevations associated with cocaine withdrawal are common during the first two weeks of treatment. Coronary spasm is hypothesized as a possible cause of the ischemic change, but the exact mechanism is unclear.

Amin *et al.* (1990) conducted a retrospective study to determine the risk of AMI in 70 patients with chest pain after cocaine use. Twenty-two (31%) of the patients developed confirmed AMI verified by elevated CK-MB (a sensitive marker of myocardial injury); nine (13%) had transitional ischemia. Coronary risk factors were not significantly different in those who did or did not have an AMI. The route of cocaine use was not a factor in AMI

Table 3.30 Coronary artery reactivity

Study	Method	Sample	Incidence	Results
Brogan et al. (1992)	Randomized double-blind, controlled clinical trial Effect of cocaine, metabolites on coronary blood flow Cineangiography; blood levels cocaine and cocaine metabolites	18 patients with chest pain (16 males, 37–65 years): 8, saline administration; 10, cocaine (2 mg/kg body weight)	Cocaine group: 30 min after administration, significant vasoconstriction ($p < 0.05$), peak cocaine blood level; at 60 min, return to baseline; at 90 min, significant vasoconstriction ($p < 0.05$), peak metabolite level	Initial vasoconstriction related to peak cocaine level; second vasoconstriction related to peak of cocaine metabolites; metabolites may have a role in vasoconstriction
Dressler et al. (1990)	Necropsy, case–control study Effect of cocaine on coronary narrowing	22 necropsy samples (17 males, 19 African American): 13 (aged 23–45 years) elevated cocaine at time of death (3.6 mg/L); 9 cocaine users, death from other causes	8/22 (36%): one or more of four major coronary arteries narrowed > 75% (atherosclerotic plaque) 12 cocaine-related death: 8% segments narrowed 76–100%; 19% segments narrowed 51–75%; 5 deaths unrelated to cocaine use: 3% segments narrowed 76–100%; 7% segments narrowed 51–75%	More atherosclerotic lesions in those with elevated cocaine levels in blood at time of death compared with those dying from unrelated causes
Flores et al. (1990)	Case–control study Intranasal administration of cocaine or saline Angiography	18 patients, 15 males, aged 35–67 years: 12 given cocaine (2 mg/kg body weight), 6 saline	No change in saline group Cocaine group: decreased lumen size in non-diseased and diseased segments (greater in diseased, $p < 0.05$)	Cocaine is a vasoconstrictor; diseased segments of coronary arteries constricted more than non-diseased segments
Kolodgie et al. (1991)	Case–control study Mast cell and lumen narrowing Autopsy review	5871 records (mean age 29 ± 2 years), 495 (8.4%) positive for cocaine; 2 controls age, gender matched	6 (1.2%) total thrombic occlusion LAD; Significantly more mast cells in cocaine-associated group	Increased number mast cells and coronary narrowing in cocaine users ($r = 0.68$ in cocaine users, $r = 0.34$ in controls); users had more vessel narrowing, plaque; mast cells may have role in vasospasm, thrombosis, sudden death
Kontos et al. (2003)	Case series Cocaine-related chest pain Angiography 5 weeks after ER visit	90 patients with cocaine-related chest pain	45 (50%) significant CAD (> 50% stenosis): 1 vessel, 32%; 3 vessel, 10%; 3 vessel, 6%; graft stenosis, 3% Significant CAD in 77% of those with AMI or increased troponin-I levels and in 35% of those without AMI, increased troponin-I	Significant CAD predicted in those with cocaine-associated AMI or increased troponin-I

Study	Design/methods	Sample	Results	Comments
Lange et al. (1989)	Case–control study. Intranasal administration of cocaine or saline. Angiography	45 admitted for evaluation of chest pain (34 males, 11 females, aged 36–67 years): given cocaine 2 mg/kg body weight	Cocaine: increased heart rate, arterial BP; decreased coronary sinus flow, decreased LCA diameter by 8–12% ($p < 0.01$); no chest pain, ischemia	Findings reversed by alpha-adrenergic blocker; no difference in those with CAD ($n = 28$) and those without CAD ($n = 17$; likely that recreational drug use will produce similar results
Majid et al. (1992)	Case series. Cocaine administration. Computer-assisted quantitative analysis	6 admitted for chest pain after cocaine use, ST T wave changes	No changes in coronary artery diameter, myocardial perfusion, left ventricular wall motion, ECG; increased heart rate and BP	Negative findings for cardiac parameters after cocaine administration; cocaine-related chest pain not associated with artery vasospasm or decreased myocardial perfusion
Moliterno et al. (1994)	Cross-sectional study. Use of intranasal cocaine (2 mg/kg body weight), cigarette smoke, or both. Measure rate–pressure product (heart rate × systolic BP)	42 smokers (28 males, aged 34–79 years): 36 with CAD	Intranasal cocaine: increased rate–pressure product, decreased lumen diameter in diseased more than non-diseased vessels. One cigarette: increased rate–pressure product, decreased lumen diameter in diseased less than non-diseased vessels. Cocaine and cigarette: greatest increase in rate–pressure product, greater vasoconstriction and more in diseased than non-diseased vessels	Combined effect of cocaine and cigarette smoking resulted in greater vasoconstriction and increased rate–pressure product
Satran et al. (2005)	Case–control study. Incidence of coronary aneurysms in cocaine users	112 cocaine users: 80% male, 95% cigarette smokers, mean age 44 years. 76 controls similar in age, risk; more atherosclerosis, diabetes mellitus, CAD	Prior AMI: cocaine group, 45% (48% non-obstructed CAD); control group, 38%. Coronary artery aneurysms: 30.4% cocaine users, 7.6% controls	Cocaine use strong predictor of coronary aneurysm development

AMI, acute myocardial infarction; CAD, coronary artery disease; ECG, electrocardiogram; ER, emergency room; LAD, left anterior descending coronary vessel; LCA, left coronary artery.

development, and cocaine use did not appear to affect any particular coronary vessel. The median onset of pain was prolonged in the cocaine users with an AMI (18 hours after cocaine use) compared with those experiencing pain but not AMI (onset within one hour of drug use). Four of the eight patients with AMI who had a coronary catheterization had significant narrowing of at least one coronary vessel.

In a four-month retrospective review of 48 cocaine users seen in the emergency room after experiencing chest pain, Zimmerman et al. (1991) found that 13 (27%) experienced chest pain in the first hour after use, and 13 (27%) experienced pain after one hour of use. Abnormalities in the ST segment were evident in 18 (37%), T wave inversion in 20 (41%), and a diagnosis of AMI made in three patients (6%). The authors concluded that the ECG changes were related to ischemia caused by chronic myocardial changes associated with chronic cocaine use.

Minor et al. (1991) studied the risk for cocaine-induced AMI in individuals with normal coronary vessels. In addition to describing three cases, the authors reviewed the literature cited in MEDLINE and Index Medicus. They found 114 cases of cocaine-induced AMI; 35 (38%) had normal coronary vessels. The average age was 32 years (range, 21 to 60). Most of the patients (77%) had left anterial ventricular wall infarctions and 68% were cigarette smokers. Vasospasm was considered a cause in two patients, and intracoronary thrombosis was found in 9 of 11 patients (82%) who had an angiogram within 12 hours of the infarct. Based on the review of the literature, the authors hypothesized that cocaine has both direct and indirect sympathetic effects on the vascular smooth muscle, particularly the large arteries and small resistance vessels of the heart. The literature also suggests that in chronic cocaine users the ability of the endothelium to release vasodilators and the development of atherosclerosis can affect vascular reactivity, and that cocaine may be a strong cardiac myocyte depressant.

In a study by Tanenbaum & Miller (1992), the ECGs of 99 cocaine abusers and 50 schizophrenic controls were compared: 11 (11%) of the cocaine users showed some evidence of AMI, ischemia, or conduction defects (bundle branch block), while none of the schizophrenic controls had ECG changes indicative of myocardial injury.

Mehta et al. (1993) studied 21 infants prenatally exposed to cocaine and 20 normal controls in a prospective case–control study. Using Holter monitoring within 48 hours after birth, 6 of the 21 cocaine-exposed infants (29%) developed transient ST segment elevation, compared with only 1 of 20 (5%) non-exposed infants (OR 7.6; 95% CI 1.14–50.64). The control infants were similar to the cocaine-exposed infants in birthweight, gestational age, and postnatal age. Although heart rates and arrhythmias were not significantly different in the two groups of infants, the cocaine-exposed infants did have increased vagal activity. The authors concluded that infants of cocaine-using mothers may experience transient myocardial ischemia postnatally.

In another study, Frassica et al. (1994) looked at the incidence of cardiac arrhythmias in 554 infants with positive urine screens for cocaine. In 13 cocaine-exposed infants, 12 developed supraventricular arrhythmias, and four ventricular ectopy; five had arrhythmias that led to CHF. Some arrhythmias persisted in the postneonatal period, including six cases of arrhythmias in five infants, including high-grade ventricular arrhythmias, with two cases of cardiopulmonary arrest. Overall, an increase in premature beats was found in cocaine-exposed infants.

In a prospective observational cohort study, Hollander et al. (1994) studied 246 cocaine-using patients evaluated for chest pain at six emergency rooms in order to identify predictive clinical characteristics associated with AMI. The cohort included 175 men (71%); 205 (83.3%) were non-white, and 205 (83.3%) were cigarette smokers. Fourteen had an AMI confirmed by elevated CK-MB levels (5.7%; 95% CI 2.7–8.7). Patients had chest pain, shortness of breath, and diaphoresis; 12 patients had arrhythmias, and four had CHF. In most cases, chest pain occurred within 60 minutes after using cocaine, and the pain lasted a median of 120 minutes. Use of the ECG to predict an AMI varied: the specificity was 89.9%, positive predictive value 17.9%, and negative predictive value 95.8%. The low positive predictive value of the ECG in identifying those with an AMI suggested to the authors that clinical tools are not adequate for ruling out AMI and, therefore, all patients should be evaluated further for this cardiac event.

Hollander *et al.* (1995a) conducted a retrospective cohort study of hospital records from 29 hospitals in order to study the mortality and complications in cases of cocaine-associated AMI. Over a six-year period, 130 patients were diagnosed with 136 myocardial infarcts; the mean age was 38 years; 94 (72%) were non-white, 118 (91%) were tobacco smokers, and 114 (88%) used cocaine in the 24 hours prior to development of chest pain. An AMI was diagnosed in 57 (44%) by ECG and ischemia in 23 (18%). Anterior and inferior infarcts occurred at the same frequency, and most (61%) were non-Q wave. Most complications occurred within 12 hours after the infarct and occurred 64 times in 49 patients (36%; 95% CI 28–44). Congestive heart failure, ventricular and supraventricular tachycardia, and brady-arrhythmias were most common. No patient deaths occurred. Based on their findings, Hollander *et al.* (1995a) concluded that the risk of mortality in cocaine-associated MI is low.

Hollander *et al.* (1995b) conducted a one-year follow-up study of individuals with cocaine-related chest pain in order to evaluate their risk of death. Mortality data were available for 203 patients, and additional clinical information available for 185. Six deaths occurred in the 408 days of data collection (98% one-year actuarial survival; 95% CI 95–100). None of the patients died from an AMI. Two patients had a non-fatal AMI (1%; 95% CI 0–2), 60% continued to use cocaine (95% CI 52–68), and 75% had recurrent chest pain. No AMIs or deaths were reported by those who indicated discontinuation of cocaine use. The authors concluded that the risk of AMI and death in those with cocaine-related chest pain is low and strategies should be directed toward drug cessation rather than immediate coronary intervention.

Another study by Hollander *et al.* (1995c) described the prevalence of cocaine-associated chest pain in patients seen in four emergency rooms. Of the 359 individuals seen, 60 (17%) tested positive for cocaine or cocaine metabolites although only 43 (72%) admitted recent use of cocaine. The likelihood of testing positive for cocaine for various age groups was as follows: 18–30 years, 29%; 31–40 years, 48%; 41–50 years, 18%; and 51–60 years, 3%. None of those aged 61 or older tested positive for cocaine use. The researchers suggested that individuals between 18 and 60 years seen in emergency rooms with chest pain should be questioned about cocaine use. However, since self-report is unreliable, testing for cocaine and cocaine metabolites would provide objective data helpful in diagnosis and treatment.

A 1999 case–control study by Mittleman *et al.* explored the risk of an AMI after cocaine use in 3946 patients; 38 (1%) had used cocaine in the year prior to their infarct, and nine used cocaine 60 minutes before their infarct. Eighty-four percent were cigarette smokers (vs. 32% for non-users; $p = 0.001$). The cocaine users with AMIs were younger than non-users (44 ± 8 vs. 61 ± 13 years; $p < 0.001$), mostly male (87% vs. 67%; $p = 0.01$), and were more likely to be minorities (63% vs. 11%; $p < 0.002$). Sixty minutes after using cocaine, the calculated risk for an AMI was 23.7 times greater than baseline (95% CI 8.5–66.3); however,

Table 3.31 Cardiac arrest outcomes in cocaine users and non-users

	Age (years)	Neurological recovery status	Deaths
Cocaine users (n = 22)	42 ± 10	12 (55%) complete recovery	10 (46%)
Randomly selected controls (n = 20)	68 ± 16	3 (15%) complete recovery	15 (75%)
Age-matched controls, non-users (n = 41)	Age matched to cocaine users	7 (17%) complete recovery	32 (78%)

this risk decreased significantly thereafter. The researchers concluded that cocaine use was associated with a rapid and immediate risk of AMI in cocaine users, but that the risk decreases within hours of use. This risk occurs in individuals who otherwise would be considered low risk.

Weber *et al.* (2000) studied 250 patients with cocaine-associated chest pain and their risk for AMI. The mean age was 33.5 ± 8.5 years; 192 (77%) were male, 210 (84%) African American, 192 (77%) smokers, 65 (26%) had hypertension, 85 (34%) had a family history of cardiovascular disease, and 100 (40%) had prior episodes of chest pain. Other cardiac risk factors were found in fewer than 8% of the patients. Cocaine had been used by 192 (77%) in the 24 hours prior to the onset of chest pain (in 85% of these, crack was used). Of the 196 patients tested, 185 (94%) tested positive for cocaine or cocaine metabolites in the urine. Using World Health Organization (WHO) criteria, 15 patients were diagnosed with an AMI (6%; 95% CI 4.1–8.9). Complications were infrequent in this group. This study supported findings in previous studies related to AMI risk.

Qureshi *et al.* (2001) used the Third National Health and Nutrition Examination Survey to determine the likelihood of developing an AMI or stroke after cocaine use. Of 10 085 adults aged 18 to 45 years, 46 developed non-fatal MIs and 33 experienced non-fatal strokes. Adjusting for age, sex, race, education, hypertension, diabetes mellitus, dyslipidemia, basal metabolic rate, and cigarette smoking, the OR for young cocaine users to develop a non-fatal MI was 6.9 (95% CI 1.3–58). No risk was determined for a stroke. The population-attributable risk percentage for a non-fatal MI in those aged 18–45 years was 25%; therefore, one out of every four non-fatal MIs in this age group can be attributed to frequent cocaine use.

Hsue *et al.* (2007) studied the risk of cardiac arrest in crack cocaine users. From a database of hospital charts from 1994 to 2006, 22 cocaine users were identified who experienced a resuscitated cardiac arrest. Two comparative cardiac arrest groups were used: a group of 20 randomly selected controls and 41 age-matched controls who were not cocaine users The results show that cocaine users were younger than randomly selected patients with cardiac arrest and were more likely to recover neurologically and survive the arrest (Table 3.31).

A study by Bansal *et al.* (2007) examined traditional risk factors and AMI in 165 cocaine users hospitalized with chest pain over a four-year period. Using WHO criteria, a diagnosis of AMI was made in 21 patients (13%). All 21 were cigarette smokers. A risk score was calculated for a number of risk factors, gender, and age. The factors found to increase the risk for AMI in cocaine users were existing CAD, age, hyperlipidemia, and a family history of CAD. The authors concluded that the risk of an AMI increases when there is an increased risk factor score in patients with cocaine-associated chest pain.

Table 3.32 summarizes these studies on chest pain, ischemia, electrocardiology changes, and acute myocardial infarction.

Table 3.32 Chest pain, ischemia, electrocardiology changes, and acute myocardial infarction

Study	Method	Sample	Incidence	Results
Amin et al. (1990)	Retrospective study Risk of AMI after cocaine use	70 patients with chest pain after cocaine use	22 (31%) confirmed AMI by CK-MB; 4/8 with AMI had narrowing of at least one vessel; 9 (13%) ischemia	AMI not predicted by route of administration of cocaine; no predilection for any particular coronary artery; those with confirmed AMI had longer time before onset of pain (18 h) after using cocaine
Bansal et al. (2007)	Chart review Traditional risk factors and AMI in cocaine users experiencing chest pain	21 (13%) of 165 patients experienced AMI (WHO criteria); all cigarette smokers	Risk score calculated on number of risks (CAD, age, hyperlipidemia, family history CAD), gender, and age	Risk of AMI increases with increased risk factor score in patients with cocaine-associated chest pain
Frassica et al. (1994)	Chart review, infants with positive urine screens for cocaine	554 infants	Arrhythmias in 13 infants, 12 supraventricular, 4 ventricular ectopy; 5 infants had six arrhythmias in postnatal period, including ventricular arrhythmias (2 cardiac arrests); 5/13 developed CHF from arrhythmia	Premature beats are common in cocaine-exposed irfants; arrhythmias can persist after neonatal period
Hollander et al. (1994)	Prospective observational cohort study Clinical characteristics leading to AMI	Data from 6 ERs for 246 cocaine-users with chest pain: 71% male, 83.3% non-white, 83.3% cigarette smokers	Chest pain most, 60 min after using cocaine; confirmed AMI by CK-MB in 14/246 (5.7%; 95% CI 2.7–8.7)	ECG predictive of AMI: specificity 89.9%, positive predictive value 17.9%, negative predictive value 95.8% Tools available inadequate in identifying those with low risk for AMI; evaluate all for AMI
Hollander et al. (1995a)	Retrospective cohort study of 29 hospitals Mortality and complications with cocaine-associated AMI	130 patients, 136 AMIs over 6-year period; mean age 38 years, 72% non-white, 91% tobacco smokers, 88% used cocaine 24 h before chest pain	By ECG, 44% AMI diagnoses, most non-Q-wave; 18% ischemia; complications, most in first 12 h: CHF, ventricular and supraventricular tachycardia, bradyarrhythmias; no deaths	Risk of mortality low in cocaine users
Hollander et al. (1995b)	Longitudinal study, 1 year follow-up Mortality with cocaine-associated AMI	203 patients; clinical information on 185; 6 non-cardiac deaths (98% 1-year actuarial survival; 95% CI 95–100)	2 non-fatal MIs (1%; 95% CI 0–2); 60% continued cocaine use; 75% recurrent chest pain	Risk of AMI and death low in those with cocaine-related chest pain

Table 3.32 *Cont.*

Study	Method	Sample	Incidence	Results
Hollander et al. (1995c)	Retrospective cohort study in four ERs	60 of 359 (17%) tested positive for cocaine or cocaine metabolites (only 43 admitted recent use)	Likelihood of testing positive for cocaine use: 18–30 years,29%; 31–40 years, 48%; 41–50 years, 18%; 51–60 years, 3%; > 60 years, 0%	In the ER, patients 18–60 years of age with chest pain should be questioned about cocaine use; self-report unreliable; use testing for cocaine for objective data
Hsue et al. (2007)	Case–control chart review, 1994–2006 Cardiac arrest in cocaine users	Resuscitated cardiac arrest: 22 cocaine users, 20 randomly selected controls, 41 age-matched non-users controls	Cocaine users younger (42 ± 10 years), more likely to completely recover neurologically (12/22), less likely to die (10/22) than randomly selected or age-matched controls	Young cocaine users with cardiac arrest more likely to recover neurologically and survive AMI than age-match controls or randomly selected controls
Mehta et al. (1993)	Prospective study Myocardial ischemia in prenatally exposed infants Holter monitoring	21 infants exposed to cocaine prenatally; 20 control infants	Transient ST segment elevation: 6 cocaine-exposed infants, 1 control infant (OR 7.6; 95% CI 1.14–50.64) Increased vagal activity in cocaine-exposed infants; no difference in heart rates, arrhythmias	Infants exposed to cocaine prenatally more at risk for ST segment elevation and possible cardiac ischemia 48 h after birth
Minor et al. (1991)	Case records (3) and literature review Cocaine-induced AMI in individuals with normal coronary arteries	3 case records, 114 cases cocaine-induced AMI in literature review; 68% cigarette smokers	Normal coronary arteries 35 (38%) (age 21–60 years); left anterior ventricular AMI 77%; vasospasm in 2; intracoronary thrombus in 9/11 with angiography 12 h after infarct	Literature findings: cocaine has direct and indirect effects on vascular smooth muscle (large arteries, resistance vessels) and endothelium (altered activity; myocardial depressant)
Mittleman et al. (1999)	Case–control study Risk of AMI after cocaine use	3946 patients; 38 (1%) used cocaine in year prior to infarct, 9 used cocaine 60 min before infarct	Cocaine users with AMIs younger than non-users (44 ± 8 vs. 61 ± 13 years; ($p < 0.001$), mostly male (87% vs. 67%; $p = 0.01$), mostly minority group (63% vs. 11%; $p < 0.002$) Risk for AMI 60 min after using cocaine, 23.7 times more than baseline (95% CI 8.5–66.3)	Risk of AMI highest within 60 min of using cocaine, substantially decreases after 1 h
Nademanee et al. (1989)	Case–control study ST and T wave changes 24-hour Holter monitoring and exercise treadmill	21 chronic cocaine users in treatment program, 42 volunteers, 119 patients with stable or unstable angina	8/21 cocaine users: frequent ST and T wave elevation first 2 weeks ($p = 0.004$, cocaine users vs. volunteers); 1/20 cocaine users positive treadmill test for ischemia	ST and T wave changes frequent in cocaine users in early weeks of withdrawal

Study	Design / Focus	Sample	Key findings	Conclusions
Qureshi et al. (2001)	Descriptive study from the Third National Health and Nutrition Examination Survey Risk of AMI, stroke after cocaine use	10 085 adults: 46 non-fatal AMIs, 33 non-fatal strokes	Adjusting for age, sex, race, education, high BP, diabetes mellitus, dyslipidemia, likelihood of developing non-fatal MI 6.9 (95% CI 1.3–58); no risk for stroke	Population attributable risk percentage for non-fatal AMI in cocaine users aged 18 to 45 years with chest pain
Tanenbaum & Miller (1992)	Case-control study ECG changes in cocaine users and schizophrenics	99 cocaine users, 50 schizophrenics	11 cocaine users had ECG changes indicating AMI, ischemia, bundle branch block; no changes in schizophrenics	
Weber et al. (2000)	Chart review Risk for AMI with cocaine-associated chest pain	250 cocaine users admitted for evaluation of chest pain: mean age 33.5 ± 8.5 years, 77% male, 84% African American, 77% smokers, 26% high BP, 34% family history of cardiovascular disease, 40% prior episodes of chest pain, 77% used cocaine in 24 h prior to pain	185 of 196 (94%) tested positive for cocaine, cocaine metabolites; using WHO criteria, 15 patients diagnosed with AMI (6%; 95% CI 4.1–8.9); complications infrequent	Study supports previous findings: relatively low incidence of AMI in cocaine users with chest pain; low mortality
Zimmerman et al. (1991)	Retrospective review Pain onset ECG changes	48 cocaine users in ER with chest pain: 34 males, age 29 ± 7.3 years	Pain within first hour of use in 13 (27%), after 1 h in 13 (27%); ST segment abnormality in 18 (37%); T wave inversion in 20 (41%); 3 confirmed AMI	Ischemic changes (ST/T wave changes) may be related to chronic myocardial changes

AMI, acute myocardial infarction; BP, blood pressure; CAD, coronary artery disease; CHF, congestive heart failure; CI, confidence interval; CK-MB, creatine kinase MB isozyme; ECG, electrocardiology; ER, emergency room; MI, myocardial infarction; OR, odds ratio; WHO, World Health Organization.

Cardiac morphological changes

Brickner *et al.* (1991) published a case–control study describing ventricular cavity size and wall motion in cocaine users. The study included 30 cocaine users, aged 34 to 44 years, residing in an inpatient treatment program. The 30 controls were age and race matched and were similar in gender, weight, height, blood pressure, and body surface area. Two-dimensional echocardiograms were conducted. Left ventricular mass index and posterior wall thickness were measured and evaluated by blind reviewers. The left ventricular mass index was greater in the cocaine users ($p = 0.0001$); the posterior wall thickness was increased in 13 (43%) of the cocaine users and in four of the controls ($p = 0.0099$).

Om *et al.* (1992) used coronary angiograms to assess left ventricular dysfunction and CAD in 33 patients with clinical indications for angiography, including chest pain (28), CHF (4), and complete heart block (1). Of the 33 patients, 26 were male; the mean age was 37 years and all were cocaine users and had cardiac symptoms. The ages and risk factors for cardiovascular disease were not significantly different in those with CAD and those with normal angiograms. The angiogram results showed that 13 (40%) had normal coronary arteries, 22 (67%) had evidence of CAD, 7 (21%) had mild vessel stenosis (< 70%), 13 (40%) had significant coronary narrowing (> 70%), and 12 (36%) had enzyme elevations indicating MI. The left ventricular ejection fraction was depressed in 18 patients (55%). All of the 12 patients with CAD and low ejection fractions had regional wall motion abnormalities. Six of the patients with normal coronary arteries and low ejection fractions had global hypokinesia.

Chakko *et al.* (1992) studied cardiac abnormalities in 50 asymptomatic long-term cocaine users in a drug rehabilitation program, 14 age-matched normal volunteers, and 14 age-matched psychiatric patients with similar smoking and alcohol histories. The ECGs of 14 (29%) of the cocaine users showed ST segment and T wave changes and evidence of an AMI. Echocardiograms showed an abnormal increase in posterior wall thickness, increased septal thickness, and an increased left ventricular mass index ($p = 0.001$ to 0.0001). Diastolic filling was not altered in those with left ventricular hypertrophy. The normal volunteers and psychiatric patients did not show similar changes. Alcohol use did not affect the findings in this study.

In a case–control study, Eisenberg *et al.* (1995) studied 20 non-hospitalized intravenous cocaine users and 20 age- and sex-matched controls to determine left ventricular function. The cocaine users had normal blood pressures, started cocaine an average of 14 years prior to the study, and used cocaine eight times a month in the preceding year. The two-dimensional echocardiogram found no significant difference between the cocaine users and the controls in left ventricular mass index, mean wall thickness, end-diastolic volume index, end-systolic volume index, or ejection fraction. None of the subjects had significant abnormal regional wall motion or an ejection fraction < 55%. The authors hypothesized that left ventricular morphological changes and dysfunction may be limited to certain high-risk cocaine users.

Karch *et al.* (1995) reported a case–control study of heart weight and atherosclerotic lesions in 32 male cocaine users who died of trauma, 26 males who died of cocaine overdose, and 51 male historical controls (World War I and the Korean and Vietnam wars). The cocaine users had larger hearts than the controls and more severe CAD. Ten (30%) of the cocaine users had disease in two or more coronary vessels ($p = 0.01$, compared with controls). Sixteen female cocaine users had no differences in heart weight or lesions compared with 17 non-cocaine-using controls. Although the degree of hypertrophy was 10% higher than normal, the authors suggested that hypertrophy may be under-reported in autopsy reports.

A more recent study by Darke *et al.* (2006) compared cardiac and cerebrovascular pathology in deaths from cocaine toxicity, opioid toxicity, or deaths from hanging (non-drug related). In this case–control study, the findings in the cocaine-related deaths were greater than in the opioid or hanging cases. There was a greater increase in left ventricular hypertrophy and ischemic heart disease. There was more atherosclerosis in the left anterior descending artery (moderate to severe), right coronary, and circumflex artery. The cocaine group also had higher levels of cerebrovascular pathology than the other two groups. The authors suggested that the changes seen were more likely to be specifically related to cocaine effects and not simply associated with a drug lifestyle.

These studies are summarized in Table 3.33.

Coagulation studies and aortic disease

Platelet activation after administration of cocaine was described in a randomized double-blind crossover study reported by Heesch *et al.* (2000). Fourteen healthy volunteers each received 2 mg/kg intranasal cocaine or a saline placebo. After each treatment, the following were measured: flow-cytometric analysis of P-selectin, platelet factor 4, β-thromboglobulin, platelet-containing aggregates and microparticles, and circulating von Willebrand factor antigen. No changes were seen in these platelet parameters after the placebo; however, there was an increase in platelet factor 4 and β-thromboglobulin 120 minutes after intranasal cocaine administration, an increase in platelet-containing microaggregates at 40 and 80 minutes after cocaine administration, and a decrease in bleeding time. The authors hypothesized that cocaine alters platelet activity and can stimulate formation of platelet thrombi, and possibly lead to ischemic events. They proposed that patients with cocaine-related ischemia receive platelet inhibitors to minimize risk of untoward events.

Two case reports suggested aortic dysfunction in cocaine users that led to renal infarction but with different causes. Mochizuki *et al.* (2003) presented a case report of a nasal cocaine user who developed aortic thrombosis and a renal infarct. Williams & Wasserberger (2006) described a crack cocaine user who binged for five days and ultimately died from severe aortic vasoconstriction that extended from the suprarenal aorta to beyond both femoral arteries. The individual died from renal failure and bowel ischemia.

Zhou *et al.* (2004) studied hospital records from a 10-year period to identify cases of acute occlusion of peripheral arteries in cocaine users. Of the 382 cases of acute arterial occlusion, five (1.3%) patients were identified as cocaine users. They included four males and one female, with a mean age of 38 years. Two used intranasal inhalants and three used crack cocaine. The mean time between using cocaine and symptoms of peripheral occlusion was 9.2 hours. The arteries affected varied: aortic thrombosis (one), superficial femoral artery thrombosis (one), iliac thrombosis (two), and popliteal artery occlusion (one). All of the patients recovered from their occlusive episode; however, one patient died later from an AMI. The authors hypothesized that cocaine use may potentiate the development of acute arterial thrombi and that prompt identification and treatment with platelet inhibitors is important.

Kolodgie *et al.* (1992) conducted a retrospective analysis to determine the degree of sudanophilia (indicating lipid deposition) in the aortas of 16 confirmed cocaine users without symptoms of atherosclerotic disease. The controls were 10 specimens from

Table 3.33 Cardiac morphological changes

Study	Method	Sample	Incidence	Results
Brickner et al. (1991)	Case–control study Ventricular cavity size, wall motion in cocaine users 2D echocardiography, blind review	30 cocaine users (age 34–44 years) inpatient treatment program; 30 controls matched for age, race, gender, height, weight, BP, body surface area	LV mass index greater in cocaine users ($p = 0.0001$); increased posterior wall thickness in 13 (43%) cocaine users, 4 (13%) controls ($p = 0.0099$)	Chronic cocaine users may experience increased LV hypertrophy, may predispose for ischemia, arrhythmias
Chakko et al. (1992)	Cross-sectional study Cardiac abnormalities in cocaine users ECG, echocardiography	50 chronic cocaine users, 14 age-matched normal volunteers, 14 age-matched psychiatric patients with similar smoking, alcohol use	Cocaine users: 29% ST segment, T wave abnormalities, evidence of AMI; echocardiogram indicated increased posterior wall thickness, septal thickness, LV mass index ($p = 0.001$ to 0.0001) No changes in normal volunteers or psychiatric patients; alcohol not a factor	ECG findings of ischemia, AMI and echocardiogram findings of LV hypertrophy more likely found in chronic cocaine users than age-matched psychiatric patients or normal volunteers
Eisenberg et al. (1995)	Case–control study Assessment of LV function 2D echocardiography	20 IV chronic cocaine users (14 years of use), 20 age/sex-matched controls	No differences in LV mass index, mean wall thickness, end-diastolic volume index, end-systolic volume index, ejection fraction; no abnormal regional wall motion, no ejection fraction < 55%	Although other studies found differences in cardiac parameters, morphological changes and dysfunction may be limited to certain high-risk cocaine users
Karch et al. (1995)	Case–control study Heart weight, atherosclerosis in cocaine users	32 male cocaine users, died of trauma, 26 males who died of cocaine overdose, 51 male historic controls (World War I, Korean, Vietnam war)	Cocaine users: larger hearts, more severe CAD, disease in 2 or more vessels (30%), ($p = 0.01$ compared with controls) Female cocaine users (16): no differences in heart weight, lesions, compared with 17 non-cocaine-using controls	Hypertrophy 10% but may be missed on autopsy; cocaine users may be more at risk for LV hypertrophy, CAD than others

Study	Design/Method	Sample	Results	Conclusions
Om et al. (1992)	Case series, convenience sample CAD and left ventricular dysfunction in cocaine users Coronary angiogram	33 cocaine users with cardiac symptoms (26 males, mean age 37 years): chest pain (28), CHF (4), complete heart block (1)	Ages, risk factors for cardiovascular disease not significantly different; 13 (40%) normal coronary arteries, 22 (66%) CAD, 7 (21%) mild vessel stenosis ($<70\%$), 13 (40%) sever stenosis ($>70\%$); 12 (36%) elevated serum enzymes, 18 (55%) LV ejection fraction depressed All 12 with CAD and low ejection fraction had regional wall motion dysfunction 6 with normal arteries and low ejection fractions had global hypokinesia	Left ventricular depression seen in chronic cocaine users withcardiovascular symptoms
Darke et al. (2006)	Case–control study Comparison of cocaine, opioid, non-drug related deaths	Pathology groups: cocaine users, opioid users, non-drug-related deaths by hanging	Cocaine users more likely than other groups to have LV hypertrophy, ischemic heart disease, moderate/severe atherosclerosis of LAD; also disease in circumflex and right cerebral artery, more cerebrovascular atherosclerosis	Cardiac, cerebrovascular changes more likely caused by cocaine use than lifestyle

2D, two dimensional; BP, blood pressure; CAD, coronary artery disease; CHF, congestive heart failure; IV, intravenous; LAD, left anterior descending coronary vessel; LV, left ventricular.

individuals with no history of drug abuse. Sudan IV was used to stain the surface lipids of the thoracic and abdominal aorta, and image analysis used to quantify the lipids. In a multilinear regressional analysis considering cocaine use, age, cigarette smoking, and lipoprotein levels, a positive association was found between cocaine use and sudanophilia in the thoracic aorta ($p < 0.002$) and abdominal aorta ($p < 0.049$). Sudan IV staining of the right coronary artery was not significant. The findings suggest that chronic cocaine use may increase lipid deposition in the aorta.

A recent article by McKee et al. (2007) described the increased risk of stent thrombosis after percutaneous transluminal coronary artery angioplasty and stent insertion. Sixty-six cocaine users were followed-up nine months after angioplasty to evaluate patency of their stents. Five of the stents (7.6%) were occluded at nine months, compared with 0.6% in the 3216 controls ($p < 0.001$). A propensity analysis was used to control for statistical bias in a non-randomized study and showed that occluded stents in 4 of 66 cocaine users versus 0 in 70 matched controls was still statistically significant ($p < 0.04$). There was no difference between the cocaine users and the controls in development of an AMI, repeat revascularization, or death. Because of the increased risk of stent occlusion, the authors proposed that healthcare providers consider more conservative treatment of coronary disease in cocaine users with chest pain.

Hsue et al. (2002) reviewed hospital charts from a 20-year period to identify aortic dissection as defined by the WHO's *International Statistical Classification of Diseases and Related Health Problems*, 9th edition. Thirty-eight cases were found, including 14 (37%) with dissection attributed to cocaine use. One of these snorted cocaine and the other 13 smoked it. The time between the use of cocaine and the onset of symptoms was 0 to 24 hours, with a mean of 12 hours. The mostly African American cocaine users were younger than non-users and had a history of untreated hypertension. The researchers concluded that aortic dissection may be a consequence of abrupt, transient, severe hypertension and catecholamine release.

Table 3.34 details these studies on coagulation disorders and aortic disease.

Comments

Thirty-five research abstracts were reviewed to assess the relationship between cocaine use and cardiovascular disease. Overall, many of the studies were small and utilized convenience samples. Consideration of confounders was not always apparent from the information available in the abstracts reviewed. Very few studies provided statistical findings that would be useful in guiding evidence-based practice or information for providers regarding the relationship between cocaine and cardiovascular dysfunction.

Further study is needed with large numbers of cocaine users to determine their cardiovascular risk factors and their statistical risks for an AMI compared with non-users. Angiographic studies of cocaine users with and without a history of CAD may help to assess the risk of myocardial dysfunction related to chronic use. The relationship of platelet and coagulation defects in cocaine users might help to determine risk of thrombi and emboli in chronic cocaine users.

Coronary artery status

Eight articles focused on the relationship between cocaine use and coronary artery status. Several of these studies used intranasal administration of cocaine at a level similar to that of cocaine-containing topical anesthetics or that typically found to produce a cocaine high.

Table 3.34 Coagulation studies and aortic dysfunction

Study	Method	Sample	Incidence	Results
Heesch et al. (2000)	Randomized double-blind crossover study. Platelet activation after cocaine administration. Flow-cytometric analysis	14 healthy volunteers, intranasal administration of 2 mg/kg body weight cocaine or placebo	No changes after placebo; changes after cocaine administration: increased platelet factor 4 and β-thromboglobulin in 120 min and platelet-containing microaggregate formation in 40 and 80 min; decrease bleeding time	Cocaine can alter platelet activity and stimulate formation of platelet thrombi; patients with cocaine-related ischemia should be evaluated for platelet inhibitors to minimize risk of ischemic damage
Hsue et al. (2002)	Chart review (20 year). Aortic dissection in cocaine users	34 cases of aortic dissection: 14 (37%) cocaine users (13 crack smoking, 1 snorting), mostly African Americans, history of untreated high BP, younger than non-users	Mean of 12 h from use of cocaine and symptoms	Aortic dissection may be a consequence of abrupt, transient, severe high BP and catecholamine release
Kolodgie et al. (1992)	Retrospective analysis. Lipoprotein analysis of thoracic, abdominal aorta. Staining with Sudan IV	26 black males aged 15–34 years; 16 (mean age 25 years) tested positive for cocaine; 10 no evidence of drug abuse	Multiple regression analysis of cocaine use, age, cigarette use, lipoprotein levels, positive association for cocaine and sudanophilia in thoracic aorta ($p < 0.002$) and abdominal aorta ($p < 0.049$)	Cocaine may increase lipid deposition in the aorta
McKee et al. (2007)	Case-control study, follow-up study. Stent thrombosis in cocaine users	Recipients of stents in percutaneous transluminal coronary artery angioplasty: 66 of 71 cocaine users, 3216 non-user controls	In 9 month follow-up, 5 (7.6%) of the stents were occluded in the cocaine users compared with 19 (0.6%) in controls ($p < 0.001$) Propensity analysis to control for bias in non-randomized study: 4/66 users vs. 0/70 controls ($p < 0.04$) No difference in AMI, repeat revascularization, death	Because of higher risk for stent occlusion in cocaine users, conservative treatment might be better choice rather than stent

Table 3.34 Cont.

Study	Method	Sample	Incidence	Results
Mochizuki et al. (2003)	Case report Aortic thrombosis, renal infarction	Nasal cocaine user	Renal infarction, aortic thrombus	Renal infarction, aortic thrombus rarely reported
Williams & Wasserberger (2006)	Case report Fatal bowel ischemia	Death of crack cocaine user after a 5-day binge	Pathology: severe aortic vasoconstriction extending from suprarenal aorta to below both femoral arteries	Vasoconstriction also associated with aortic dysfunction
Zhou et al. (2004)	Chart review, 10 years Acute occlusion of peripheral arteries in cocaine users	382 with acute occlusion; 5 (1.3%) cocaine users	Mean duration from cocaine use to occlusion, 9.2 h; arteries affected, aorta, superficial femoral, iliac (2), popliteal; all recovered but one later died from acute myocardial infarction	Cocaine may potentiate development of acute arterial thrombi; prompt identification and treatment important; consider platelet inhibitors

BP, blood pressure.

One of four cardiac perfusion studies did not confirm the decrease in coronary artery diameter, changes in perfusion, or coronary sinus flow seen in the other three. One other study did find that the combination of cocaine and cigarette smoking resulted in a greater degree of vasospasm than use of either alone. Another study found that vasoconstriction after cocaine administration was bimodal: there was a peak of vasoconstriction at 30 minutes (presumably from cocaine and circulating catecholamines), a return to baseline at 60 minutes, and a second peak of vasoconstriction at 90 minutes. They attribute the second vasoconstriction to a corresponding increase in cocaine metabolites in the blood. In general, these studies involved small numbers, but most did include both cocaine users and healthy volunteers.

Two of three other studies in the coronary artery subsection were autopsy reports on the degree of atherosclerosis in the coronary vessels. Both small studies found atherosclerotic lesions or total thrombic occlusion in the coronary vessels. A third study looked at the predisposition for coronary artery aneurysms and found an increase in aneurysms in cocaine users compared with non-users.

These coronary artery studies support other studies that found that cocaine and associated catecholamine increase contribute to vasoconstriction in users soon after administration of cocaine. The necropsy studies suggest that this is also true in chronic users. It is unclear from the information available whether the subjects were cigarette smokers or had other risk factors that might affect the results.

Chest pain, injury, electrocardiology changes, and acute myocardial infarction

Fifteen articles explored the relationship between chest pain after cocaine use and subsequent development of an AMI. Several also discussed the use of an ECG to confirm or predict an MI. Several studies looked at ST and T wave changes in individuals who had used or been exposed to cocaine. In one study of cocaine users in withdrawal, 8 out of 21 users experienced ST and T wave changes within the first two weeks of withdrawal, suggesting some degree of ongoing ischemia. Another study found ST and T wave changes in 57% of cocaine users after experiencing chest pain; however, only three patients (6%) actually had an AMI. In infants exposed to cocaine in utero, ST and T wave changes were found in 29%. In another study, cardiac arrhythmias occurred in infants and persisted for several weeks after birth. One study did explore the specificity and predictive value of the ECG and determined that the ECG had a low positive predictive value in determining the likelihood of developing an AMI, and that the incidence of AMI in cocaine users is relatively low. Few of the studies used troponin-I or enzyme studies (CK-MB) and none reported use of myoglobin or other cardiac biomarkers to confirm a diagnosis of an AMI.

Several studies reported on risk factors for an AMI in cocaine users. In many studies, the cardiovascular risk factors were similar in those cocaine users experiencing an AMI soon after using cocaine and in chronic cocaine users, non-drug-using controls, and non-drug users with CAD. One study that used WHO criteria for AMI diagnosis found 14% of cocaine users developed an AMI soon after use. However, other risk factors were also identified, including existing CAD, a family history of CAD, hyperlipidemia, and older age. One large study found the risk of AMI in cocaine users was 23.7 times greater than in non-users. In another large study, cocaine use was attributed to one of every four occurrences of a non-fatal AMI in young adults, with an OR of 6.9 in persons under the age of 45 years. That study also found that there was almost no risk of developing a stroke after cocaine use.

Studies also reported on risk of complications and death after AMI. In most cases, the AMI was non-fatal. In some cases where death occurred, the deaths were not attributed to recent cocaine use but to other factors. In one study looking at outcomes after a cardiac arrest, the younger cocaine users tended to have no neurological dysfunction after the arrest and were more likely to survive than the non-cocaine-using controls.

Overall, it appears that the risk of an AMI in individuals experiencing chest pain after cocaine use is relatively low. Most infarcts were non-Q wave (likely subendocardial) and resulted in few complications. Death from an AMI was infrequent. In studies that reported tobacco use, the range of smokers was 77 to 100%. The concurrent use of cocaine and cigarettes may increase the likelihood of chest pain and evaluation for an AMI. However, in most cases, it appears that the risk of AMI and subsequent death after cocaine use is relatively low.

Cardiac morphology

Five small case–control studies reported on cardiac parameters in cocaine users. Echo-cardiography showed increases in left ventricular mass, increased wall and septal thickness, and decreases in left ventricular ejection fraction. Some subjects had CAD and prior infarcts. However, one study found no difference in cardiac parameters in cocaine users. Further studies are needed with a large number of cocaine users to determine the risk of abnormal cardiac function and cardiac changes over time. One case–control study compared pathology findings from cocaine, opioid, and non-drug-related deaths and found greater cardiac and cerebrovascular pathologies in cocaine users. More studies are needed to strengthen the findings in these studies.

Coagulation defects and aortic disease

Several studies reported on the incidence of thrombus formation and vascular occlusion associated with cocaine use. In a randomized double-blind crossover study, intranasal administration of cocaine was followed by an increase in platelet markers, platelet aggregates, and platelet thrombi. In a chart review of patients with peripheral arterial occlusion, 5 of 382 cocaine users had significant thrombi in major peripheral vessels. Another study found that 6.2% of cocaine users experienced stent occlusion after percutaneous trans-luminal coronary artery angioplasty. Coupled with the incidence of thrombi in cocaine users evaluated for chest pain and AMI, and thrombi identified on autopsy, assessment of platelet factors and coagulability in cocaine users experiencing chest pain may be valuable in guiding treatment, including the administration of platelet inhibitors.

The two case studies demonstrate the variability of cocaine's effect on the vasculature. In one patient, aortic thrombosis was found, while in the second severe vasoconstriction resulted in death. In other autopsy analyses, it may not be possible to determine which of the two effects caused the pathology.

Dermatological disease

Two articles were found in the PubMed literature published between 1988 and 2008 related to epidemiological studies on cocaine use and skin conditions (Table 3.35). Feeney & Briggs (1992) described lesions found on the hands of crack cocaine users. Multiple lesions, some circular, on the palmar surface of the fingers and palms appeared blackened and hyper-keratotic. These lesions appeared primarily in the dominant hand and were caused by contact with the hot glass cocaine pipe.

In their review of dermatological manifestations of cocaine use, Brewer et al. (2008) described formication, a common side effect of cocaine use. This paresthesia typically

Table 3.35 Dermatological disease

Study	Method	Sample	Incidence	Results
Brewer *et al.* (2008)	Literature review Dermatological lesions		Discussion of cutaneous conditions seen in cocaine abuse, including vasculitides, infections, formication (delusional parasitosis)	
Feeney & Briggs (1992)	Descriptive, case series	Multiple cases of skin lesions caused by contact with the hot glass cocaine pipe	Multiple blackened hyperkeratotic lesions of the dominant hand, primarily on the palmar surface of the fingers and palm	

involves the sensation of insects crawling on or under the skin, which may be perceived as biting or stinging. It is considered a delusional parasitosis. The authors suggested that patients with chronic skin lesions and vague medical histories be screened for possible cocaine use.

Comments

Only two studies were identified that related to dermatological conditions and cocaine use. More studies are needed to clarify whether the findings of these two can be generalized to a larger population

Nutritional and metabolic disease

Several epidemiological articles appeared in the PubMed literature between 1988 and 2008 related to nutritional and metabolic conditions associated with cocaine use. Studies found related to diabetes mellitus are included in the section below on endocrine disorders.

Nutritional studies

In 1990 Mohs *et al.* published a review article on the nutritional effects of a number of abused drugs, including marijuana, heroin, cocaine, and nicotine. Cocaine is one of several drugs that affect food selection and intake during illicit drug use and withdrawal. Cocaine is typically seen as an appetite depressant, leading to weight loss.

Rosse *et al.* (2005) studied whether BMI is related to cocaine-induced psychosis (CIP). Forty patients with CIP and 29 cocaine users (controls), all in a research substance abuse unit, participated in the study. Height, weight, and BMI were determined. The study showed that those with CIP had statistically lower BMIs than individuals without CIP ($p = 0.003$). The percentile ideal body weight was also different in the two groups. The authors suggested that a low BMI might be associated with an increased risk in developing CIP, or that a high BMI is protective against developing CIP. They also suggested possible mechanisms for the low BMI in the CIP group, including cocaine's effect on tumor necrosis factor (an anorexigenic cytokine), the cocaine-and-amphetamine-regulated transcript (CART), or suppression of neuropeptide Y (an appetite-stimulating peptide), and defects in nicotinic cholinergic neural transmission. All four of these are associated with appetite and body weight but are also implicated in having a role in idiopathic psychoses.

Comments

As reported by Mohs *et al.* 1990 and others, cocaine and other illicit drugs can affect food intake and nutritional status. Cocaine use may be associated with changes in appetite and inadequate nutritional intake; however, very little has appeared on this topic in the PubMed literature in the past 20 years.

More studies are needed to determine the relationship between BMI and CIP, as described by Rosse *et al.* (2005). Some recent research (Hubert *et al.* (2008; Jaworski & Jones 2006; Rogge *et al.* 2008; Vicentic & Jones 2007) has described the action of CART and provides some insight into the relationship of this neurotransmitter and cocaine. Although CART is widely distributed throughout the body, in the CNS it has a predominant role in the ventral tegmental area (part of the mesolimbic dopamine system), the nucleus accumbens (where CART blunts cocaine's effects and may oppose an increase in dopamine signaling), and the ventral pallidum. The CART family is thought to regulate food intake, aid in maintaining body weight, and have a role in the reward and motivation effects of food and psychostimulants. The CARTs may also have a role in endocrine function.

Metabolic disorders and cocaine use

Five articles related to metabolic disorders and cocaine use published between 1988 and 2008 were reviewed that addressed plasma cholinesterase levels, adrenergic crisis, urinary CK, and acid–base balance associated with cocaine use. A number of studies were also reviewed that addressed hyperthermia, rhabdomyolysis, acute cocaine toxicity, and excited delirium. This last group of studies is discussed at the end of this section. Two studies by Hoffman *et al.* examined the role of cocaine and plasma cholinesterase activity. Hoffman *et al.* (1992) looked at the relationship of plasma cholinesterase (pseudocholinesterase) and life-threatening cocaine toxicity. All patients ($n = 187$) presenting in an emergency room with cocaine toxicity during a three-month period were included in this case–control prospective study. The cases were separated by severity into a life-threatening group or a non-life-threatening group based on certain criteria. A third group of non-cocaine users comprised the controls. Plasma cholinesterase levels were measured electrometrically and the levels for the three groups were analyzed. The lowest level of the enzyme (in Michel units per liter [U/L]) was found in the life-threatening toxicity group (mean, 682 ± 277 U/L), and the highest level in the controls (mean, 1058 ± 385 U/L). The group with non-life threatening cocaine toxicity fell between these (mean, 904 ± 279 U/L). In an ANOVA analysis, all three groups were statistically significantly different from one another ($p < 0.05$). The authors hypothesize that the risk of life-threatening cocaine toxicity was associated with a low plasma cholinesterase level.

In a subsequent study, Hoffman *et al.* (1998) further explored whether plasma cholinesterase levels were a factor in developing life-threatening cocaine toxicity, a consequence of cocaine use, or a confounding variable. Nine patients who used approximately 2 g of cocaine for at least one year prior to the study were enrolled in this study. After being drug free for two days, the subjects smoked cocaine for four days (≤ 405 mg in five hours/day) and then were drug free for two more days. Blood for plasma cholinesterase measurement was drawn at 9 am and 4 pm daily; there was no difference in the daily plasma cholines-terase between these two times. The baseline plasma cholinesterase was 265–930 U/L. From day one to day 8, the plasma enzyme level increased by 112 ± 100 U/L ($p = 0.025$). There were no differences between the plasma cholinesterase levels on the days of high cocaine use and those of low use. Hoffman *et al.* suggested that because the enzyme level did not change as the result of cocaine use, but did increase during the time the patients participated in the study, cocaine studies conducted in inpatient settings may be affected by a rise in pseudocholinesterase.

Merigian *et al.* (1994) reported on five cases of adrenergic crisis precipitated by crack cocaine use. All five patients presented with adrenergic crisis after a latent period and after using cocaine in a variety of amounts and routes of intake. Symptoms typically were hypertension, tachycardia, hyperthermia, agitation, and generalized seizures. Some patients had ECG changes suggestive of cardiac ischemia but plasma CK-MB was normal. Patients were treated with a rapid acting benzodiazepine and adrenolysis with a cardioselective β_1-blocker. One patient died from complications related to status epilepticus. The authors suggested that prompt treatment is needed when cocaine-using patients present with adrenergic crisis.

In a retrospective analysis, Warrian *et al.* (1992) studied urinary CK in healthy heavy crack users. Urine samples were collected for 20 days and once weekly for 12 weeks from 36 African American males. Average CK levels for the 464 samples collected was 397 IU/L (SD, 784) and 19% of the samples were > 500 IU/L. If the subjects had medical conditions that could interfere with the CK samples or were taking other drugs concurrently, their urine samples and CK data were excluded. When samples from alcohol users were excluded from the remaining samples, a significant relationship was found between the urine cocaine metabolites and an elevated CK level. The authors suggested that crack cocaine is associated with significant quantitative effect on CK levels.

One study assessed acid–base balance in 156 patients with cocaine toxicity admitted to emergency departments (Stevens *et al.* 1994). Arterial blood gases were within the normal range (pH 7.35–7.45) for 81 (52%), indicated acidosis (pH 6.4–7.35) in 51 (33%), and indicated alkalosis (pH > 7.45) in 23 (15%). Of the acidotic patients, 33 had metabolic acidosis (bicarbonate 14 ± 6 mmol/L) and 18 had respiratory acidosis with hypoventilation. The patients with alkalosis had primarily respiratory alkalosis, with tachypnea and a low partial pressure of carbon dioxide. Signs and symptoms seen in these patients included chest pain, shortness of breath, a depressed mental state, trauma, and seizures. The authors concluded that acid–base imbalances occur commonly with cocaine toxicity, regardless of the route of cocaine administration, and arterial blood gases should be assessed in the toxic patient.

These studies on metabolic disorders are given in Table 3.36.

Comments

Five studies were reviewed that covered four different topics. The two studies on plasma cholinesterase had small sample sizes (five and nine patients each). More studies are needed to determine the patterns of plasma cholinesterase in cocaine users (e.g., bingers, chronic users) to learn more about the variations in this enzyme. Since plasma cholinesterase converts cocaine to ecgonine methyl ester (a mild vasodilator), it would be interesting to determine whether the decrease in blood pressure after cocaine use is related to increased cocaine metabolism and ecognine methyl ester production. Further study comparing cocaine users might provide more epidemiological support for the role of plasma cholinesterase and hypotension seen in some users.

The single study on adrenergic crisis in crack cocaine users also had only five subjects, who appeared to have signs and symptoms similar to those seen in hypertensive crisis, preeclampsia, and renal disorders (see above). The signs and symptoms may result from the

Table 3.36 Nutritional and metabolic disorders

Study	Method	Sample	Incidence	Results
Hoffman et al. (1992)	Cohort prevalence study Cocaine toxicity and plasma cholinesterase Measurement of plasma cholinesterase	Life-threatening cocaine toxicity, cocaine users without life-threatening cocaine toxicity, non-cocaine users	Lowest level of plasma cholinesterase in those with life-threatening toxicity, highest level in controls; three groups differed statistically ($p < 0.05$)	Cocaine use did not change enzyme level
Hoffman et al. (1998)	Convenience sample, descriptive study Fluctuations of plasma cholinesterase in cocaine smokers	9 healthy cocaine users, 2 g cocaine/week for at least 1 year: drug-free day 1 and 2, smoked cocaine for 4 days, drug-free for 2 more days	No difference between 9 am and 4 pm levels of the enzyme during 8 days; baseline level of enzyme increased from day 1 to day 8	
Merigian et al. (1994)	Case series Adrenergic crisis and cocaine use	5 cocaine users	Signs/symptoms: hypertension, tachycardia, hyperthermia, agitation, generalized seizure activity; 1 death from complications of status epilepticus	Prompt treatment of cardiovascular, neurological signs/symptoms necessary
Mohs et al. (1990)	Literature review Nutritional effects of illicit drugs		The effects of a number of illicit drugs on nutrition are described; cocaine can affect food selection and is an appetite suppressant	
Rosse et al. (2005)	Case-control study BMI and CIP Height, weight, BMI measurements	Cocaine users: 40 with CIP, 29 without CIP	BMI lower in CIP group than controls (23.1 vs. 25.4 kg/m^2; $p = 0.003$); percentile ideal body weight also different in the two groups	Low BMI may lead to CIP-prone condition, or high BMI may be protective
Stevens et al. (1994)	Descriptive study Blood gas analysis in cocaine users	156 cocaine users in ER for chest pain, shortness of breath, decreased mental state, trauma, seizures	81 (52%) pH normal (7.35–7.45), 51 (33%) acidosis (< 7.35) (33 metabolic acidosis, 18 respiratory acidosis), 23 (15%) alkalosis, respiratory with tachypnea	Acid–base imbalances common with cocaine toxicity regardless of route of administration
Warrian et al. (1992)	Retrospective analysis Urinary CK in asymptomatic cocaine users	36 African American men, 464 urine samples	Mean CK 397 IU/L (SD, 784); 19% > 500 IU/L. Excluding samples from alcohol users, significant association between urine cocaine metabolites and urine CK	Crack cocaine may significantly affect CK levels

BMI, body mass index; CIP, cocaine-induced psychosis; CK, creatinine phosphokinase; ER, emergency room.

vasoconstrictive properties of cocaine and stimulation of the dopaminergic and sympathetic nervous systems.

Urinary levels of CK were evaluated in 36 heavy crack users. From the findings in this study, it appears that chronic crack users may have elevated levels of CK. This might have implications in diagnostic testing for rhabdomyolysis, renal pathology, or cardiac ischemia. Further studies of CK levels in larger samples of cocaine users might help in understanding the implications of these elevated levels.

The last study, on acid–base imbalances in cocaine toxicity, reflects on the effects of large doses of cocaine. Acidosis could be related to vasoconstriction and decreased tissue oxygenation and depressed respiratory function. Alkalosis could be reflective of the tachypnea in agitated cocaine intoxication. Health practitioners should be aware of likelihood of these imbalances when treating patients with cocaine toxicity.

Hyperthermia, rhabdomyolysis, excited delirium, and cocaine toxicity

Crandall et al. (2002) studied the mechanisms that lead to cocaine-induced hyperthermia in humans. In a randomized, double-blind placebo-controlled crossover study carried out in a cardiovascular physiology laboratory, seven healthy cocaine-naive individuals each received intranasal cocaine (2 mg/kg body weight) and a lidocaine placebo (2 mg/kg) during passive heat stress. The physiological measurements were esophageal temperature monitoring, skin blood flow assessment, and measurement of sweat rate. The subjects' perception of heat was also recorded. The findings showed that during heat stress, cocaine significantly increased esophageal temperature ($p < 0.001$), demonstrated by a rightward shift in the temperature threshold for cutaneous vasodilatation (37.37 °C for cocaine, 37.06 °C for lidocaine; $p = 0.01$). A rightward shift in temperature threshold also occurred for sweating (37.38 °C for cocaine, 37.07 °C for lidocaine; $p = 0.002$). Cocaine also impaired the subjects' perception of thermal discomfort. The authors concluded that cocaine's mechanism of increased body heat in passive heating situations was related to impaired compensatory vasodilation and sweating. Altered heat perception could also impair cocaine-exposed individuals' ability to make appropriate adjustments when in environments of high heat.

Menaker et al. (2008) described a case of cocaine-induced excited delirium with hyperthermia in which the individual survived and was neurologically intact after aggressive efforts to lower the individual's body temperature. Ice packs, gastric lavage, and bilateral chest cavity lavage with chest tubes were used to lower the core temperature, which was 42.6 °C at the time of hospitalization. The patient did have a positive toxicology screen for cocaine and did develop rhabdomyolysis, renal failure, and coagulation abnormalities.

Blaho et al. (2000) studied the prevailing hypothesis that hyperthermia may accelerate cocaine metabolism and decrease the drug's half-life. In two patients with hyperthermia, agitation, and cardiovascular abnormalities, serial cocaine blood levels were measured with mass spectrometry. However, using pharmacokinetic modeling, they found no significant change in the half-life of cocaine in the presence of hyperthermia.

Tanvetyanon et al. (2001) described a case of a risperidone-treated schizophrenic patient who developed hyperthermia and chronic pancerebellar syndrome after cocaine use. Since cocaine had been reported to cause hyperthermia, the authors hypothesized that use of cocaine induced the hyperthermia and cerebellar dysfunction.

Occurrences of rhabdomyolysis were discussed above under urological disease as this condition is related to renal failure associated with cocaine use. However, a variety of conditions can be associated with rhabdomyolysis, including trauma, such as crushing

Table 3.37 Cocaine-related conditions involving hyperthermia and rhabdomyolysis

	Cocaine-associated rhabdomyolysis	Excited delirium	Acute cocaine toxicity
Typical signs, symptoms	Delirium, excitement, hyperthermia	Delirium, excitement, hyperthermia	Agitation, hypertension, hyperthermia, seizures, tachycardia
Additional signs, symptoms		Aggressive behavior, bizarre/violent behavior, paranoia, respiratory collapse, unexpected strength	
Route of ingestion	Smoking, injection	Smoking, injection	Not limited to any one route
Demographics	Chronic cocaine user, male, obese, young age	Chronic cocaine user, male, obese, young age	
Associated with			Cocaine overdose, rupture of ingested or body-stuffed packets
Physiological mechanism	Altered dopamine processing	Altered dopamine processing, hyperdopaminergic state	Cocaine toxic effects, increased adrenergic response
Blood cocaine levels	Significantly lower than in cocaine overdose	Significantly lower than in cocaine overdose	Elevated cocaine and benzoylecgonine
Also known as		Excited delirium (fatal, cocaine-related), agitated delirium, cocaine-induced psychosis	

injury; immobilization; exercise, particularly intense exercise; extremes in environmental temperature leading to hypo- and hyperthermia; infection, including those caused by influenza virus, Epstein–Barr virus, and cytomegalovirus; drugs, including illicit drugs, statins, alcohol, and antipsychotic drugs; and toxins, including those associated with some bee stings, snake, and spider bites.

Rhabdomyolysis has also been linked to hyperthermia found in several cocaine-related conditions, including cocaine-associated rhabdomyolysis, fatal excited delirium, and acute cocaine toxicity. Fatal excited delirium was mentioned above under urological diseases as a condition that can lead to rhabdomyolysis and ARF in some cocaine users. Table 3.37 illustrates the typical findings in each of these three conditions.

The relationship among three conditions (cocaine-associated rhabdomyolysis, fatal excited delirium, and acute cocaine toxicity) is inconclusive. However, among the articles reviewed, there is some agreement on the possible causes of the signs and symptoms associated with each condition. Hyperthermia may be caused by downregulation of cell membrane dopamine transporters, which, in some chronic cocaine users, increases the risk of excited delirium. The dopamine D_2 receptors that are associated with lowering the body temperature are particularly vulnerable, leading to excessive dopamine in the synapse. The deficit of D_2 receptors in the temperature-regulating centers and the abundance of synaptic dopamine lead to an increase in D_1 receptor activity and an elevated body temperature. Other risk factors include a high environmental temperature and an elevated BMI.

Long-term (chronic) use of cocaine is a risk factor for the development of both cocaine-associated rhabdomyolysis and excited delirium. Acute cocaine toxicity is related to the toxic effects of excessive levels of the drug, leading to CNS, cardiovascular, and respiratory complications. Adrenergic stimulation has a major role in these outcomes.

Ruttenber *et al.* (1999) hypothesized that cocaine-associated rhabdomyolysis and fatal excited delirium are different stages of the same syndrome. They both differ from acute cocaine toxicity by the absence or rare occurrence of seizure activity.

Wetli and Fishbain (1985) were among the first to describe CIP as a syndrome with paranoia, hyperthermia, and bizarre violent behavior accompanied by unexpected strength, and often death within an hour of physical restraint. This condition is often seen in police-related situations where violent individuals are restrained and subsequently die without evidence of internal trauma or police abuse. Of seven individuals described by the authors, five died. Blood cocaine levels were 10 times lower than the cocaine level frequently found in cocaine toxicity. Subsequently to publication of this article, a number of descriptors have been used for this condition, including Bell's mania, fatal excited delirium, cocaine-related excited delirium, and agitated delirium.

Similar syndromes with mental excitement include "exhaustive mania," first described in 1849 by Luther Bell (Kraines 1934), who reported on over 40 cases of death related to mental excitement. Neuroleptic malignant syndrome was the name used to describe a syndrome associated with fatal reactions to the administration of dopamine antagonists or withdrawal of dopamine agonist drugs (Levinson & Simpson 1986). However, one characteristic of this syndrome is muscle rigidity. Although individuals with excited delirium may also have rigidity, the rigidity is typically brief and often precedes respiratory collapse. Excited delirium, neuroleptic malignant syndrome, and exhaustive mania may be variants of the same syndrome. Besides cocaine, methamphetamines and MDMA have also been linked to excited delirium.

A 1997 study by Ruttenber *et al.* compared 58 individuals with excited delirium with 125 patients who died from accidental cocaine overdoses. The individuals with excited delirium were more likely to die in police custody and receive medical treatment before their death, were frequently younger than cocaine overdose victims, were obese males, experienced hyperthermia, and died in the summer. The serum levels of cocaine and benzoylecgonine were not significantly different in the patients seen in the emergency department and those dying from accidental cocaine overdose. The authors hypothesized that the emergency department deaths were related to dopamine dysfunction associated with chronic cocaine use.

Ross (1998) reviewed 61 cases of excited delirium that occurred between 1988 and 1997. All deaths occurred within one hour of restraint because of violent behavior. Death often occurred during transport to medical facilities or at the scene of the disturbance that precipitated the initial police response. Ross hypothesized that acute cocaine toxicity could have contributed to the altered behavior and deaths in some of these individuals.

Stratton *et al.* (2001) described 18 individuals who died after being restrained because of violent behavior. After struggling, the individuals stopped struggling, displayed agonal breathing, and had a cardiopulmonary arrest. Stimulant drug use, chronic disease, and obesity were commonly associated with these individuals. Although various cardiac abnormalities occurred, the most common was ventricular tachycardia (but with the absence of ventricular fibrillation) followed by cardiac standstill. All 18 were associated with out-of-hospital physical restraint.

These studies are summarized in Table 3.38.

Table 3.38 Nutritional and metabolic disorders: hyperthermia, rhabdomyolysis, excited delirium, and cocaine toxicity

Study	Method	Sample	Incidence	Results
Blaho et al. (2000)	Serial concentration study: half-life of cocaine Serum cocaine, metabolites Mass spectrophotometry	Two patients with excited delirium: hyperthermia, agitation, cardiovascular abnormalities	Pharmacokinetic modeling used to show half-life of cocaine not affected by hyperthermia; one patient died	Hyperthermia did not alter half-life of cocaine; amount and route of drug administration not associated with catastrophic outcomes
Crandall et al. (2002)	Random, double-blind, placebo-controlled crossover trial Hyperthermia mechanisms	7 healthy cocaine-naive volunteers given 2 mg/kg body weight intranasal cocaine or 2 mg/kg lidocaine as placebo	Cocaine increased esophageal temperature during heat stress ($p < 0.001$); rightward shift in ETT for onset of cutaneous vasodilation (cocaine 37.37 °C, lidocaine 37.06 °C; $p = 0.01$); rightward shift in ETT for sweating (cocaine 37.38 °C, lidocaine 37.07 °C; $p = 0.002$)	Hyperthermia related to impaired heat dissipation: impaired sweating and vasodilation, impaired heat perception
Kraines (1935)	Descriptive study, Bell's mania	Description of Bell's case from 1849	Bell's mania: sudden onset, excessive overactivity, profound sleepiness, rapid speech, delusions, transient hallucinations; often fatal outcome; can last 3 to 6 weeks	Also known as typhomania, acute delirious mania, delirium grave, acute delirium, specific febrile delirium, collapse delirium Not necessarily associated with cocaine use
Levinson & Simpson (1986)	Case series Neuroleptic malignant syndrome	39 patients divided into 3 groups: those with medical problems that could cause fever, those with medical problems less likely related to fever, those with other medical disorders	Extrapyramidal symptoms associated with dehydration, infection, pulmonary embolus, rhabdomyolysis; 3 patients died	Hypotheses for development of fever: psychiatric illness, altered dopaminergic thermoregulation, peripheral and central effects associated with muscle contraction Suggests many causes of extrapyramidal symptoms with fever, not all neuroleptic malignant syndrome
Menaker et al. (2008)	Case report	41-year-old cocaine user with cocaine-induced agitated delirium with hyperthermia (rectal temperature, 42.6 °C); positive cocaine toxicology screen	Cooling techniques: ice packs, gastric lavage, bilateral chest cavity lavage with multiple chest tubes	ER and critical care teams, aggressive approach successful in decreasing core temperature; patient survived neurologically intact

Reference	Study type	Sample	Findings	Conclusions
Merigian et al. (1994)	Case series; Adrenergic crisis	5 patients, crack cocaine ingestion	Adrenergic crisis: hypertension, tachycardia, hyperthermia, agitation, generalized seizure activity; ECG showed cardiac ischemia without CK-MB elevation; one death (status epilepticus)	Crack cocaine toxicity underappreciated; prompt treatment needed to reverse cardiovascular, neurological signs and symptoms
Ross (1998)	Literature review; Excited delirium	Review of 61 deaths from excited delirium deaths reported in the literature	All fought with, were restrained by police; all died during transport or at crime scene; survival time frequently < 1 h	Physical restraint and acute cocaine toxicity may have contributed to deaths
Ruttenber et al. (1997)	Descriptive study; Evidence for mechanism of cocaine toxicity	Review of all cocaine-related deaths from 1969 to 1990 in Dade County FL: 58 excited delirium, 125 accidental cocaine overdose	Excited delirium decedents: likely to be younger, more males than overdose deaths; also received medical treatment before death, survived longer, had hyperthermia, died in the summer Blood levels of cocaine, benzoylecgonine not statistically different between the two groups	Findings consistent with hypothesis that dopamine dysfunction in chronic cocaine users is likely to lead to agitation, delirium, hyperthermia, rhabdomyolysis, sudden death
Ruttenber et al. (1999)	Literature review; Rhabdomyolysis and excited delirium	Review of cases: 150 rhabdomyolysis, 58 FED, 125 fatal acute cocaine toxicity	Decedents from rhabdomyolysis and FED similar in demographics, signs and symptoms Rhabdomyolysis victims were not similar to fatal acute cocaine toxic victims in demographics, signs and symptoms	Concluded that cocaine-associated rhabdomyolysis and FED were the same syndrome but at different stages of the illness; hypothesized that dopamine dysfunction in chronic cocaine users was the cause of the syndrome, and not cocaine toxicity
Stratton et al. (2001)	Case series; Identification, ranking of factors associated with excited delirium	18 sudden deaths, wrists and ankles bound, restrained behind back; 196 survivors of excited delirium	Sudden death associated with victim struggle, cessation of struggling and development of respiratory distress, then cardiopulmonary arrest (ventricular tachycardia but not ventricular fibrillation); 78% also positive for stimulant drugs; 56% had chronic disease; 56% were obese	Concluded that death in excited delirium is not infrequent outside of hospital; associated factors leading to death are predictable

Table 3.38 *Cont.*

Study	Method	Sample	Incidence	Results
Tanvetyanon et al. (2001)	Case report Hyperthermia and pancerebellar syndrome	1 chronic schizophrenic taking risperidone (dopamine antagonist)	After using cocaine, developed hyperthermia, abnormal motor function and chronic pancerebellar syndrome	Both neuroleptics and cocaine associated with hyperthermia; cocaine may have caused hyperthermia, pancerebellar syndrome in this case
Wetli & Fishbain (1985)	Case series Cocaine-induced psychosis and sudden death	7 recreational cocaine users with excited delirium	Symptoms: bizarre/violent behavior, intense paranoia, hyperthermia, exaggerated strength Sudden respiratory collapse, often within 1 h of restraint Serum cocaine levels 10 times lower than that found in acute cocaine deaths	Excited delirium may be related to acute cocaine toxicity; victims require prompt treatment, including cocaine antagonists, and respiratory support

CK-MB, creatine kinase isozyme; ECG, electrocardiogram; ER, emergency room; ETT, esophageal temperature threshold; FED, fatal excited delirium.

Comments

The study on hyperthermia by Crandall *et al.* (2002) provides a possible physiological explanation for the altered normal body response to an elevated temperature. The study by Tanvetyanon *et al.* (2001) suggested that cocaine was the cause of hyperthermia that occurred in a risperidone-treated patient. However, risperidone is a strong dopamine antagonist that has a high affinity for D_2 receptors and some serotonergic receptors. The combination of this neuroleptic and cocaine may have been the trigger for the hyperthermic response.

The studies on hyperthermia, rhabdomyolysis, and deaths related to chronic cocaine use demonstrate similar signs and symptoms. There is some evidence that cocaine-associated rhabdomyolysis, excited delirium, and neuroleptic malignant syndrome are variants of the same syndrome. The downregulation of D_2 receptors in the temperature control center and the overstimulation of D_1 receptors by excessive synaptic dopamine appear to be common pathophysiological features in these conditions. Acute cocaine toxicity, however, is more commonly associated with excessive blood levels of cocaine and its metabolites and is associated with an increased adrenergic response. In all of these conditions, fatal outcomes are possible.

Endocrine system disease

Four epidemiological studies (two on prolactin and two on diabetic ketoacidosis [DKA]) were found in a review of PubMed publishing between 1988 and 2008. The two prolactin studies provide contradictory data for the relationship between prolactin levels and treatment outcomes. The first study, by Kranzler & Wallington (1992) found elevated prolactin levels in 13 of 33 patients (39%) in an inpatient treatment program. The prolactin levels were not significantly correlated with cocaine use or craving. The authors suggested that hyperprolactinemia is not an outcome of the dopamine depletion seen with chronic cocaine use. However, hyperprolactinemia was associated with an early treatment discharge, while gender, use of other drugs or alcohol, and antisocial personality disorder were not.

In a case–control study by Patkar *et al.* (2004), prolactin levels of 141 African American cocaine users were compared with 60 similar controls. The Addiction Severity Index (ASI) was used to assess drug use. Subjects were tested during a 12-week treatment program and at a 6-month follow-up visit. The basal level of prolactin was higher in the cocaine users than in the controls (9.28 ± 4.13 vs. 7.33 ± 2.94 ng/mL; $p < 0.01$). The basal prolactin level in cocaine users was positively correlated with composite scores on the ASI-drug ($r = 0.38$; $p < 0.01$), ASI-alcohol ($r = 0.19$; $p < 0.05$), and ASI-psychological ($r = 0.25$; $p < 0.01$). The baseline prolactin level was also positively correlated with the amount of cocaine use ($r = 0.18$; $p < 0.05$). Basal prolactin levels in the cocaine users were not significantly correlated with treatment days, sessions attended, dropout rate, or negative drug screens. Nor were prolactin levels associated with ASI scores during the drug treatment program or at the 6-month follow-up visit. Prolactin levels were not a predictor of treatment outcomes. The researchers concluded that prolactin levels may be affected by cocaine use but were not useful in predicting outcomes.

Two studies reported on risk factors for DKA. Warner *et al.* (1998) carried out a retrospective case–control study with 27 cocaine users and 85 non-users hospitalized for DKA. The 27 cocaine users were admitted for DKA 102 times (mean, 3.78) while the 85 non-users were admitted 154 times (mean, 1.81); the difference was significant at $p = 0.03$.

The cocaine users were less likely than the non-users to have a precipitating illness ($p < 0.001$) and were more likely to have missed taking insulin ($p < 0.001$). Although the cocaine users had higher blood glucose on admission (5.934 mg/L vs. 5.311 mg/L), the severity of DKA and treatment outcomes were not different. Based on the findings, a risk factor for DKA appears to be cocaine use. The underlying reason is unclear; however insulin deficit or effects of other hormones may be a cause; non-compliance with treatment could also explain the onset of DKA.

In a 2007 retrospective analysis, Nyenwe *et al.* studied 168 patients, average age 38.6 ± 14.8 years, admitted over a three-year period for DKA; 54 (32%) had type 2 diabetes and 44 (26%) were newly diagnosed. There were 219 episodes of DKA. There was a statistically significant difference ($p < 0.0001$) in recurrence rate for DKA in the active cocaine users (169%) compared with non-users (39%). Active cocaine use (OR 4.38; $p = 0.001$), non-compliance (OR 1.96; $p = 0.05$), and Hispanic ethnicity (OR 0.40; $p = 0.005$) were identified as risks for recurrent DKA. Non-compliance (44%) and infections (26%) were the most common precipitating causes of DKA. Cocaine use, marijuana use, and cigarette use were most commonly associated with non-compliance. The authors recommend that patients with recurrent DKA be screened for illicit drugs.

Table 3.39 summarizes these studies on prolactin and DKA.

Comments

The two prolactin studies provide some evidence that prolactin levels are correlated with cocaine use. Both studies showed higher basal levels of prolactin in cocaine users. This finding supports the laboratory research and mechanism of prolactin release from the prolactin-releasing cells in the anterior pituitary. Prolactin release is normally suppressed by dopamine (a prolactin-inhibitory factor). Chronic drug use may cause dysregulation of the hypothalamus and alter normal regulatory patterns. Hyperprolactinemia can result in low testosterone levels, with resulting decreased libido and sexual potency in males. In females, hyperprolactinemia can suppress ovulation and increase risk of bone loss because of lower estrogen levels. The two studies provide some contradictory findings: prolactin is not correlated with cocaine use or craving, prolactin levels increased with the quantity of cocaine use; hyperprolactinemia was associated with early discharge from treatment, prolactin was not a predictor of treatment outcomes. More research is needed to determine whether prolactin can be used as a marker for determining the effectiveness of treatment and the role cocaine has in prolactin secretion. Use of other drugs such as opiates and selective serotonin-reuptake inhibitors can also cause hyperprolactinemia, as well as stress, chronic renal failure, and epileptic seizures. These conditions need to be controlled for in studies related to prolactin levels and cocaine use.

The two studies on DKA in cocaine users support the risky behavior seen in cocaine users – in this case, failure to comply with treatment (insulin use). Diabetic cocaine users were much more likely to be hospitalized with recurrence of DKA than non-users, and were less likely to have concurrent illnesses that would precipitate DKA. Assessment of cocaine use in patients with recurrent DKA may be helpful in identifying drug users and guide treatment.

Immune system disease

One case report was found in the PubMed database published between 1988 and 2008 describing the relationship between the immune system and cocaine use. This is a 1998 case

Table 3.39 Endocrine disorders

Study	Method	Sample	Incidence	Results
Kranzler & Wallington (1992)	Descriptive study Prolactin levels and early treatment discharge Serum prolactin	33 inpatients in cocaine addiction treatment program	13 (39%) cocaine users with elevated prolactin levels; no correlation found between elevated prolactin and cocaine use or craving; elevated prolactin related to early discharge	More studies needed to identify etiology of elevated prolactin
Nyenwe et al. (2007)	Retrospective study Cocaine use and DKA	168 diabetics with 219 episodes of DKA (96 males, 72 females, age 38.6 ± 14.8 years): 54 (32%) type 2 diabetes mellitus, 44 (26%) new-onset diabetes	Recurrence rate for DKA 169% in cocaine users and; 9% in non-users ($p < 0.0001$); risk for recurrent DKA: active cocaine use (OR 4.38, $p = 0.001$); non-compliance (OR 1.96; $p = 0.05$); Hispanic (OR 0.40; $p = 0.005$) Non-compliance associated with cocaine use ($p = 0.008$), marijuana use ($p = 0.04$), cigarette use ($p = 0.01$)	Strong association between cocaine use and DKA; patients with recurrent DKA episodes should be screened for cocaine use
Patkar et al. (2004)	Case–control study Prolactin levels and treatment outcomes Basal prolactin, Addiction Severity Index	141 African American cocaine users, 60 African American controls	Basal prolactin level: cocaine users 9.28 ± 4.13 ng/mL, controls 7.33 ± 2.94 ng/mL ($t = 3.77; p < 0.01$) Correlation studies ASI: drug, $r = 0.38$, $p < 0.01$; alcohol, $r = 0.19$, $p < 0.05$; psychiatric symptoms, $r = 0.25$, $p < 0.01$ Prolactin level and quantity of cocaine use: $r = 0.18, p < 0.05$	Cocaine may influence prolactin levels; prolactin is not a predictor of treatment outcomes
Warner et al. (1998)	Retrospective case–control study Cocaine use and DKA	27 cocaine users, 85 non-users	Cocaine users compared with non-users: admissions for DKA, 102 (mean 3.78) vs. 154 (mean 1.81) ($p = 0.03$); have concurrent illness, 14.7% vs. 33.1% ($p < 0.001$); not taken insulin, 45.1% vs. 24.7% ($p < 0.001$)	No differences in severity of illness or treatment outcomes; cocaine use a risk factor for DKA (missed insulin or other hormonal factors)

ASI, Addiction Severity Index; DKA, diabetic ketoacidosis; OR, odds ratio.

report of a 46-year-old male who was a heavy cocaine user and developed scleroderma complicated by scleroderma-related renal crisis (Attoussi *et al.* 1998). No other studies related to cocaine use and sclerodermas have been identified.

Although a number of animal and in vitro cell studies have been carried out, very few controlled, longitudinal epidemiological studies have been done to clarify the association between cocaine use and changes in immune system function. However, for up to 9.5 years, Minkoff *et al.* (2008) studied the role of cocaine in the risk of detection of prevalent and incident oncogenic human papillomavirus infection in over 3100 HIV-seropositive and HIV-seronegative women. Using multivariate analyses, they found that use of crack/cocaine was associated with the viral infection (OR 1.30; 95% CI 1.09–1.55) in both HIV-sero-positive and HIV-seronegative women. There was also an increased risk for positive squamous intraepithelial lesions (OR 1.70; 95% CI 1.27–2.27) in these two groups of women.

In a longitudinal analysis of men who had sex with men, Chao *et al.* (2008) found no clinically meaningful association between drug use (including cocaine) and CD4 and CD8 T cell counts in HIV-infected or uninfected men, or the rate of conversion from HIV-negative status to HIV positive.

Irwin *et al.* (2007) studied the ability of monocytes exposed to cocaine to respond to a bacterial challenge. Macrophages of cocaine-dependent men had a decreased expression of two inflammatory cytokines: tumor necrosis factor-alpha and interleukin-6. After an injection of cocaine, there was a decreased response to lipopolysaccharide. An increase in sympathetic nervous system response (increased heart rate) was associated with decreased monocyte expression of tumor necrosis factor-alpha. Their study suggested that cocaine decreased the function of the innate immune system.

In a review of the literature, Cabral (2006) found that sigma-1 receptors may play a role in the immune modulation seen with cocaine use, and that many illicit drugs exert their effects on the immune system by altering cytokine and chemokine release from T helper cells type 1 (proinflammatory) and type 2 (anti-inflammatory). Cocaine is thought to be a weak agonist for sigma receptors.

Table 3.40 summarizes these studies on the immune system.

Comments

These studies provide some insight into the role of cocaine and an altered immune system. Several additional studies using cultured alveolar macrophages obtained from non-smokers, cigarette smokers, marijuana smokers, and crack cocaine smokers by Roth *et al.* (2004) showed that macrophages from marijuana and cocaine users were less likely to demonstrate antimicrobial activity than other smokers. They found that nitric oxide function in the macrophages of these smokers was depressed and suggested that the role of nitric oxide as an antimicrobial agent is altered in marijuana and cocaine smokers. In an earlier study, Baldwin *et al.* (1997) showed that alveolar macrophages from marijuana and cocaine smokers were less able to kill bacteria and cancer cells than macrophages from non-smokers or cigarette smokers. This finding was presumed to reflect decreased levels of tumor necrosis factor-alpha, granulocytic–macrophage colony-stimulating factor, and interleukin-6 in the macrophages.

Despite the significant findings in the studies cited, more studies are needed to clarify the role of cocaine in immune system function. It appears that there are complex nervous system and hormonal actions that might influence immunity, and these actions may need

Table 3.40 Immune system

Study	Method	Sample	Incidence	Results
Attoussi et al. (1998)	Case report Scleroderma precipitated by cocaine use	46-year-old male, heavy cocaine user	Developed scleroderma and scleroderma renal crisis after cocaine use	
Cabral (2006)	Literature review Drugs of abuse and immune modulation	Review of articles on illicit drug use and immune function	Cocaine: sigma (1) receptors may have a role in cocaine alteration of the immune system	Few epidemiological studies available for cocaine effect on immunity
Chao et al. (2008)	Longitudinal analysis of the Multicenter AIDS Cohort Study Drug use and CD4, CD8 T cells	Men having sex with men: HIV positive, HIV negative	No effect of cocaine or other illicit drugs on CD4, CD8 cell counts after adjusting for confounders	No clinical meaningful association between illicit drug use and CD4, CD8 cell counts, change from HIV-negative to HIV-positive status
Irwin et al. (2007)	Case–control study Effect of cocaine on monocyte cytokine expression Measurement of TNF-α, IL-6	Cocaine-dependent subjects, controls	Cocaine users compared with controls: monocytes of cocaine users less likely than controls to express TNF-α, IL-6; lipopolysaccharide infusion showed decreased response in monocytes in cocaine users; increase in heart rate (sympathetic nervous system) with decrease in TNF-α	Cocaine alters autonomic activity, decreases innate immune function
Minkoff et al. (2008)	Longitudinal study HPV infections in HIV-positive and HIV-negative women who use cocaine Follow-up 6 months to up to 9.5 years PAP smear, cervicovaginal lavage samples, health/behavior questionnaires	2278 HIV-seropositive women, 826 high-risk but HIV-seronegative women	Cocaine use associated with HPV (OR 1.30; 95% CI 1.09–1.55) and HPV-positive squamous intraepithelial lesions (OR 1.70; 95% CI 1.27–2.27)	Cocaine associated with prevalent and incident oncogenic HPV infection and intraepithelial lesions

CI, confidence interval; HIV, human immunodeficiency virus; HPV, human papillomavirus; IL-6, interleukin-6; OR, odds ratio; TNF-α, tumor necrosis factor-alpha.

to be clarified before epidemiological studies can be carried out to determine meaningful risks for cocaine users.

Environmental disease

A number of epidemiological studies were reviewed that focused on trauma and illicit drug use, including cocaine, and also provided information about body stuffers and packers and consequences of packet rupture. These studies are discussed in the following subsections.

Trauma

Twenty-six studies reported on trauma situations that involved cocaine use. Most of the studies were prospective cross-sectional studies, chart reviews, retrospective analyses, or a review of the literature. In the literature review, Macdonald *et al.* (2003) examined a variety of studies describing injury risk in cocaine and cannabis users. They found that both drugs are associated with intentional injuries and injuries in general. However, while cannabis users tended to have similar proportions of users involved with fatal and non-fatal injuries, collisions, violence, and injuries in general, cocaine users tended to have significantly more intentional injuries (28.7%) than motor vehicle injuries as the driver (4.5%).

In a chart review of 114 deaths where the subject tested positive for cocaine (Budd 1989), 70 (61.4%) died a violent death, with 48 (68%) of these dying from a shooting or stabbing. He also found that 20% of those not dying from a violent death had acted violently prior to their death. Budd concluded there was an association between cocaine use and violent behavior.

In a chart review of 452 patients visiting the emergency room with trauma and 160 victims of trauma from the medical examiners' records, Rivara *et al.* (1989) studied the association between trauma and drug use. Drug screens were positive for marijuana, cocaine, opiates, benzodiazepines, and alcohol. One-third of all the patients tested positive for alcohol. Marijuana was the most common drug for patients from both settings. Alcohol and drugs were most commonly found in males, younger persons, and victims of assault or traffic accidents.

Sloan *et al.* (1989) studied 623 toxicology screens of patients admitted to a trauma center: 86% were positive, with 53% positive for ethanol, 37% positive for cannabis, and 34% positive for cocaine. The OR for illicit drug use by blacks before trauma was 1.9–4.2 ($p < 0.005$); for those aged 17–40 years, the OR for positive urine toxicity screens was 4.7–16.8 ($p < 0.001$).

Clark & Harchelroad (1991) conducted a retrospective analysis of 177 trauma patients and their toxicology screens. They found positive toxicology screens in 127 (72%); of these 20% tested positive for ethanol only, 45% for drugs other than alcohol, 21% for cocaine; and 35% for alcohol and at least one other drug.

McGonigal *et al.* (1993) conducted a review of medical examiners' records to study trends in firearm deaths over a five-year period in Philadelphia. In 1985, 145 firearm homicides occurred, compared with 324 in 1990 (a 123% increase). In 1990, the homicides primarily involved young, black males. In 90% of the deaths, handguns were used. There also were differences in intoxication of the victims: in 1985, 54% were intoxicated, while 61% were intoxicated in 1990. The major drug of abuse in 1990 was cocaine (39%).

A prospective age-matched control study by Loiselle *et al.* (1993) found that 65 adolescents with trauma tested positive for alcohol or illicit drugs. The average age was 15.4 years. Ethanol was detected in eight patients, benzodiazepines in eight, cocaine in five, and cannabinoids in four. More positive drugs screens were found in patients with intentional injury (21/71) than in unintentional injury (1/63).

Over a 37-month period, 854 patients were hospitalized for serious injury, according to a study by Stoduto *et al.* (1993). Drug screens were carried out on 474. Of drivers involved in motor vehicle accidents, 339 (41.3%) tested positive for drugs and 78 (16.5%) tested positive for drugs and alcohol. The most commonly found drugs were cannabinoids (13.9%), benzodiazepines (12.4%), and cocaine (5.3%). There were no differences found in the severity of injury in the trauma victims based on substance abuse.

Bailey (1993) conducted a chart review of plasma levels of cocaethylene, cocaine, and ethanol in 15 trauma patients. He found cocaethylene in all but two of the patients. He also determined that there was a statistically significant correlation between cocaethylene concentrations and cocaine ($p < 0.01$). When looking at the half-lives of cocaethylene and cocaine, he found that the plasma half-life of cocaethylene is longer than that of cocaine (reported at one hour) with cocaethylene found at 3.5, 4.5, and 5.5 hours in three patients. (Cocaethylene is the compound formed in the liver from cocaine and alcohol. Actions are similar to cocaine and may produce a greater euphoria than cocaine alone.)

A chart review by Marzuk *et al.* (1995) looked at cocaine use in fatal injuries. Of 14 843 fatal injuries in New York City over a three-year period, cocaine use was found in 18.3% of the victims and benzoylecgonine in 26.7%. From 1990 to 1992, fatal injury cocaine use was listed as one of the five leading causes of death in those aged 14–44 years in New York City. Two-thirds of cocaine-positive victims died from traumatic injury.

Of the 85 (68%) positive drugs screens in 125 adolescent trauma patients, 21 (25%) tested positive for alcohol, cocaine, or opiates (Gordon *et al.* 1996).

Regidor *et al.* (1996) carried out an interview survey of 4261 individuals in the general population, 369 cocaine users, and 215 heroin users, and assessed the prevalence of injury. They found the annual prevalence in the general population was 7.9%; in cocaine users, the prevalence for injury was 10.8%, and in heroin users the prevalence was 35.2%. They also found a statistically significant association for injury in cocaine users who also used non-heroin opiates.

Parry *et al.* (2005) carried out a cross-sectional study of drug use trends among trauma patients. Trauma admissions during four weeks in three separate years were tested for illicit drugs. Over one-half of the victims experienced violent injuries. During the three study times, 33 to 62% of the 1565 patients tested positive for at least one drug, including cocaine. The most commonly abused drugs were cannabis and methaqualone. During the third year of the study (2001) more trauma patients tested positive for illicit drugs than in the previous two years, and more violently injured patients tested positive for drugs.

Blondell *et al.* (2005) carried out a cross-sectional study looking at drug abuse in trauma patients. Alcohol and cocaine were independently associated with violence-related injuries, while opiates were independently associated with non-violence-related injuries and burns.

Siegal *et al.* (2006) studied charts and participant drug-use self-report of crack cocaine users seen in an emergency room over a three-year period: 211 individuals were seen on 643 occasions. Injury and poisoning were the most common cause of the visits (29.5%). An increased odds of visiting an emergency room was associated with times in drug treatment (OR 1.04; 95% CI 1.10–1.09), chronic disease (OR 1.46; 95% CI 1.06–1.99), and a high ASI score (OR 1.62; 95% CI 1.15–2.29).

Ch'ng *et al.* (2007) studied the drug use in individuals involved in motor vehicle accidents. Of 436 blood samples, 66% were positive in males and females between the ages of 15 and 44. Cocaine was found in 1.4%. The most commonly found drug was cannabis (46.7%), with benzodiazepines found in 15.6%, and opiates in 11%. They also found that benzodiazepines were more likely to be found in the older victims.

Narongchai et al. (2007) studied the incidence of drug abuse in individuals dying unnatural deaths in Thailand. The mean age of 153 individuals was 34 years (range, 10–76) and 92% were male. Although a variety of drugs were detected, cocaine, heroin, and morphine were not found.

In a 2001 retrospective review of a clinical toxicology database of 53 338 patients, Soderstrom et al. (2001) looked at trends in drug use in trauma victims over a three-year period. They found a 212% and 543% increase in cocaine-positive and opiate-positive patients, respectively, over the three-year period ($p < 0.001$). At the same time, there was a 152% increase in non-violent crime associated with cocaine use, and a 226% increase in violent crime associated with cocaine use. During this period, there was a decreasing trend for alcohol use.

Lindenbaum et al. (1989) studied a random sample of 169 trauma patients: 81 were involved in violent crime, with 80.3% testing positive for illicit drug use and 6.2% testing positive for alcohol. The greatest number of all trauma patients tested positive for cocaine (54.4%), with cannabis (37.2%) and ethanol (35.5%) also found in many patients.

Trauma related to specific causes

Five studies looked at drug abuse in specific situations. In a prospective study, Levy et al. (1996) explored drug use in patients with orthopedic trauma over a two-year period. Alcohol and illicit drugs were positive in 430 (56%) of the 767 patients: alcohol in 25%, cocaine in 22%, and marijuana in 21%. Those with orthopedic trauma who were also drug users had more severe injuries and longer hospitalizations than non-drug users.

Barillo & Goode (1996) conducted a retrospective analysis of fire victims and drug use. Over a seven-year period, 727 fatalities were tested for substance abuse including cocaine. Drug use was positive in 78 of 534 patients, with 75% of those drug positive being between 21 and 50 years of age. The authors suggested that, in this age group, there is a high risk of death from fire in substance abusers because of impaired functioning associated with drug use.

McGill et al. (1995) also studied substance abuse in burn injury. Positive drug screens (including a cocaine screen) were found in 161 of 398 patients with burns. Substance abusers were more likely to have a greater burn area, more inhalation injury, and increased mortality than non-drug users.

Galea et al. (2002) also conducted a trend study using medical examiners' records for an eight-year period for firearm deaths in New York City. Positive drug screens were available for 50% of the victims, and were mostly positive for cocaine, marijuana, opiates, and alcohol. In year 8, minorities were three times more likely to die from violence. Most deaths occurred in cocaine- and opiate-using Latinos and marijuana-using African Americans.

In a study by Reis et al. (2006), almost 17% of trauma victims testing positive for substance abuse tested positive for cannabis and cocaine. Cannabis was found in 33 (13.6%) of the 243 tested; cocaine was found in eight (3.3%). Benzodiazepines were detected in seven (4.2%) of those tested for this drug.

Related trauma studies

Two other studies looked at drug reporting compliance and accuracy of a rapid point-of-collection drug-testing device. Brookoff et al. (1993) conducted a retrospective study of drug reporting compliance at a hospital in line with guidelines for reporting to the US Federal Drug Abuse Warning Network (DAWN). During the time of the study, 520 patients were treated for trauma; 217 (42%) tested positive for drugs, including 82 (38%) who tested positive for cocaine. Fifty-seven victims of violent assault tested positive for cocaine. Of the 102 motor vehicle accident victims, 20 (20%) were positive for cocaine; 30% of those under the age of 40 years were cocaine-positive. The researchers found that only 48 hospital visits were reported to DAWN, indicating a significant non-compliance with reporting guidelines.

Walsh *et al.* (2004a) used a point-of-collection drug-testing device with 322 motor vehicle crash victims. The point-of-collection results correlated well with the hospital laboratory results.

These studies on trauma are summarized in Table 3.41.

Comments

It is evident that cocaine is associated with a variety of trauma situations. Cocaine was identified among the top five illicit drugs found in most of the trauma studies, especially violent death, non-violent trauma, motor vehicle accidents, firearm deaths, and severe orthopedic injuries. However, cocaine often was low (percentage) compared with the most frequently used drugs. Since the studies were published between 1989 and 2006, the use of cocaine has changed throughout these 17 years. Seven countries contributed to the research reported, including five European countries and one Asian country. The availability and use of cocaine may vary in these countries and account for some of the variance in the risk for trauma associated with cocaine use.

Body stuffers and packers

Fourteen articles were reviewed that addressed body stuffing and body packing. Four retrospective studies, including one chart review, and 10 case reports describe body stuffing, where drugs are ingested or inhaled to escape detection by law enforcement officers or other authorities, and body packing, where drugs are concealed in the body as a mode of transport. Body "pushers" have also been described who "push" drugs into the vagina or rectum. In this review, body pushers will be classified as body packers.

The first retrospective cohort study was published by Sporer & Firestone (1997). From 75 000 emergency room visits over a three-year period, 98 cases of crack cocaine body stuffing were detected. Most of the stuffers were male and under age 30. Through self-report, the crack was wrapped in plastics bags (29%) or stuffed unwrapped (28%). One to fifteen rocks were generally stuffed in one individual. Four percent of the stuffers developed seizures within two hours after ingesting the crack cocaine. More common symptoms included tachycardia without dysrhythmias (54%), high blood pressure (23%), agitation (22%), and the need for sedation (19%). No deaths were reported.

A 2002 chart review by Gill & Graham (2002) reported on 50 body-packer deaths occurring in New York City over a 10-year period. Most of the packers were 19–57 years of age (mean, 37.1), male (82%), Hispanic (66%), or black (24%). The average number of recovered packets was 46, with a range of 1 to 111. Each bag averaged 377 g, with a range of 9.4 to 1200 g/bag. Most of the deaths occurred because of acute intoxication ($n = 42$); intestinal obstruction or bowel perforation occurred in five patients. One death was related to intracerebral hemorrhage as a result of hypertension. Most of the deaths were in packers transporting opiates (42/50), while four deaths occurred in those carrying cocaine.

129

Table 3.41 Trauma

Study	Method	Sample	Incidence	Results
Bailey (1993)	Chart review Plasma levels cocaethylene, cocaine, ethanol	15 male trauma patients	Cocaethylene found in all but 2 patients; concentration significantly correlated with cocaine intake ($p < 0.01$); cocaethylene plasma half-life longer than that of cocaine (1 h); cocaethylene detected in 3 patients: 3.5, 4.5, 5.5 h	
Barillo & Goode (1996)	Retrospective analysis Fire victims and drug use	727 fatalities tested over 7 year period	Blood alcohol positive in 215/727 (29.5%); drugs positive in 78/534 (14.6%); alcohol and drugs in 36; in those aged 21 to 50 years, 75% drug positive; 58% alcohol positive	There is a high risk of death from fire in middle-aged substance abusers
Blondell et al. (2005)	Cross-sectional study Drug abuse and trauma		Alcohol and cocaine independently associated with violence-related injury; opiates independently associated with non-violence-related injuries and burns	
Brookoff et al. (1993)	Retrospective study of reports to the US Federal Drug Abuse Warning Network (DAWN) Drug reporting compliance	520 patients treated for trauma	217 (42%) tested for drugs, 82 (38%) positive for cocaine; 102 motor vehicle accidents, 20% positive for cocaine; 30% under age 40 years tested positive for cocaine; 57 victims of violent assault positive for cocaine	Only 48 hospital visits reported to DAWN; under-reporting occurred despite compliance with system guidelines
Budd (1989)	Chart review, medical examiners' offices Drug use and violent behavior	114 coroner's cases positive for cocaine	70 (61.4%) died violent death, 68% shootings, stabbings; 14 (20%) behaved violently before death	Connection found between cocaine use and violent behavior
Ch'ng et al. (2007)	Chart review, blood samples Drug use in motor vehicle accidents	436 blood samples: positive drug screen in 66% of tests from males and females 15–44 years of age	Drugs found: cannabis 46.7%, benzodiazepines 15.6%, opiates 11%, amphetamines 4.1%, methadone 3%, cocaine 1.4%	Substantial substance abuse found in trauma victims; older persons more likely to use benzodiazipines
Clark & Harchelroad (1991)	Retrospective analysis Trauma patients and toxicology screen	177 trauma patients	127/177 (72%) positive toxicology screen: 26 (20%) ethanol only, 57 (45%) drugs other than ethanol; 35% alcohol and at least one other drug Drugs: alcohol 55%, marijuana 24%, cocaine 21%, pharmaceuticals 9%	

Study	Method/focus	Sample	Findings	Conclusion
Galea et al. (2002)	Medical examiner record review 8-year period (New York City). Trends in firearm deaths		Positive drug screens in 50%; mostly cocaine, marijuana opiates, alcohol. Latino: cocaine, opiates; African American: marijuana. Minorities 3 times more likely to die from violence than whites in year 8. Most deaths: Latino, African American	Complex role of illicit drug use and firearm deaths
Gordon et al. (1996)	Chart review. Drug screen of adolescent trauma patients	125 adolescents admitted to trauma center	85 (68%) screened: 21 (25%) positive for alcohol, cocaine, opiates	
Levy et al. (1996)	Prospective study. Orthopedic trauma patients and drug use. Blood alcohol and urine drug screens	All orthopedic patients in 2-year period: screens for 767 patients	Alcohol, drugs positive in 56%: alcohol 25%, cocaine 22%, marijuana 21%	Drug-users with orthopedic trauma have more severe injuries, longer hospitalizations
Lindenbaum et al. (1989)	Random sample trauma patients. Alcohol, drug use in trauma patients	169 trauma patients	Cocaine 54.4%, cannabis 37.2%, ethanol 35.5% violent crime 81 (47.9%) (80.3% positive for illicit drugs, 6.2% for alcohol)	Illicit drugs, alcohol major factors associated with accidental and crime-related trauma
Loiselle et al. (1993)	Prospective age-matched controlled study. Adolescent trauma and drug use	Pediatric ER setting, 134 trauma patients: 22/65 positive for alcohol or illicit drugs	Average age 15.4 years for positive drug screen; of 22 testing positive, ethanol 8, benzodiazepines 8, cocaine 5, cannabinoids 4	More positive drug screens in trauma patients than controls; more positive drug screens in intentional (21/71) vs. unintentional (1/63) injury ($p < 0.001$)
Macdonald et al. (2003)	Literature review. Cannabis and cocaine use: injury risk	Studies reviewed: laboratory studies, descriptive and analytical epidemiological studies, non-clinical studies, clinical samples of drug users	Cannabis: similar proportions test positive in fatal, non-fatal injuries, collisions, violence, injuries in general. Cocaine: different proportions found (e.g., 28.7% intentional injuries; 4.5% injured drivers)	Cannabis and cocaine both associated with intentional injuries, injuries in general
Marzuk et al. (1995)	Chart review in New York City. Cocaine and fatal injuries	14 843 fatal injuries in 3 years	Cocaine in 18.3%, benzoylecgonine in 26.7%	Cocaine use one of five leading causes of death in those aged 15–44 years in New York City (1990–1992)
McGill et al. (1995)	Retrospective analysis. Thermal injury and substance use	398 with burns	161 positive drug screen (cocaine included); substance users compared with non-users: greater burn area (25% vs. 17%), more likely to have inhalation injury (29% vs. 7%), increased mortality (14% vs. 3%)	Best independent predictors of death: age, inhalation injury, percentage body burned, ethanol use

Table 3.41 Cont.

Study	Method	Sample	Incidence	Results
McGonigal et al. (1993)	Medical examiner record review (Philadelphia) Trends in firearm deaths	Firearm homicide victims over 5 year period	1985: 145 firearm homicides; 1990: 324 firearm homicides, mostly young, black, males; 90% handguns 1985: 54% victims intoxicated; 1990: 61% victims intoxicated, cocaine most common abused substance (39%)	1985: 145 firearm homicides; 1990: 324 firearm homicides, mostly young, black, males; 90% handguns
Narongchai et al. (2007)	Chart review Drug abuse and unnatural deaths	Incidence of drug abuse in 153 persons, mean age 34 years (range, 10–76), 92% male	Causes of death: traffic injury 33%, gun shot 26%, other 41%; manner of death: accidental 40%, homicide 28% 9% positive for methamphetamine or derivatives	No cocaine, heroin, 6-monoacetyl morphine, morphine detected
Parry et al. (2005)	Cross-sectional study Trauma patients and drug use	Trauma unit admissions in 4-week period over 3 years.	Over 50% experienced violent injuries; 33–62% positive for at least one drug including cocaine (n = 1565), mostly cannabis, methaqualone	Drug positivity greater in last of the 3 years studied
Regidor et al. (1996)	Interview survey, general population	Subjects aged 16–40 years: 4261 general population, 369 cocaine users, 215 heroin users	Prevalence for injury: 7.9 general population, 10.8 cocaine users, 35.2 heroin users	Positive statistical association for injury in cocaine users with the use of non-heroin opiates
Reis et al. (2006)	Prospective cross-sectional study ER trauma victims and drug use	353 patients over 3-month period: drug use assessed by WHO questionnaire, self-administered questionnaire, drug abuse screening test, urine drug screen, blood alcohol level	242 positive drug screen for cannabis/cocaine, 166 positive for benzodiazepines, 39 elevated blood alcohol (33 [10%] intoxicated) Most abuse drugs: cannabis (13.6%), cocaine (3.3%), benzodiazepines (4.2%)	Substantial substance abuse found in trauma victims
Rivara et al. (1989)	Chart review, medical examiners' office, ER Drug use in trauma victims Screened for marijuana, cocaine, opiates, benzodiazepines, alcohol	452 in ER, 160 in medical examiners' office	151 (33%) positive for alcohol; 40.3% positive for one drug at ER; 18.7% positive for one drug at MEO; marijuana most common drug in both groups	Alcohol, drugs most commonly found in younger persons, males, victims of assault or traffic accidents

Study	Method	Sample	Results	Conclusion
Siegal et al. (2006)	Chart review, participant self-report; Crack use and ER visits	211 persons, 643 ER visits in 3 year period	Injury and poisoning most common cause for visit (29.5%); Increased risk of visiting ER: times in drug treatment (OR 1.04; 95% CI 1.01–1.09), chronic disease (OR 1.46; 95% CI 1.06–1.99), high Addiction Severity Index score (OR 1.62; 95% CI 1.15–2.29)	In addition to drug use, other factors may affect ER use by crack users
Sloan et al. (1989)	Chart review; Drug screen of patients in trauma center	623 toxicology screens: mostly black males, mean age 32 ± 22 years	536 (86%) positive screens: ethanol 53%, cannabis 37%, cocaine 34% OR 1.9–4.2 for illicit drug use at time of trauma ($p < 0.005$); OR 4.7–16.8 for age and illicit urine screen ($p < 0.001$)	Alcohol found mostly in older trauma patients
Soderstrom et al. (2001)	Retrospective review of clinical toxicology database; Trends in drug use in trauma victims	53 338 patients in database over 3-year period	Increase in positive results over 3 year period: 21.2% for cocaine and 543% for opiates ($p < 0.001$); Increase in non-violent crime: cocaine 152%, opiates, 640%; Increase in violent crime: cocaine 226%, opiates 258%	Epidemic increase in cocaine and opiate use in trauma patients; mostly in victims of violent crime; decreasing trend for alcohol use
Stoduto et al. (1993)	Chart review; Seriously injured patients and alcohol and drug use	854 patients admitted over 37-month period	32% motor vehicle accidents: 35% drivers positive for alcohol; 474 drug screens, 339 drivers: 41.3% positive for drugs, 16.5% positive for drugs and alcohol; Drugs: cannabinoids 13.9%, benzodiazepines 12.4%, cocaine 5.3%	Blood alcohol positive drug-screened drivers more likely to be male, involved in single vehicle collision, not wearing seat belt, ejected from vehicle, traveling at high speeds; no differences in injury severity of trauma victims
Walsh et al. (2004a)	Chart review; Use of rapid POC drug testing device	322 motor vehicle crash victims: comparison of POC results with clinical urine specimens in hospital laboratory	Drug-only use greater than alcohol use (33.5% vs. 15.8%); 9.9% tested positive for drug and alcohol use	POC test results correlated well with laboratory results; POC results facilitated rapid intervention/treatment

CI, confidence interval; ER, emergency room; OR, odds ratio; POC, point-of-collection; WHO, World Health Organization.

Schaper *et al.* (2007) conducted a retrospective study to develop a treatment algorithm to use in German/French airports and a poison center. The rectum and vagina were used by 312 pushers, while 4660 packers were also identified. There was equal ratio of men and women transporting the drugs. Life-threatening signs and symptoms of cocaine toxicity as a result of packet rupture were seen in 64 packers. Twenty individuals had packets removed surgically, and 44 died prior to surgery.

The most recent retrospective study was by de Beer *et al.* (2008). Seventy individuals were identified as body packers over a five-year period. Most of the packets were removed surgically by enterostomies, although three required a partial small bowel resection. One person died from postoperative disseminated intravascular coagulation. Although the incidence of fascia dehiscence was typical of non-cocaine surgical events (2.9%), the wound infection rate (32.9%) was much higher than expected.

Comments

Based on the studies reviewed, body stuffing and packing carries an increased risk of cocaine intoxication caused by rupture of cocaine packets or ingestion of the packets without wrapping. The risk of death appears to be low (44 out of 4972 individuals reported here), and may be caused by cocaine toxicity, obstruction or perforation of the small or large intestine, or cerebral hemorrhage associated with severe hypertension. Cocaine intoxication was more often seen in the packers and stuffers, with signs and symptoms including tachycardia, high blood pressure, and agitation.

The packers and stuffers also appear to be creative in their mode of hiding cocaine in spaces besides the digestive system. Some inhaled the packets or pushed the packets in the vagina or rectum. Some found that putting small packets in a single larger packet did not necessarily protect them from the consequences of packet rupture.

Although males were more often reported as body packers and stuffers, females and pregnant women were also transporters. Individuals under the age of 30 were often packers and stuffers; Hispanics and African Americans were frequent carriers.

Table 3.42 summarizes all the studies reviewed here on body stuffing and packing.

Other pathological conditions

Five studies were found in the PubMed database published between 1988 and 2008 and related to pathology and cocaine use. However, a number of other studies demonstrating pathological findings are discussed in other subsections of this chapter, including the sections on the nervous system, female genitalia and pregnancy, and cardiovascular disorders.

In order to determine the integrity of cerebral neurons in cocaine-using individuals, Lim *et al.* (2002) used diffusion tensor imaging (DTI) to study the white matter of 12 cocaine users and 13 age-similar controls. This technique can be used to estimate and locate damage to nerve fibers and is able to visualize and map subtle anatomical changes. Fractional anisotropy (FA) was also used to determine the shape of organization of the nerve tracts. Lim *et al.* (2002) found decreased FA, reflecting decreased frontal white matter. They suggested that this decrease in the orbitofrontal area of the brain may explain some of the decision-making deficits seen in chronic cocaine users.

A recent study by Lim *et al.* (2008) used DTI and FA to show that cocaine users ($n = 21$) had lower FA than controls ($n = 21$) in the inferior frontal region of the cerebrum. The cocaine users also had a smaller gray/white matter volume than the controls. There was a correlation between the length of cocaine use and severity of brain damage.

Table 3.42 Body packers and body stuffers

Study	Method	Sample	Incidence	Results
Chang et al. (2006a)	Case report Body stuffer	Trauma patient with abnormal chest radiography	Exploratory bronchoscopy; packet ruptured during removal from right lower lobe bronchus; developed pneumonitis	
Ciszowski et al. (2005)	Case report, review Body smuggling (packer)		During hospital stay (37 h) passed packets (500 g) without evidence of cocaine intoxication	
Cobaugh et al. (1997)	Case report Body stuffer	39-year-old male with cocaine balloon aspiration	Numerous packets removed from oropharynx; packet removed by bronchoscopy from right lower lobe of lung	Body stuffing can include pulmonary system as well as digestive
Cordero et al. (2006)	Case report Body stuffer/packer	Pregnant female	Perimortum cesarean section after rupture of cocaine packet	Special protocols are needed for pregnant body stuffers/packers
de Beer et al. (2008)	Retrospective study Body packing	70 patients over 5-year period	Surgical removal of packets: most enterostomies, 3 partial small bowel resections Wound infection 32.9%, fascia dehiscence 2.9%, 1 death (postoperative disseminated intravascular coagulation)	Low mortality; high rate of wound infection
Eng et al. (1999)	Case report False negative CT scan	Body stuffer with abdominal pain; ingested large packet containing small packets of cocaine	Negative abdominal CT scan without contrast	CT scan not completely reliable in identifying ingested packets
Fineschi et al. (2002)	Case report Body stuffer	17-year-old dealer	Died after ingesting plastic bag of cocaine	
Furnari et al. (2002)	Case report Body packer	27-year-old cocaine user ingested 99 packets of cocaine powder (10 g 86% cocaine per packet)	Died from acute cocaine intoxication after rupture of 4 packets Autopsy: edema; organ congestion; high levels cocaine, benzoylecgonine in blood, urine, bile, vitreous humor, brain, hair	Cocaine and metabolites found in various body fluids in cocaine user

Table 3.42 Cont.

Study	Method	Sample	Incidence	Results
Gill & Graham (2002)	Chart review Deaths of body packers	50 deaths from open or leaking drug packets in New York City over 10 years; most packers were 19–57 years old (mean, 37.1), 82% male; 66% Hispanic, 24% black	4 carrying cocaine, 42 carrying opiates Recovered number of packets: 1 to 111 (average 46); 9.4–1200 g/bag (average, 377 g) Deaths: 42 acute intoxication, 5 intestinal obstruction or bowel perforation, 1 intracerebral hemorrhage from high BP	
Koehler et al. (2005)	Case report Body packer		Death from cocaine intoxication	
Malbrain et al. (1994)				Reported on treatment options for individuals with ruptured packets
Norfolk (2007)	Case report Body stuffer	50-year-old female	Died 10 h after swallowing plastic-wrapped cocaine	
Schaper et al. (2007)	Retrospective study to develop treatment algorithm at airports, poison center	312 pushers (vagina, rectum), 4660 packers: sex ratio 1:1	After packet rupture, 64 developed life-threatening signs and symptoms of cocaine toxicity, 20 had packets removed surgically, 44 died before surgical intervention	
Sporer & Firestone (1997)	Retrospective cohort study Crack cocaine body stuffers	98 stuffers: 75 000 ER visits in 3 years	Mostly males < 30 years; self-report 1–15 rocks (29% wrapped in plastic bag; 28% unwrapped) Seizures in 4% within 2 h of ingestion; 54% tachycardic (no arrhythmias), 23% high BP, 22% agitated, 19% required sedation	

ER, emergency room; BP, blood pressure; CT, computer tomography.

Moeller *et al.* (2007) studied the effect of cocaine on myelin function in 13 cocaine users and 18 healthy controls. Diffusion tensor eigenvalues (comparing diffusion along fiber tracts with that perpendicular to the fiber tracts) indicated that altered myelin in the corpus callosum was more common in cocaine users than in non-users. This study supported other similar studies that found cocaine-induced alterations or damage to myelin that increased diffusion perpendicular to the tracts. Neuronal loss or damage to axonal tracts are possible explanations for these findings.

Two studies looked at placental pathology in cocaine users. Mooney *et al.* (1998) studied placentas from 29 cocaine users and 15 non-using controls. Drug use was verified by urine tests. Both groups showed some evidence of chorioamnionitis: 58% of the placentas from cocaine users, 66% of the placentas from non-users. However, only the cocaine users' placentas showed some evidence of edema (17%) and chorionic villus hemorrhage (17%). The authors hypothesized that edema and chorionic villus hemorrhage may be associated with cocaine use even if placenta abruptio had not occurred.

The second study (Cejtin *et al.* 1999) also reported on cocaine's effect on the placenta. This study controlled for gestational age and tobacco use and compared the placentas from 26 cocaine users with those from 26 non-users. Chorioamnionitis and funisitis were more common in the non-cocaine exposed placentas than cocaine exposed (10 vs. 6, chorioamnionitis; 4 vs. 1, funisitis). The cocaine-exposed placentas showed an infarct, chronic villitis (three), and segmental necrosis (one). One decidual vasculopathy and one thrombus were found in the control placentas. There was one incidence in each of the two groups for a thrombus in a fetal vessel. This study showed that cocaine use did not statistically increase the incidence of typical pathological findings in placentas.

Table 3.43 summarizes these studies on pathological conditions.

Comments

Two studies were found describing altered myelin tract organization in cocaine users. Other studies are reported in the literature regarding FA, which reflects white matter tract organization in other types of pathology. Use of FA and DTI, along with other neuro-imaging techniques, may be helpful in identifying the location and intensity of cerebral abnormalities in cocaine users. Studies are needed to compare findings in users with different experiences in terms of amount and length of drug use, and perhaps to identify confounders or polydrug combinations associated with cocaine use and altered white matter. More studies on the etiology of altered myelin tracts are also needed that might give insight into the mechanisms for development of the changes.

The two studies on placental abnormalities in cocaine users provide some additional information about the possible pathologies that might be associated with fetal outcomes in cocaine-using women. The development of edema and chorionic villus hemorrhage in some placentas in the study by Mooney *et al.* (1998) needs to be confirmed by other placental studies.

Cocaine: summary and overview

Epidemiological studies on the effect of cocaine on various health conditions have been describe in the preceding subsections based on epidemiological research published between 1988 and 2008. Studies published prior to 1988 demonstrated that cocaine had adverse drug effects in a number of body systems, including the nervous system (strokes and seizures), head and neck disease (destructive bone and cartilaginous lesions),

Table 3.43 Other pathologies

Study	Method	Sample	Incidence	Results
Cejtin et al. (1999)	Case-control study Cocaine and placental pathology	Placentas from 26 cocaine users (no other drug use), 26 controls	Higher incidence of chorioamnionitis and funisitis in controls than cocaine users: chorioamnionitis, 10 vs. 6; funisitis, 4 vs. 1 Cocaine users only: 1 infarct, 3 chronic villitis, 1 segmental necrosis Controls only: 1 decidual vasculopathy, 1 thrombus Both: 1 fetal vessel thrombus	No statistically significant differences; cocaine use not likely cause of any of the 15 features of placental dysfunction analyzed
Lim et al. (2002)	Case-control study DTI in cocaine users:	12 cocaine users, 13 age-similar controls	Cocaine users compared with controls: decreased FA in frontal white matter	Area of decreased white matter may explain deficits in decision making in some cocaine users
Lim et al. (2008)	Case-control study DTI and FA studies	21 cocaine users (mean age 42.5 years, average 18.9 years of cocaine use), 21 age/gender-matched controls	Cocaine users compared with controls: lower FA in inferior frontal white matter; smaller, not significant, gray–white matter volume	Length of cocaine use was associated with severity of brain abnormalities
Mooney et al. (1998)	Case-control study Placental pathology and cocaine use	Placentas from 29 cocaine users, 15 controls	Chorioamnionitis in cocaine users (58%) and controls (66%); only cocaine-exposed placentas had edema (17%) and chorionic villus hemorrhage (17%)	Edema and chorionic villus hemorrhage may occur in cocaine users even without placenta abruptio

DTI, diffusion tensor imaging; FA, fractional anisotropy.

ophthalmic disorders (corneal abrasions), cardiovascular dysfunction (AMI, endocarditis, tachyarrhythmias), pulmonary complications (barotrauma, exacerbation of asthma, eosinophilia [crack lung], and talc granulomatosis), genitourinary dysfunction (sexual), and damage to the musculoskeletal system (rhabdomyolysis). However, for this review, the earlier studies were not critiqued, and the basis (laboratory or clinical research) of cocaine's relationship to medical disease was not explored. However, in some cases, these pathologies continue to be researched and risk to cocaine users identified. Consequently, additional pathologies are emerging in long-term cocaine users that can help to identify risks for chronic users.

Recent laboratory and epidemiological studies have helped to clarify the role of cocaine in various pathological findings and found that, in some situations, it is not the cocaine that is damaging to body tissue or fetal development but rather the effects of risky sexual behavior, use of unsafe drug paraphernalia, and poor lifestyle choices. More recent epidemiological studies are beginning to determine the cocaine user's risk for pathophysiological changes. Although much more can be done to clarify the role and risk of cocaine use and pathological conditions, many of the clinical research studies are beginning to describe the association between cocaine use and body system dysfunction. However, much research still needs to be done, particularly epidemiological research linked to findings in laboratory studies, to provide a research basis on which to practice evidence-based medicine.

Table 3.44 at the end of this section indicates the various topics under major body systems and the evidence available in the epidemiological research published from 1988 to 2008. The text that follows is a brief summary of the topics and evidence supporting an association between cocaine and the specific topic. More detailed critique of the research is found in the individual summaries in the preceding subsections.

Infections

Bacterial infections. Several of the studies relating to bacterial infections and cocaine use were case reports describing sepsis after splenic infarct, and endocarditis related to needle licking prior to injection. Two large studies (140 to 150 patients) identified the presence of S. aureus in the nasal cavity of 35% of the cocaine users, and the need for incision and drainage of abscesses associated with subcutaneous or intramuscular injection of cocaine. Two studies demonstrated the risk for syphilis in cocaine users. One study found that TB booster testing (two-step testing) could identify 5% more cases of TB than a single TB screen.

Mycoses. One case of endocarditis and systemic fungal sepsis was found in the review of the literature. Fungal sepsis is rare in non-immunocompromised individuals; however, in the report, the immune status of the individual was not given.

Parasitic infections. Risky sexual behavior was linked to an increase in the spread of trichomoniasis in one study.

Viral (non-HIV) infections. Intravenous drug use, needle sharing, and risky sexual behavior were associated with cocaine use in six studies reporting on HAV, HBV, and HCV infections. Most of the studies were large (151 to 1512 subjects) and indicated that cocaine users were more likely to acquire or spread hepatitis viral infections through risky behavior. The one study of HSV showed that over 60% of the 462 subjects tested positive for the virus.

Overall association: supported by some evidence

Most of these studies demonstrate an association between cocaine use and infections, but do not establish a cause and effect relationship. These infections are more likely a result of other behaviors associated with cocaine use and may have been avoided by safer sex practices, use of sterile needles, and limited sharing of other drug paraphernalia.

Clinical implications

Identification and treatment of those infected with STDs, herpes and hepatitis viruses, and TB might help to control the spread of these infections. Appropriate vaccination of uninfected drug users might also help to limit the number of new cases in the future. Teaching drug users the need for clean/sterile equipment and discouraging needle and paraphernalia sharing might also help to decrease the number of newly infected individuals.

Neoplastic disease

Overall association: supported by some evidence

Only two studies were found for neoplastic conditions and cocaine use. A chart review of 198 individuals with pancreatic cancer found that 6% were under the age of 40 years. A total of six persons (3%) had a history of cocaine or marijuana use. In a case–control study of 378 patients with NHL, the risk of developing NHL was higher in males using illicit drugs, especially cocaine. With only two studies, one on each type of cancer, there is insufficient information to support a strong risk of these cancers with cocaine use.

Musculoskeletal system disease

Discussion of rhabdomyolysis was included in the renal subsection of Urological diseases; crack dancing was discussed in the section on the CNS.

Digestive system disease

Overall association: supported by strong evidence

Although most of the eight studies discussed were case reports of 13 patients, one retro-spective study demonstrated that almost one-third of 78 patients with perforated ulcer disease used crack cocaine prior to developing an acute abdomen. Pathological specimens in these studies generally showed no evidence of atherosclerotic or thrombotic lesions in the vessels to the stomach, duodenum, ileum, or colon. Cocaine and cocaine's metabolites are known vasoconstrictors that have been shown to cause vasospasms in a variety of vessels. Coupled with the increase in alpha-adrenergic stimulation by norepinephrine and the close association between the last use of cocaine and onset of clinical symptoms, it is possible that cocaine use increases the risk of an acute abdomen.

Clinical implications

Although recall bias may be a factor, all of the studies showed that there was a temporal relationship between the time of use of cocaine and the onset of clinical symptoms. Individuals seeking healthcare for an acute abdomen should be assessed for recent cocaine use, particularly those under the age of 40 years.

Stomatognathic disease

Discussion of the oral cavity and jaw was included in the section on otorhinolaryngological disease.

Respiratory system disease

Asthma

Overall association: supported by strong evidence

Three studies looked at the association of cocaine with asthma. One small retrospective study found that 14 of 23 out-of-hospital deaths were attributed to asthma in illicit drugs users. Cocaine was one of several drugs that were associated with the deaths. One cross-sectional study found that cocaine users had a three-fold increase in new bronchospasms or a recurrence of asthma symptoms. One cross-sectional study found that 22% of patients hospitalized for asthma were cocaine users. The patients also had a longer hospital stay than the non-illicit drug users.

One very small study of bronchial washings in cocaine users did show increased alveolar macrophages and elevated endothelin-1. Endothelin-1 or cocaine itself may contribute to the bronchospasm and/or inflammation seen in asthma. Some researchers suggest that these changes may occur in cocaine users prior to the onset of respiratory signs and symptoms.

Respiratory changes

Overall association: supported by strong evidence

Two large case–control studies by the same research group found an increase in respiratory symptoms in crack cocaine users (177 and 202). Signs and symptoms included an increase in cough and black sputum production, obstructive disease of the large airways, and a mild change in alveolar diffusion capacity. An increase in chest pain and cough was found in one-third of the subjects. One small prospective cohort study found that 10 cocaine users had no hemoptysis and had normal spirometry tests. However, bronchial washings showed an increase in alveolar macrophages (also seen in cigarette smokers) and elevated endothelin-1.

There are limited studies on the respiratory changes associated with cocaine use. It is possible that the 177 subjects in one study are also included in the second study by the same research group. Some of the subjects were also cigarette smokers, so the effect of smoking cigarettes could also cause some of the respiratory symptoms seen in the subjects even though smoking was considered in the statistical analyses.

More studies with larger numbers of subjects are needed to provide more evidence for respiratory changes in cocaine users, who also might be exposed to environmental hazards that might contribute to respiratory dysfunction.

Otorhinolaryngological disease

Sensory changes

Overall association: supported by strong evidence

Two studies suggest that cocaine use is a risk factor for alteration of olfaction and hearing. A cross-sectional study with 50 participants found that cocaine and alcohol users had smaller olfactory evoked potentials compared with cigarette smokers and non-drug users. The other study was a case report of a cocaine user who developed bilateral sensorineural hearing loss after using cocaine.

Oral lesions

Overall association: supported by some evidence
Only one case report found that local application of cocaine to the gums and teeth was associated with rapid gingival recessional and dental erosion. In this unusual case, it is possible that the vasoconstrictive effect of cocaine and adrenergic neurotransmitters is a direct cause of the injury. Reports of apoptotic effects of cocaine also suggest a link to this case of oral damage.

Nasal signs and symptoms

Overall association: supported by strong evidence
A large survey of non-intravenous drug-using adolescents in outpatient treatment programs in five geographic regions provides some evidence of nasal symptoms in drug users. Cocaine users were more likely than others to have sniffling, sinus problems, and diminished olfaction. Daily cocaine users often had nasal crust and recurrent epistaxis.

Although one study was reported on nasal signs and symptoms in non-intravenous cocaine users, the 336 individuals reporting use of cocaine were young adolescents from five different geographic areas. The signs and symptoms reported could be precursors of more severe midline nasal–sinus lesions described below. Further studies are needed to increase the research evidence of early respiratory pathology in snorters and smokers.

Midline nasal lesions

Overall association: supported by strong evidence
Eight case reports, describing 62 patients, were found in the epidemiological literature over the past 20 years. The lesions included nasolacrimal duct destruction, nasal septal destruction, turbinate destruction, necrotic inflammation, perforation of the hard palate, and extensive cartilage and bone destruction. Two case–control studies were carried out to help determine differential diagnoses and diagnostic markers for CIMDL. These studies found similar findings in patients with WG, lymphoma, and sarcoidosis. Use of ANCA, proteinase-3, and caspase 3 and 9 has varying ability to differentiate the cause of the destructive lesions. One study suggested that use of HNE-ANCA was a more specific marker for cocaine-related lesions.

It is likely, based on the case–control studies and numerous case reports, that snorted and smoked cocaine can cause destructive midline lesions. There appears to be a time and dose-dependent increase in injury and apoptotic changes to a variety of cells, including epithelium, cartilage, and bone.

Clinical implications
Health care providers seeing midline lesions should consider cocaine use in their differential diagnosis. Other possible causes include WG, lymphoma, and sarcoidosis.

Thermal injury

Overall association: supported by some evidence

Two reports of epiglottitis in 11 cocaine users were found in the literature. In one report, three cocaine users sustained epiglottic burns when metal pieces of crack pipes were inhaled. The other report described mucosal burns of the upper airway in seven individuals, two of whom required tracheotomies.

Thermal injury can occur in non-intravenous cocaine users; however, this appears to be either an under-reported situation or a rare event.

Nervous system disease

Cerebrovascular disease

Overall association: supported by some evidence

Five small studies reported on cerebrovascular changes with cocaine administration. In all studies, vasoconstriction occurred. There also was also evidence of hypoperfusion in dopamine-rich areas of the brain. More studies are needed with larger numbers of cocaine users to confirm the finding of an apparent cumulative effect of cocaine use on the cerebrovascular reactivity.

Strokes and subarachnoid hemorrhage

Overall association: supported by strong evidence

Twenty studies describe the occurrence of strokes, including SAHs, in cocaine users. The studies included case reports, and case–control, retrospective, cross-sectional, and pathology studies. Overall, they show that CVAs occur more often in young cocaine users, that there is a strong temporal relationship between cocaine use and the onset of signs and symptoms, and that hemorrhagic stroke is more often seen in individuals with aneurysms or arterial-venous malformations. Although there appears to be a higher mortality in cocaine users with aneurysmal SAHs, those with ischemic strokes have fewer complications and decreased mortality. Some of the studies showed that cerebral vessel involvement was diffuse and not specific to a certain cerebral vessel, and that the cause of the CVA could be attributed to vasospasm, elevated blood pressure, or occlusive disease. Polydrug use, especially the use of amphetamines, was seen in many studies.

It is likely, based on the studies, that cocaine use is a risk factor for ischemic and hemorrhagic strokes, despite the report of three studies that there was no association between strokes and cocaine use. Since cocaine alters uptake of the alpha-adrenergic neurotransmitters, the likelihood of vasospasm or vasoconstriction occurring after cocaine use is high. With some of the metabolites of cocaine also having vasoconstrictive properties, the occurrence of delayed stroke signs and symptoms could be attributed to the pharmacological responses of the metabolites. Young cocaine users with undiagnosed berry aneurysms or arterial-venous malformations appear to be at greater risk for SAHs and poorer outcomes than those users with strokes from other causes.

Clinical implications

Because of the relationship between cocaine use and the occurrence of strokes, young individuals with strokes should be screened for drug use. Since the incidence of SAH appears to be related to existing anatomical lesions, and also has poor outcomes, prompt recognition is important in treatment.

Autonomic nervous system dysfunction

Overall association: supported by strong evidence

The four studies described all involved newborns or seven-month-old infants exposed to cocaine in utero. Two were large studies that looked at the risk for ANS outcomes in infants. One study found that the 717 cocaine users and 92 cocaine/opiate users were more at risk for ANS/CNS alterations. The second study found that the 717 infants of cocaine users were more likely to be jittery, irritable, have tremors and a high-pitched cry, have an excessive suck, and demonstrate hyperalertness. In an experimental study, 21 cocaine-exposed babies were more tachycardic before and after a tilting experience simulating orthostatic stress, and had a slower increase in heart rate and longer return to baseline. In a fourth study, after exposure to positive and negative affective tasks, 7-month-old infants exposed to cocaine in utero had heart rates that were slower to respond to the stimuli than the control infants.

Although the research is limited, the three newborn studies suggest that the ANS may have altered regulation related to cocaine use. More studies are needed to further describe the types of behavior seen in infants exposed to cocaine and determine other factors that might also influence behavior. As one group of researchers pointed out, smoking cigarettes also increases the risk of ANS dysfunction and, because more pregnant women smoke cigarettes than use cocaine, the attributable risk associated with tobacco smoking is greater.

The one study on responses to affective tasks was carried out on infants seven months after in utero exposure. The results of this type of study may be distorted by the inability to control the infants' environment from birth to seven months. The effect of maternal interaction with the infant and exposure to other drugs or toxins all may influence outcomes.

Central nervous system atrophy

Overall association: supported by some evidence

Two research reports by the same group described diffuse brain atrophy in cocaine users who also had seizures. The long-term cocaine users also appeared to have more cerebral atrophy.

Central nervous system: seizures

Overall association: supported by strong evidence

Four large studies explored the incidence of seizures in cocaine users who were seen in an emergency room, were hospital inpatients, or experienced acute cocaine toxicity. Seizures appear to be a rare event in cocaine users but may be seen in those using intravenous, nasal, or smoked cocaine. The prevalence of seizures in cocaine users ranged from 2.8 to 10.3% and occurred in first-time users as well as habitual users. The seizures were focal or generalized and often occurred within 90 minutes of cocaine use.

It appears likely that seizures may occur in cocaine users and that the seizures are directly related to the drug. Cocaine appears to lower the threshold for seizures, both in first-time users and in cocaine users with unrelated seizure disorders. In cocaine toxicity or with massive doses of cocaine, the seizure risk increases. However, there are other potential causes of the seizures, including non-compliance with medication (in persons with a seizure disorder), poor diet, or poor sleep habits; all of these could be consequences of illicit drug use.

Central nervous system: crack dancing

Overall association: supported by some evidence

The phenomenon of crack dancing includes the presence of abnormal motor movements, such as choreoathetosis, akathisia, and Parkinson-like tremors. Two case reports were found in the literature; however, this condition may be under-reported. The altered motor function can occur several days after cocaine use and, though transient, can last for as long as seven days.

It is likely that crack dancing appears more often than reported. It could be explained by the altered dopamine function in cocaine users.

Demyelinating studies: white and gray matter changes

Overall association: supported by some evidence

Three small epidemiological studies suggest alterations to myelin in cocaine users. White and gray matter volumes differed between cocaine users and non-using controls. Changes were found in the corpus callosum, premotor, orbitofrontal, and thalamic areas of the brain. Cerebellar changes in both gray and white matter were also seen in one study. One study found increased white matter hypersensitivity. These changes were attributed to vasoconstriction, neuronal loss, or axon tract damage.

Too few studies are available to confirm the effect of cocaine on the white and gray matter of the CNS structures.

Neurological manifestations

Overall association: supported by some evidence

A number of small case–control and cross-sectional studies were reviewed in which children exposed to cocaine in utero and adult cocaine users were evaluated for neuropsychological manifestations. One study showed that children who were exposed to marijuana and alcohol had the same changes in growth and development or behavior as those children exposed to cocaine. Another study with older children found those under the age of five years were more likely to experience seizures, while those older than 10 years were more likely to experience delirium, dizziness, drooling, and lethargy. Both studies are limited in the research methodology and in the conclusions that can be drawn based on exposure to a drug in the past.

Five small studies used a variety of psychological tests to evaluate cognitive function, learning, and executive function in adult cocaine users. Since the tests used in these studies all varied and there were differences in abstinence rates, the results are difficult to compare. In some of the studies, the cocaine users also used other substances, so it was difficult to attribute the findings to cocaine use alone.

As indicated above, these are small studies with many confounders. Results from these studies alone would not be sufficient for evidence-based practice.

Sleep

Overall association: supported by some evidence

One review of the literature on sleep patterns in cocaine users and several small case–control and case reports were found in the review of epidemiological research and cocaine use. Most of the studies used polysomnography to record sleep patterns and interviews or self-report to determine the quality of sleep. Overall, there appears to be a discrepancy between actual sleep patterns and the perceived quality of sleep reported by the cocaine abuser. Several studies suggest the "sleep homeostat" is disrupted by cocaine use and abstinence. More studies are needed to confirm the findings in these studies.

Ocular disease

Corneal changes

Overall association: supported by some evidence

Five studies described 147 cases of corneal disease in cocaine users. Infectious keratitis was seen in many patients and caused by a mix of bacterial and fungal organisms, including *S. aureus*, *Candida albicans* and *Streptococcus* and *Pseudomonas* spp. Several cases of sterile keratitis were also reported. Some occurred when cocaine users rubbed their eyes vigorously after use. In some cases, ulceration of the cornea occurred. Some individuals were also heroin users.

Based on the number of cases reported, it seems likely that cocaine can act as an irritant in contact with the cornea and predispose individuals for infection or ulceration.

Retinal damage

Overall association: supported by some evidence

Microtalc retinopathy was reported in 61 cocaine users, particularly those inhaling cocaine. Magnesium silicate and other impurities in the cocaine mixtures can form microemboli, which can travel through the retinal vessels and cause rake and slit retinal damage leading to neovascularization. Visual field changes similar to glaucoma can also occur.

Microtalc retinopathy has been reported by two research groups. Larger studies are needed to determine whether this phenomenon occurs in all forms of cocaine use and whether certain users are more susceptible than others. Since the macula receives a dual blood supply, damage to this area can cause chronic vision problems. It is feasible that talc emboli could lodge not only in the retinal microvasculature but in other microvessels in other organs as well.

Iritis

Overall association: supported by some evidence

Only one case of iritis was described in an intranasal cocaine user. Too little information is available to suggest this was only related to cocaine use.

Color vision changes

Overall association: supported by some evidence

Only one small case–control study reported that blue–yellow color loss occurred more often in cocaine users than in matched controls. Since there is a role for dopamine in color vision signaling, cocaine use could have a role in color vision distortion, but further study is needed to evaluate color vision changes in cocaine users.

Acute-angle-closure glaucoma

Overall association: supported by some evidence

Two incidences of acute-angle-closure glaucoma were reported. One female developed glaucoma 24 hours after application of a 2% cocaine paste to her nasal cavity as part of a surgical procedure. One male nasal cocaine user also developed glaucoma. Since cocaine and alpha-adrenergic neurotransmitters can cause pupil dilation, acute-angle-closure glaucoma is a possibility in some susceptible individuals with shallow anterior chambers. More studies are needed to quantify the risk of this type of glaucoma in cocaine users.

Male urological disease

Genital ulcer disease

Overall association: supported by some evidence

Several studies, including descriptive and retrospective studies, describe the risk for GUD in cocaine users. In all studies and a review of the literature, cocaine-associated GUD was associated with high-risk behavior that leads to development of STDs.

Although there is an increased risk of GUD in cocaine users, the risk is primarily related to risky sex practices and prostitution rather than a direct cause and effect relationship between GUD and cocaine.

Sexual dysfunction

Overall association: supported by some evidence

A descriptive study of users of a combination of alcohol and cocaine indicated, by self-report, that the drug users experienced sexual dysfunction. Further study of cocaine users not abusing other drugs or alcohol would help to identify the risk for sexual dysfunction in this population.

Priapism was described in six cocaine users. Laboratory studies showed that although alpha-adrenergic function was normal, long-term use of cocaine could deplete the sympathetic nervous system norepinephrine, leading to priapism. More studies are needed to identify the risk of priapism in cocaine users.

Renal dysfunction

Overall association: supported by strong evidence

Several fairly large studies found that illicit drugs users in general had an increased risk of declining renal function over time, as reflected in rising serum creatinine and urea nitrogen levels. Those cocaine users who ultimately developed ESRD tended to develop renal failure at a younger age than their non-cocaine-using counterparts.

Some of those with renal disease had hypertension, but in most studies the hypertension was acute and most likely the result of vasoconstriction from recent cocaine use or the effect of alpha-adrenergic neurotransmitters. Some studies also found that hypertensive renal tissue changes occurred despite normal blood pressures in cocaine users.

Several pathological findings were reported in cocaine users with renal disease, including renal hemodynamic changes, altered glomerular matrix synthesis and degradation, evidence of oxidative stress, and atherogenic vessel changes. Fibrinoid glomerular necrosis and thrombic macroangiopathy also were found and renal infarcts have been reported. Rhabdomyolysis appeared to be associated with renal failure in some cases, although other studies found no evidence of elevated myoglobin levels or associated renal pathology. The presence of antibodies against the GBM was found in several case studies, suggesting an autoimmune renal component in some.

It appears that there is an association between cocaine use and declining renal function; however, the cause of this decline is not clear. Renal disease may occur with or without evidence of chronic hypertension, although renal hypertensive changes may be seen in normotensive cocaine users. Renal insufficiency may be caused by ischemia related to thrombosis or vasoconstriction. Rhabdomyolysis may occur and can cause renal failure. Rhabdomyolysis may be caused by vasoconstriction and the pyrogenic effect of cocaine. Cocaine may also have a direct toxic effect on the renal tissue. Microtalc deposits from cocaine fillers may contribute to the development of microangiopathy. Overall, it appears that cocaine users are at higher risk of developing renal disease than non-users. Polydrug users may be at even a greater risk.

Clinical implications

Monitoring renal function in cocaine users prior to development of renal signs and symptoms may be helpful in identifying those individuals at risk for renal failure with continued use of cocaine. Rhabdomyolysis needs to be considered as a cause in ARF in young individuals and they should also be screened for illicit drug use.

Female genital and neonatal/congenital disease

Female genital disorders

Overall association: supported by some evidence

In addition to the studies described under male urological disease, two other studies suggest that drug users tend to engage in risky sexual practices that can lead to PID in women or atypical genital ulcers caused by a variety of pathogens.

Pregnancy complications

Overall association: supported by some evidence

In the 18 studies of pregnancy complications discussed, the most commonly cited outcomes include (in descending order): preterm labor, LBW, placenta abruptio fetal death, small for gestational age, decreased length, IUGR, small head circumference, and placenta previa. Many of these outcomes are also seen in infants of mothers who abuse alcohol, tobacco, and other illicit drugs during their pregnancies. Associated with cocaine users is a decrease in appetite, decreased or absent prenatal care, and non-compliance with prenatal instructions.

One case report described a pregnant woman with symptoms of pre-eclampsia who had a positive drug screen for cocaine. However, she had no positive tests for pre-eclampsia and her signs and symptoms resolved quickly after admission; it was thought that her symptoms were likely caused by cocaine use.

The lack of prenatal care and the appetite-depressant capability of cocaine and decreased nutritional intake could also contribute to some of the findings in this section. Many cocaine users also abuse tobacco, alcohol, and other drugs. This could also affect infant outcomes, including decreased intrauterine growth, LBW, and small stature.

Collectively, it is difficult to compare some of the studies because of methodological differences. The definition of prematurity varied in several studies, and different methods were used to assess cocaine use in the mothers and infants. The lack of prenatal care, early detection of possible complications, and lack of compliance of the mothers are also factors that could influence maternal and infant outcomes.

Cardiovascular infant studies

Overall association: supported by strong evidence

A number of studies, including large case–control and cross-sectional studies found some alterations in umbilical vessels and transient arrhythmias and other cardiovascular events in newborns exposed to cocaine. Umbilical artery flow was normal in those women with placenta abruptio but abnormal in those with preterm labor, and in infants small for gestational age and LBW. A study on umbilical coiling found cocaine use was associated with hypercoiling and premature delivery.

Since cocaine can affect blood vessel diameter, changes in umbilical vessels could occur in cocaine-using pregnant women. These changes could affect blood flow to the fetus, resulting in decreased growth parameters.

Cardiac arrhythmias were more common in cocaine-exposed newborns, including respiratory sinus arrhythmia, increased vagal tone, cardiac arrest, and transient ST segment changes. Cardiac consultations also were more frequent for cocaine-exposed newborns.

Cocaine is known to cause ECG changes by blocking sodium and potassium channels. Along with excess catecholamine stimulation, supraventricular and ventricular arrhythmias can also occur. Bradyarrhythmias can occur, particularly in cocaine overdoses. If the mother had recently used cocaine, her newborn could be at higher risk for a variety of arrhythmias during the postnatal period.

Congenital syphilis

Overall association: supported by some evidence

Four studies, including two large studies, found that maternal cocaine use was associated with congenital syphilis in newborns. However, two of the studies found no association between cocaine and syphilis. Congenital syphilis was associated with lack of maternal prenatal care and failure to comply with syphilis treatment. One retrospective study of 73 infants with congenital syphilis showed a large stillbirth rate, and most of the viable infants were asymptomatic for the disease. As the rate of cocaine use increased, the prevalence of congenital syphilis increased – suggesting risky behavior and non-compliance on the part of pregnant cocaine users.

Congenital anomalies

Overall association: supported by some evidence

Two studies were reviewed. One study found an increased risk of subependymal cysts in infants of cocaine-using mothers. However, these cysts are also found more often in premature infants and are generally benign. In a large study, there appeared to be an increased risk of urinary anomalies in cocaine-exposed newborns, but no increase in genital anomalies.

Cardiovascular disease

Coronary artery disease

Overall association: supported by strong evidence

The studies reviewed focused on atherosclerosis risk and vasoconstrictive effects associated with cocaine use. Several small studies found increased coronary vessel narrowing by atherogenic lesions in one or more vessel. In an autopsy study of 495 cocaine-related deaths, only 1.2% of the coronary vessels showed total thrombic occlusion. Other studies showed that the combination of cigarette and cocaine use increased the risk of atherosclerosis in these users.

Vasoconstriction caused by cocaine administration was confirmed on several vascular studies. One study was able to reverse the increased heart rate and blood pressure, and decreased coronary sinus flow, using alpha-adrenergic blockers. One of the few random, double-blind controlled studies found a bimodal temporal vasoconstrictive effect when individuals were administered cocaine. The first vasoconstrictive event occurred 30 minutes after cocaine administration, coinciding with the peak cocaine blood level. At 90 minutes after cocaine administration, a second vasoconstrict event occurred, coinciding with the peak of cocaine metabolites.

Most of the vascular studies confirm the vasoconstrictive properties of cocaine.

Chest pain, ischemia, electrocardiography changes, and acute myocardial infarct

Overall association: supported by strong evidence

Several studies of ST segment changes in infants and adults exposed to or using cocaine were reviewed. As noted in the previous subsection, use of cocaine can alter sodium and potassium channels, which would result in changes in the action potentials and be manifested in ECG changes. In the case of infants and adults in withdrawal, the ST segment changes were transient and not necessarily associated with ischemia or were chronic changes in cocaine users.

Chest pain is a common symptom in cocaine users. However, in studies exploring the relationship between cocaine, chest pain, and AMI, most found that the incidence of AMI was relatively low. In a large case–control study of 3946 patients with AMI, 1% used cocaine in the prior year. Some experienced pain within 60 minutes of cocaine use, while others had a delayed onset of pain. Overall, those cocaine users were younger than other patients with AMI, had fewer complications, and were more likely to completely recover. It appears there is a low risk for AMI and an even lower mortality risk.

Although many of these studies need to be carried out with larger numbers of cocaine users and taking into account confounders (including tobacco use and use of other illicit drugs), there is some evidence that certain high-risk cocaine users may be more vulnerable to experiencing ischemia and AMI after cocaine use. Chronic users may be more at risk than young, recreational users.

Cardiac morphology changes

Overall association: supported by some evidence

Five relatively small studies reported on changes in left ventricular mass, cardiac hypertrophy, and depressed cardiac function. There is some limited evidence that left ventricular hypertrophy is more common in cocaine users than in others, but other studies found no differences in ventricular size or ejection fraction. Larger studies are needed.

Coagulation studies

Overall association: supported by strong evidence

There is good evidence that cocaine use can alter platelet activity and increase the risk of thrombi formation. One of the few randomized double-blind studies reviewed showed increased platelet factors, thromboglobulin, and microaggregates after cocaine administration. Numerous cases have been reported of thrombi formation and occlusion of various arterial systems that led to ischemic organs and limbs. Along with a known vasoconstrictive risk and a possible atherogenic effect, cocaine use increases the risk of ischemic and thrombic events in these drug users.

Dermatological disease

Overall association: supported by some evidence

Two published articles describe an association between cocaine use and dermatological conditions: one reporting hyperkeratotic lesions associated with contact with hot glass cocaine pipes, and a second describing skin paresthesia, referred to as formication and possibly a delusional parasitosis. No other dermatological studies were found in the literature review.

Nutritional and metabolic disease

Nutrition

Overall association: supported by some evidence

Too few studies were found to suggest that BMI affects the development of CIP. The relationship between BMI and the development of psychosis is unclear. More studies are needed to determine the risks of nutritional problems in cocaine users.

Metabolic disorders

Overall association: supported by some evidence

Too few studies were found to suggest that cocaine use alone causes changes in plasma cholinesterase and information about the effect of cocaine on the development of acidosis or alkalosis is also limited. More studies are needed to determine the risks of metabolic problems in cocaine users.

Hyperthermia, rhabdomyolysis, excited delirium, and cocaine toxicity

Overall association: supported by strong evidence

There is evidence that cocaine is related to the development of hyperthermia in cocaine users. Based on the research reviewed, it also appears that cocaine is associated with rhabdomyolysis and excited delirium. These conditions appear to be related to chronic cocaine use and altered function of the dopaminergic system, resulting in overstimulation of the temperature center and leading to an increase in core temperature. Accompanying this rise in body temperature is alteration in the normal body response to an elevated temperature by a decrease in sweating and lack of vasodilation. The altered dopaminergic function is also associated with the signs and symptoms of excited delirium.

The mechanism for cardiovascular, CNS, and respiratory responses to cocaine toxicity is thought to be different from that seen in excited delirium. Although dopaminergic dysfunction has a role in cocaine toxicity, other adrenergic neurotransmitters also have a major effect. Additionally, in those deaths associated with cocaine toxicity, the serum levels of cocaine and its metabolites are significantly elevated, while in excited delirium and cocaine-associated rhabdomyolysis, at least one study found a significant decrease in cocaine levels.

Endocrine disease

Overall association: supported by some evidence

Only two epidemiological studies were reviewed related to cocaine use and prolactin levels. Both focused on treatment outcomes and not the effects of prolactin on body function. Numerous laboratory studies have been published regarding cocaine and prolactin; however no other epidemiological studies were found in the literature.

Two studies of cocaine use and DKA suggest cocaine-using diabetics are more at risk for DKA, probably because of treatment non-compliance or possible hormonal imbalances. However, more studies are needed in this area to determine whether, and to what effect, non-compliance and other factors are associated with DKA.

Immune system disease

Overall association: supported by some evidence

Too few studies were found relating cocaine to immune dysfunction. A few case reports describe development of scleroderma or anti-GBM antibody formation in cocaine users, but these situations may be limited to a susceptible group of individuals. One study identified decreased monocytic function in cocaine users; however more studies involving immunity are needed.

Environment disease

Trauma

Overall association: supported by strong evidence

Based on the studies reported, cocaine appears to be one of the major drugs associated with motor vehicle accidents, both violent and non-violent injury, and increased risk of death or severe injury.

Body stuffing and packing

Overall association: supported by strong evidence

Based on the evidence, cocaine, along with heroin, is frequently hidden in body spaces to prevent detection by law enforcement personnel or to transport the drug illegally. Although death from rupture of the packets is rare according to the studies reviewed, the risk of cocaine intoxication is high if the packets rupture or crack cocaine rocks are ingested unwrapped. It also appears that the digestive tract is the major body system used but the respiratory tract, vagina, and rectum are also used by the packers and stuffers.

Other pathological conditions

Placental pathology

Overall association: supported by some evidence

Only two small studies on placental pathology were reviewed. One study found no significant difference between placentas from cocaine users and controls. Another study found some evidence of edema and chorionic villus hemorrhage in cocaine users.

Brain pathology

Overall association: supported by some evidence

Two small studies by the same researchers suggest that chronic cocaine use is associated with a decrease in gray and white matter brain volume.

Research concerns

While the research described in this chapter provides some evidence that cocaine use carries a risk for some health problems, questions can be raised about the research methodology and the results reported, particularly in abstracts. Most of the research studies were case reports or case–control studies. Convenience samples were used in many studies, particularly subjects in inpatient treatment centers. Retrospective chart reviews and some prospective studies were also reported. Very few cohort or randomized control studies were found. Lack of controls in some studies weakens the validity of the findings, and selection bias makes generalization of the findings difficult. Few studies used similar methodology and measurement tools (e.g., different cognitive tests to assess higher brain function; different length of abstinence to determine cocaine effect on sleep). As pointed out in the subsection on strokes, the terminology used to describe the cerebral vascular events was inconsistent. Many of the abstracts lacked the statistical measures needed to make wise practice decisions. Many studies reported probability statistics rather than risk statistics and 95% CI values.

In many studies, determination of cocaine or other drug use was by self-report. Self-report can be unreliable for many reasons, including lack of truth telling and recall bias. Some studies used urine toxicology tests to confirm cocaine use; however, urine tests may not be as accurate as blood tests, testing hair samples, and meconium testing in newborns.

Some studies identified confounders and controlled for them in the statistical analyses. However, not all studies controlled for similar demographic variables, other illicit drug use, and alcohol and tobacco use, while some studies only controlled for some of these

Table 3.44 Cocaine summary

Body system	Topic and evidence of association
Infections	Bacterial, mycoses, parasitic, viral (all some)
Neoplastic	Non-Hodgkin's lymphoma (some), pancreatic cancer (some)
Musculoskeletal	See nervous system for crack dancing, renal system for rhabdomyolysis
Digestive	Perforated ulcer, gastrointestinal ischemia and infarct (strong)
Stomatognathic	Included with otorhinolaryngological
Respiratory	Asthma (strong), respiratory changes signs and symptoms (strong)
Otorhinolaryngological	Oral lesions (some); nasal, including olfaction (strong); midline lesions (strong)
Nervous	Cerebrovascular (some); strokes, subarachnoid hemorrhage (strong); autonomic nervous system in newborns (strong); central nervous system atrophy (some), seizures (strong), crack dancing (some), demyelination (some), neuropsychological (some), altered sleep patterns (some)
Ocular	Corneal (some), retinal (some), iritis (some), altered color vision (some), acute-angle-closure glaucoma (some)
Urological	Genital ulcer disease in males (some); male sexual dysfunction, priapism (some); renal (strong)
Female reproductive and congenital/neonatal	Genital ulcer disease, pelvic inflammatory disease (some); pregnancy complications (some); infant cardiovascular conditions (strong); congenital syphilis (some); congenital anomalies (some)
Cardiovascular	Coronary artery studies (strong); chest pain, acute myocardial infarction, electrocardiogram changes (strong); cardiac morphology (some); coagulation defects (strong)
Dermatological	Lesions (some)
Nutritional and metabolic	Altered plasma cholinesterase (some), body mass index and cocaine-induced psychosis (some), acid–base imbalance (some), hyperthermia (strong), rhabdomyolysis (strong), excited delirium (strong), cocaine toxicity (strong)
Endocrine	Altered prolactin (some), diabetes mellitus and ketoacidosis (some)
Immune	Autoimmune diseases (some), monocyte dysfunction (some)
Environment	Trauma (strong), body stuffers/packers (strong)
Other pathologies	Placental pathology (some), brain pathology (some)

confounders. In the studies of pregnancy outcomes, use of cigarettes and alcohol and lack of prenatal care could have a significant effect on infant outcomes, so studies comparing cocaine users with controls with similar prenatal care and cigarette and alcohol use might help to identify pregnancy risks in cocaine users. Longitudinal studies of children exposed to cocaine in utero may be difficult to perform because of the difficulty in controlling for environmental exposure to drugs in infancy and childhood. If a child grows up in a home where there is use of illicit drugs and alcohol and tobacco use, what effect does the exposure to these conditions have on development of juvenile hypertension or cognitive defects? If children grow up in a depressed socioeconomic environment and chaotic home, what effect does this have on health outcomes in later childhood and adolescence?

While this chapter describes a number of good epidemiological research studies on the relationship of cocaine to health problems in children and adults, more cohort and randomized control studies are needed to identify risks and to generalize to a larger population. The studies also need larger sample sizes and to be replicated by other researchers in order to increase the reliability and validity of the findings. Linking appropriate laboratory research to clinical studies may also help to strengthen the findings and enhance the use of the research to generate evidenced-based practice guidelines.

Table 3.44 summarizes the association of cocaine with research covering various body systems described in this chapter. The Topic column indicates the condition described, followed by the rating for the evidence of association in parentheses. The term "strong" suggests there is a significant body of knowledge supporting a direct or indirect association between cocaine and the condition (e.g., a significant number of studies, cohort or case-controlled studies, clinical laboratory studies, or a single seminal study). "Strong" suggests the clinician may find this condition in a cocaine user. "Some" suggests that there are some studies supporting a direct or indirect association between cocaine and the condition (e. g., a smaller number of studies, case–control or case reports, or a study reporting a rare or under-reported condition). In many cases, "some" suggests more evidence is needed to support a strong association with a condition.

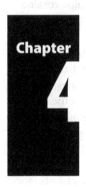

Results: marijuana

Introduction

Marijuana is the most frequently used illegal drug in the USA and is used worldwide. While much is known about the psychological effects of the drug, less is known about the effects of marijuana on various body systems. Although the acute effects have been observed and studies have been done to evaluate the function of individuals "high" on marijuana, less is known about the long-term effects of the drug. Because marijuana is currently used in medical situations, it is important to know about the long-term effects of the drug being prescribed. The focus of this chapter is to explore the epidemiological research on marijuana use and diseases of the body systems.

Over 150 abstracts were initially reviewed that were selected from the Medline database covering 1988 to 2008. The abstracts were selected from epidemiological research, case studies, and reviews of the literature on marijuana use and human disease. The abstracts are classified in MeSH categories as subsections. In some cases, the abstracts could be classified in several categories, but the "best fit" was chosen for discussion. At the end of the discussion of the research, a summary of the marijuana research is presented. All research articles are listed in the References.

Background

The physiological chemicals in marijuana are phytocannabinoids from the *Cannabis sativa* plant, which grows worldwide. Three classes of cannabinoid are found: the phytocannabinoids from *Cannabis* and the *Echinacea* plant, the endocannabinoids (ECs) that are inherent in mammals and other animals, and the synthetic agonists used medically and in research.

The EC include arachidonyl ethanolamide (anandamide) discovered in 1992; 2-arachidonyl glycerol, *n*-arachidonyldopamine, and virodhamine (*O*-arachidonoylethanolamine). A fifth possible EC is 2-arachidonyl glycerol ether (nolandin ether/norepinephrine). The ECs are intercellular messengers derived from arachidonic acid. As lipophilic compounds, they are integral to the cell membrane and are found in the central and peripheral nervous systems and other body tissue, where they interact with cannabinoid receptors (CB1 and CB2) and other cell receptors.

The EC receptors are G-protein-coupled receptors and are found on postsynaptic cells in most tissues of the body. The ECs function through a retrograde signaling mechanism where they are released from the postsynaptic cell and then interact with the EC receptor on the terminal axon of the presynaptic cell. Upon binding to the EC receptor, they inhibit the release of the presynaptic transmitter. If an inhibitory transmitter is decreased, the EC-releasing cell is excited; if a stimulatory transmitter is decreased, the excitability of the EC-releasing cell is decreased.

The cannabinoid receptors are found throughout the body: CB1 receptors are primarily associated with the CNS but are also found in adipose tissue, the gastrointestinal tract, liver, pancreas, heart, blood vessels, and skeletal muscle; CB2 receptors are primarily found in peripheral tissue, but especially in those cells involved in inflammation and immunity, including T helper types 1 and 2 cells, B lymphocytes, natural killer cells, and macrophages. The CB2 receptors modulate the release of cytokines and may be involved in differentiation of B and T cells.

The ECs have important functions in the human body, including fetal and early childhood development and development of the immune system. Several EC–receptor systems have been described. The EC–CB1 receptor system primarily functions in the CNS, where a large number of receptors are found on the basal ganglia, limbic system, nigrostriatal path, and prefrontal cortex. A gut–brain system functions to control satiety and metabolite–energy balance. An endogenous cardiac cannabinoid system has been identified in animals and may also function in humans as a cardioprotective system.

The main source of phytocannabinoids is the marijuana plant. Over 60 cannabinoids have been identified; however, the three most abundant and most-studied are Δ^9-tetrahydrocannabinol (THC), cannabindiol, and cannabinol. The psychoactive phytocannabinoid is THC, which is a partial agonist for CB1 and CB2 receptors. Cannabindiol has no psychotropic effects. Cannabinol is a degradation product of THC and has a mild psychotropic effect. The phytocannabinoids can enter the body through a variety of portals, including smoking, vaporization, intravenous injection, sublingually, and rectally. The chemicals are broken down in the liver by the cytochrome P450 oxidases. Some metabolites may remain in the body for several weeks and can be stored in adipose tissue.

Medicinal cannabinoids are found in drugs available in the USA and worldwide. Dronabinol is an oral medication containing THC and is a Schedule III drug used for appetite stimulation. It is also an antiemetic and analgesic. Nabilon is a Schedule II synthetic analog of dronabinol. It is an oral preparation that interacts with the CB1 receptors and is used to treat nausea and vomiting. Sativex, an oral spray, contains THC and cannabindiol and has been used to treat neuropathic pain. Rimonabant is a selective CB1 receptor antagonist and is currently being studied as an anti-Parkinson drug. It is also used as an antiobesity drug and as a smoking inhibitor. Rimonabant has been associated with reducing body weight, hyperlipidemia, insulin resistance, and decreasing high density lipids and hemoglobin A1c.

Infections

Bacterial infections

Seven citations were found on a PubMed search for bacterial infections and marijuana, including two reviews, four case series on infectious outbreaks, and a cross-sectional study.

The review article by Friedman *et al.* (2006) reported on studies describing the mechanisms by which drugs of abuse modify immune mechanisms. Alcohol, nicotine, opiates, cocaine, and marijuana were the target of the studies reviewed. Marijuana and opiates were found to bind with receptors on immune cells and on presynaptic neurons in the CNS and peripheral nervous system. Immune cell activity was decreased, suggesting that use of these drugs can lead to an increased susceptibility to a wide range of infections.

Klein *et al.* (1998) reviewed research looking at marijuana and immunity. Animal, human, and in vitro studies of immune cells showed that marijuana/cannabis modulates the T helper cells types 1 and 2, B lymphocytes, natural killer cells, and macrophages. The cannabinoids modulate the acute phase of inflammation and the release of cytokines associated with inflammation and immunity. The review describes the role of the cannabinoids in suppressing the inflammatory response and immunity, and in decreasing host resistance to various infectious agents.

Two case series described outbreaks of TB in marijuana users. Munckhof *et al.* (2003) reported marijuana users and a TB outbreak in Queensland, Australia. Active TB was found in five individuals who shared a water pipe. The same TB isolates were found in all five individuals; 149 contacts were identified, and 114 were screened. Of those screened, 57 (50%) had significant tuberculin skin tests. Of 45 contacts who shared a water pipe with the infected five individuals, 29 (65%) had positive tuberculin skin tests. The OR for TB transmission was found to be 2.22 (95% CI 0.96–5.17). However, in addition to the risk of sharing of marijuana water pipes, close household contacts with positive tuberculin skin tests were found to be a more important risk in these individuals (OR 4.91; 95% CI 1.13–20.70).

In a second TB case series, Oeltmann *et al.* (2006) reported on an outbreak of TB in Seattle, USA in 2004. Eleven young patients with TB were found to have been "hot boxing" – smoking marijuana in a closed car in order to re-inhale exhaled smoke. The same TB isolates were found in all 11 individuals. Twenty-two of their friends were also screened for TB and 14 (64%) also had positive TB tests. The authors suggested that TB can be transmitted in socially linked marijuana users.

In a study of the role of social networks and marijuana smoking in a community outbreak of *Neisseria meningitides* (meningococcus), Krause *et al.* (2001) interviewed nine new meningitis patients and their contacts. Of the nine patients tested, seven isolates of the bacteria were identical. The patients and their contacts were interviewed and linked to marijuana use. There was no report of meningococci in the contacts. The authors suggested that studying social networks and marijuana use might help to prevent secondary infections by identifying close contacts of patients.

Finn *et al.* (2001) reported on a cluster of three adolescents and young adults developing meningococcal infections after attending a party where alcohol and marijuana use occurred. The serotype C meningococcus was found in all three. Four controls who also attended the party tested negatively for meningococcus. The authors suggested that transmission of the bacterium occurred at the party where marijuana and alcohol was used and that modifying these risky behaviors could decrease the incidence of meningococcal disease.

One cross-sectional study found an association between STDs and use of condoms and marijuana. Liau *et al.* (2002) reported on 522 African American female adolescents tested for STD infection and marijuana use. Since self-report may be unreliable, marijuana use was confirmed by laboratory testing in this study. Those who used marijuana (28 [5.4%]) were more likely than non-marijuana users to have *Neisseria gonorrheae* infections (AOR, 3.4) and *Chlamydia trachomatis* infections (AOR, 3.9). The marijuana users were also less likely to use a condom than their counterparts (AOR, 2.9 for previous 30 days; AOR, 3.6 previous six months). The authors suggested that that STDs and risky sexual behavior may co-occur with marijuana use.

Table 4.1 summarizes these studies.

Table 4.1 Increased risk of bacterial infection with marijuana use and close contact with infected individuals

Study	Method	Sample	Incidence	Results
Finn et al. (2001)	Case–control study Meningococcal outbreak after party where alcohol and marijuana present	3 patients serogroup C meningococcus; 4 controls	3 patients confirmed by laboratory analysis to have identical meningococcal subtypes	Transmission of bacterium is possible in gatherings where alcohol and marijuana use occurs
Friedman et al. (2006)	Review of research Immunomodulation associated with drugs of abuse, including marijuana and opiates	Research using animal models, in vitro studies with immune cells		Studies show an increase in susceptibility to infectious disease with use of abused drugs; marijuana and opioid use associated with receptor interaction on immune and nervous system cells
Klein et al. (1998)	Review of research Marijuana and immunity, infection			Research suggests cannabinoids in marijuana modulate immune cell function, including T cells, B cells, natural killer cells, and macrophages; changes occur in acute phase, and as secondary response: decreased activity of cytokines; macrophages, T helper function
Krause et al. (2001)	Case study Patients in community outbreak of Neisseria meningitides infection	9 patients and their contacts	Laboratory results for patients confirmed 7 positive cultures with identical isolates	All patients linked to contacts and marijuana use
Liau et al. (2002)	Cross-sectional study	522 female African Americans	5.4% positive for marijuana use; users more likely to test positive for N gonorrheae (AOR 3.4) and Chlamydia trachomatis (AOR 3.9), less likely to use condom in last month (AOR 2.9) or last six months (AOR 3.6)	STDs and sexual risk behavior may be associated with marijuana use
Munckhof et al. (2003)	Case report TB outbreak in marijuana users and use of water pipe	5 with active TB, same bacterial isolates	149 contacts identified, 114 (77%) completed screening; 57 (50%) TB test positive; sharing water pipe risk of TB transmission (OR 2.22; 95% CI 0.96–5.17); most important risk was close household contact with a person with TB (OR 4.91; 95% CI 1.13–20.70)	Use of inhaling cannabinoids in vapors may contribute to transmission of TB; household contact with infected individuals also an important risk factor
Oeltmann et al. (2006)	Case series TB outbreak in Seattle USA 2004	11 young TB patients with same isolates	14/22 (64%) friends also with TB	Transmission of Mycobacterium tuberculosis may occur during hotboxing (rebreathing exhaled marijuana smoke in closed car)

AOR, adjusted odds ratio; STD, sexually transmitted disease; TB, tuberculosis.

159

Table 4.2 Mycoses

Study	Method	Sample	Incidence	Results
Darling *et al.* (1990)	Case–control study Candidal oral lesions in drug- and non-users Imprint culture technique for *Candida* diagnosis	58 marijuana–methaqualone–tobacco users; 50 age- and sex-matched controls	Marijuana–methaqualone–tobacco users had an increased prevalence and density of *C. albicans* compared with non-smokers; 2 subjects had oral multifocal candidiasis	There was no difference in the prevalence of candidiasis in subjects and controls

Comments

Very few studies explore the relationship between various bacterial infections and marijuana use. Most of the epidemiological studies (four of the five) are case series with small numbers of subjects and lack of controls. One study is a cross-sectional design involving a fairly large number of subjects (522). In all but one study, the use of marijuana was self-reported and not laboratory verified. This may significantly affect the validity of the studies if self-report of marijuana use is low, as suggested by Liau *et al.* (2002). None of the studies indicate the length of prior use of marijuana in the individuals with the bacterial infections. Since cannabinoids can diminish the inflammatory and immune responses, length of time of marijuana use prior to exposure to the infectious agent may be a significant risk factor.

The two reviews of the scientific literature related to the cannabinoids and the inflammatory and immune responses suggest that marijuana use can diminish the normal protective mechanisms to mount an effective inflammation and immune response to infectious agents. The literature reviewed included articles from human and animal studies, as well as in vitro cell culture studies.

Mycoses

Only one epidemiological study published between 1988 and 2008 explored the relationship between marijuana and the presence of *Candida* in the oral cavity. Darling *et al.* (1990) studied the effect of marijuana smoking along with methaqualone and tobacco use and the presence of *Candida albicans* in the oral cavity; 58 tobacco smoking, methaqualone, and marijuana users were age and sex matched with 50 non-smokers. The marijuana–methaqualone–tobacco users had a higher prevalence and density of oral *Candida* than the non-smokers. However, there was no difference in the incidence of candidiasis (*Candida* infection) in either subjects or controls. Multifocal candidiasis was found in two subjects (Table 4.2).

Comments

Since only one epidemiological study was published since 1990, more studies are needed to show whether marijuana users are more at risk for candidal overgrowth and candidiasis. Besides marijuana use, the subjects also used methaqualone and tobacco. Cross-sectional studies comparing marijuana, methaqualone, and tobacco users with non-users would help to determine the effect of each illicit drug on the growth of *Candida* in the oral cavity. Considering other confounding variables (age, sex, alcohol use, duration and amount of marijuana use) would strengthen the results of future studies.

Viral infections

Two epidemiological studies were found in a review of PubMed from 1988 through 2008 on the association between viral infections (not HIV) and marijuana use. Both were published in 2008 and both explored risk of developing severe steatosis (fatty degeneration) and fibrosis in the liver with marijuana use.

Hézode et al. (2008) studied 315 patients with untreated chronic hepatitis C infection who underwent liver biopsy. Marijuana use, alcohol consumption, and tobacco use were assessed through patient histories. Liver biopsies were carried out and evaluated by the Metavir scoring system by two pathologists. Metavir is a diagnostic tool that grades and stages the amount of inflammation and fibrosis or scarring on tissue obtained by liver biopsy. A Metavir score of 30% or more was used to define marked steatosis. There were three groups of patients in this study: non-marijuana users (63.5%), occasional marijuana users (12.4%), and daily marijuana users (24.1%). Multivariate analysis was used to identify predictors of marked steatosis: daily marijuana use (OR 2.1; 95% CI 1.01–4.5), activity grade equal to or over A2 (OR 2.1; 95% CI 1.0–4.3), genotype 3 (OR 5.4; 95% CI 2.6–11.3), hyperglycemia or diabetes mellitus (OR 5.1; 95% CI 1.8–15.0; 5), BMI > 27 kg/m^2 (OR 2.1; 95% CI 1.0–4.3), and serum HCV RNA load(OR 1.7; 95% CI 1.0–2.9). Marked steatosis was more often seen in daily marijuana users than occasional users (p = 0.03), and more often seen in daily users than in non-users (p = 0.008) when HCV genotype and alcohol use was considered in the analysis. These findings concur with research showing that ECs bind with CB1 receptors in the liver and promote steatosis in experimental conditions. Hézode et al. (2008) concluded that daily use of marijuana is an independent predictor of steatosis in persons with chronic HCV infection.

A prospective cohort study by Ishida et al. (2008) showed that daily marijuana use is associated with moderate to severe fibrosis in 204 patients with chronic HCV infection. The participants had a median age of 46.8 years, more were male (69.1%), 49% were white, and were most likely to develop chronic HCV infection through intravenous drug use (70.1%). Alcohol lifetime use was 29.1 years, 1.94 drinks/day. Marijuana use was daily in 13.7%, occasional in 45.1%, and never in 41.2%. The Ishak method was used to determine liver fibrosis (F, staged from 1 to 6), which evaluates the degree of pathology in liver cells, including necrosis, inflammation, and fibrosis. A significant association was found between daily marijuana use and moderate (F1–F2, 55.4%) and severe (F3–F6, 17.2%) fibrosis. Using univariate analysis, the OR was 3.21 (95% CI 1.20–8.56; p = 0.02); multivariate analysis showed an OR of 6.78 (95% CI 1.89–24.31; p = 0.003). Development of portal tracts and long-term moderate to heavy alcohol use were also identified as independent predicators of stage F3 to F6 fibrosis.

Table 4.3 summarizes these studies.

Comments

Both studies show a strong association between daily marijuana use and moderate to severe steatosis and fibrosis in persons with chronic HCV infection. Confounders, including alcohol use, were considered in data analysis. Both studies suggest that individuals with chronic HCV infection should refrain from use of marijuana because of the likelihood of developing severe steatosis and fibrosis.

These studies support laboratory studies that indicate cannabinoids can bind to CB1 receptors in the liver and cause steatosis. Further studies are needed to identify the role of other confounders identified in the Hézode study, including concurrent diabetes mellitus, hyperglycemia, and an elevated BMI, in increasing the risk of steatosis in marijuana users

Table 4.3 Viral (non-HIV) infections

Study	Method	Sample	Incidence	Results
Hézode et al. (2008)	Case–control study Identification of predictors for steatosis and fibrosis in chronic HCV infection Liver biopsy; pathology assess by Medtavir scale	315 with untreated chronic HCV infection undergoing liver biopsy	Multivariate analysis identified 6 predictors of steatosis: daily marijuana use (OR 2.1; 95% CI 1.1–4.5), activity grade ≥ 2 (OR 2.1; 95% CI 1.0–4.3), genotype 3 (OR 5.4; 95% CI 2.6–11.3), hyperglycemia or diabetes mellitus (OR 5.1; 95% CI 1.8–15.0), BMI > 27 kg/m² (OR 2.1; 95% CI 1.0–4.3), serum HCV RNA load (OR 1.7; 95% CI 1.0–2.9) With adjustment for HCV grade (3 vs. non-3) or alcohol intake (< 30 g/day vs. > 30 g/day), marked steatosis more frequent in daily marijuana users compared with occasional ($p = 0.03$) and non-users ($p = 0.008$)	Marijuana smoking is a novel independent predictor of steatosis severity in chronic HCV infection; research supports laboratory studies showing cannabinoid binding to CB1 receptors in liver, leading to steatosis; marijuana use should be discouraged in those with chronic HCV infection
Ishida al. (2008)	Prospective cohort study Chronic HCV infection and degree of liver fibrosis Pathology assessed by Ishak method	204 with chronic HCV infection: median age, 46.8 years; 69% male; 49% white Infection route: intravenous drug use, 70.1%; alcohol use, 29.1 years, 1.91 drinks/day; cannabis use daily 13.4%; cannabis use occasionally 45.1%; cannabis use never 41.2%	Fibrosis in daily marijuana users, univariate OR, 3.21 (95% CI 1.20–8.56; $p = 0.02$; multivariate OR, 6.78 (95% CI 1.89–24.3; $p = 0.003$); other independent predictors of severe steatosis: 11 or more portal tracts (OR 6.92; 95% CI 1.34–35.7; $p = 0.021$); lifetime duration of moderate to heavy alcohol use per decade (OR 1.72; 95% CI 1.02–2.90; $p = 0.044$)	Daily marijuana use strongly associated with moderate to severe liver fibrosis; Persons with chronic HCV infection should be encouraged to abstain from marijuana use

BMI, body mass index; CB, cannabinoid; CI, confidence interval; HCV, hepatitis C virus; OR, odds ratio.

Neoplastic disease

Twelve abstracts of epidemiological studies on neoplasms and marijuana smoking published between 1988 and 2008 were reviewed. Five studies were review articles published since 2000. Six were case–control studies involving cancer of the mouth, airway, upper digestive tract, and urinary bladder. One study was a retrospective study of respiratory tract cancer. All of the studies looked at the relationship between marijuana use and cancer development.

Carriot & Sasco (2000) reviewed literature associated with marijuana smoking and cancer. An increased risk was found for head and neck cancers in marijuana users who were frequent smokers over an extended period of time. However, interactions were found with cigarette smoking and alcohol use. The reviewers suggest that THC, a major phyto-cannabinoid in marijuana, may have a different carcinogenic effect to that of other chemicals associated with smoking.

Mehra *et al.* (2006) reviewed literature from 1966 to 2005 that was associated with marijuana smoking and lung changes leading to cancer; 19 studies were selected for review. Although marijuana smoking was associated with changes in alveolar macrophage and bronchial mucosal function, the observational studies failed to show a significant association between marijuana use and lung cancer when adjusted for tobacco use. The reviewers noted methodological limitations in many of the reviewed studies, including selection bias, small sample size, limited generalizability, and lack of adjustment for tobacco smoking. Since premalignant changes and cancer development may take some time to develop, the young age of many of the studies' subjects could be a confounding factor in the results of the studies.

The first of two reviews by Hashibe *et al.* (2002) included laboratory studies that described the antitumor and tumor-promoting properties of marijuana. Although THC may have protective apoptotic properties, the chemical has also been shown to suppress immune function and increase tumorigenic reactive oxygen species. According to the review, marijuana tar contains similar carcinogens to the tar in cigarettes, and marijuana smokers tend to inhale and retain more smoke than cigarette smokers. Cell changes in the bronchial mucosa were described in the reviewed literature. Several case studies suggested a relationship between marijuana use and oral, head, and neck cancer. However, one prospective cohort study showed no apparent increased risk in marijuana smokers compared with cigarette smokers in an eight-year follow-up.

The second review article by Hashibe *et al.* (2005) described two cohort studies and 14 case–control studies. The cohort studies explored the association between marijuana use and adult-onset gliomas and lung, colorectal, prostate, and cervical cancer. The case–control studies explored the association between marijuana use and a variety of cancers. Many of the studies had conflicting results or lacked a statistically significant association between marijuana use and cancer. The review pointed out some limitations of the studies, including possible under-reporting of self-marijuana use, small sample size, and confounders such as concurrent tobacco smoking. The reviewers suggested that more studies are needed that focus on marijuana use and tobacco-related cancers, that give more detailed information about the marijuana users and their smoking habits, that have larger numbers of patients and controls so can be expanded to a larger population, and that control for concurrent tobacco use by the marijuana users.

Nieder *et al.* (2006) reviewed the literature on transitional cell bladder carcinoma as part of a case report of a 45-year-old heavy marijuana user who developed this form of cancer.

Since this type of cancer is associated with long-term smoking, the authors also reviewed related literature.

A case–control study by Zhang *et al.* (1999) studied 173 subjects with squamous cell cancer of the head and neck along with 176 cancer-free controls. Using a questionnaire addressing tobacco, alcohol, and marijuana use, and controlling for age, sex, race, and passive smoking, the researchers found that marijuana users had an increased risk for squamous cell cancer compared with non-marijuana smokers (OR 2.6; 95% CI 1.1–6.6). Interaction effects were found with marijuana use and cigarette smoke, mutagen sensitivity, and use of alcohol. The findings also suggest that marijuana users may have an increased risk of head and neck cancer, especially with a dose–response association with marijuana smoking over a long period of time.

Rosenblatt *et al.* (2004) studied the association between marijuana use and oral squamous cell cancer. In this population-based case–control study, 407 individuals with newly diagnosed oral squamous cell cancer were compared with a control group of 615 individuals randomly recruited by phone. The patients with oral cancer ranged in age from 18 to 65 years. Marijuana use was similar in both groups (AOR 0.9; 95% CI 0.6–1.3). With adjustments for sex, education, birth year, alcohol use, and cigarette use, there was no significant association between oral squamous cell cancer risk and marijuana use.

A case–control study by Chacko *et al.* (2006) examined a convenience sample of 52 men aged 59 years or younger diagnosed with transitional cell bladder cancer (TCBC) and 104 age-matched controls with no history or signs and symptoms of TCBC. The subjects completed a questionnaire assessing past exposure to known TCBC carcinogens and marijuana use. Forty-six (88.5%) of the men with TCBC acknowledged habitual marijuana use, and 72 (69.2%) of the controls habitually used marijuana. The researchers noted there was a statistically significant difference ($p = 0.0008$) between the number of habitual marijuana users with TCBC and the habitual marijuana-using controls. They also found a significant correlation between marijuana use and the stage, grade, and recurrence of the cancer. Although a large number of both those with TCBC and those without TCBC were habitual marijuana users, the authors suggested that marijuana smoking increased the risk of TCBC. No risk data were provided, and it is not clear whether confounders such as cigarette smoking were considered in this study.

Hashibe *et al.* (2006) studied 1212 patients with lung and upper aerodigestive cancer and 1040 cancer-free controls. The subjects and controls were matched for age, gender, and place of residence. This population-based case–control study involved a questionnaire that gathered information about marijuana use in joint-years (where 1 joint-year was one joint per day per year). The results of the study showed a positive association between long-term marijuana smokers ($\geq$ 30 joint-years) with the types of cancer studied, but not a significant relationship when adjusted for confounders that included cigarette smoking. Comparing with 0 joint-years, the AORs for $\geq$ 60 joint-years and various cancers were 1.1 (oral), 0.84 (laryngeal), and 0.62 (lung), while the AOR for $\geq$ 30 joint-years was 0.57 for pharyngeal cancer and 0.53 for esophageal cancer. They concluded that there was not a strong relationship between marijuana use and these cancers. Similar limitations were cited for this study as for those described in the Hashibe review articles (Hashibe *et al.* 2002, 2005), including selection bias, measurement errors including lifetime exposure, and accuracy of information about confounders (e.g., cigarette smoking, exposure to known carcinogens) in patient and control subject histories.

A paper published by Voirin *et al.* (2006) described a case–control study of lung cancer in marijuana users, comparing 149 hospitalized patients with lung cancer with 188 controls.

For tobacco smokers and development of lung cancer, the OR was 3.9 (95% CI 1.4–10.9) in former smokers and 17.1 (95% CI 6.3–46.3) in current smokers with a history of over 35 years of cigarette smoking. A linear relationship was found with increased risk of lung cancer and increased number of years the subjects smoked ($p = 0.0001$). When adjusted for age, tobacco use, and occupational exposures, the OR for past use of marijuana and development of lung cancer was 4.1 (95% CI 1.9–9.0). Although the use of marijuana may be a risk factor for the development of lung cancer, this study did not show a dose–response relationship between lung cancer development and the intensity or duration of marijuana use.

In a case–control study by Aldington *et al.* (2008), individuals were interviewed to assess risk factors for lung cancer. Seventy-nine individuals with lung cancer (aged 55 or younger) were compared with 324 randomly selected controls. The subjects were matched by five-year age intervals and location of residence. After adjusting for cigarette smoking and other confounding variables, for each joint-year of cannabis smoking there was an 8% increased risk of developing lung cancer (95% CI 2–15). When using cigarette pack/year and adjusting for marijuana use, there was a 7% increased risk of developing lung cancer (95% CI 5–9). Heavy marijuana users were identified and risk assessed. After adjusting for cigarette smoking, this group had an RR of 5.7 (95% CI 1.5–21.6) of developing lung cancer. These results showed an increased risk of lung cancer with long-term use of marijuana.

A retrospective study by Taylor (1988) involved a review of surgical pathology reports of patients with respiratory cancer. The use of marijuana was studied in 10 patients aged 40 years or younger with respiratory cancer. Five were heavy users and two were regular users of marijuana. The findings suggested that regular marijuana use was an additional risk for developing respiratory cancer.

These studies are summarized in Table 4.4.

Comments

A relatively small number of epidemiological studies concerning marijuana's association with neoplastic diseases were found in the literature reviewed from 1988 and 2008. Five studies were reviews, six were case series or case–control studies, and one study was a retrospective chart review. Four of the studies (with the number of patients ranging from 7 to 173) suggest that there is an increased risk of head, neck, and lung cancer with marijuana smoking. Two of the four studies considered confounders that might increase the risk of cancer.

Four reviews found conflicting results and, in general, found either no association or a weak association between marijuana smoking and the development of head, neck, or lung cancer. Three of the case–control studies found either no association or a weak association between marijuana use and the development of oral, upper aerodigestive, lung cancers, or TCBC. One study found no dose–response relationship in the development of lung cancer and marijuana use.

Several limitations in these studies make it difficult to make generalizations that would indicate a significant association between marijuana use and cancer development. Most of the studies were case–control studies, although one study described cancer development in one marijuana user, and one study was a prospective study of eight years' duration. Most of the case–control studies were based on convenience samples (hospitalized patients or chart review), and controls were often selected randomly from the general population. The number of subjects with the cancer being studied ranged from 1 to 1212, with all but one

Table 4.4 Increased risk of cancer

Study	Method	Sample	Incidence	Results
Aldington et al. (2008)	Case–control study Association between lung cancer and marijuana smoking	79 adults, 55 years or younger, with lung cancer; 324 controls randomly selected from electoral role	Increased risk joint-year adjusted for cigarette smoking: 8% (95% CI 2–15); increased pack-year adjusted for marijuana smoking: 7% (95% CI 5–9); heavy marijuana users risk of lung cancer RR 5.7 (95% CI 1.5–21.6)	Both tobacco smokers and marijuana smokers have increased risk of lung cancer; there is an increased risk of lung cancer with long-term heavy cannabis use
Carriot & Sasco (2000)	Literature review Cannabis and cancer	Not identified		In individuals 40 years old or younger, there may be an increased risk of SCC in the upper airway, tongue/larynx; an increased dose response seen with frequency and duration; there is interaction with cigarette smoking and alcohol use
Chacko et al. (2006)	Case–control study Marijuana and bladder cancer	52 with TCBC, 104 age-matched controls	46 (88.5%) marijuana users had TCBC; 72 (69.2%) controls also marijuana users ($p = 0.0008$, significant)	Marijuana use may be an increased risk factor for the development of TCBC; although a large percentage of those with TCBC smoked marijuana in the study, so also did a large percentage of the controls
Hashibe et al. (2002)	Literature review Marijuana smoking and head and neck cancer	Not identified		Laboratory studies show THC may have antitumor properties and also tumor-promoting properties; similar carcinogens in marijuana and cigarette smoke; bronchial mucosa cell changes occur; one prospective study (8-year) showed no increased risk of cancer in marijuana vs. cigarette smokers
Hashibe et al. (2006)	Population-based case–control study in Los Angeles Marijuana use and lung, upper aerodigestive cancer	1212 with cancer; 1040 cancer-free controls matched for age, gender, neighborhood	Marijuana smokers ≥ 30 joint-years, positive association with cancer, but not when adjusted for confounders (cigarette smoking): 60 vs. 0 joint-years, AOR 1.1 (oral), 0.84 (laryngeal), 0.62 (lung); 30 vs. 0 joint-years, AOR 0.57 (pharyngeal), 0.53 (esophageal)	There is an association, but not strong, between marijuana use and cancer
Hashibe et al. (2005)	Literature review Marijuana use and cancer risk	2 cohort studies, 14 case–control studies	Cohort studies: no association between lung, colorectal cancer, and marijuana smoking; increased risk of prostate and cervical cancer in non-tobacco smokers; increased risk of glioma in tobacco and non-tobacco users	Conflicting results in studies reviewed; insufficient number of studies to conclude an association between marijuana smoking and cancer risk

Reference	Study type	Sample	Results	Conclusion
Mehra et al. (2006)	Literature review; Marijuana smoking and premalignant lung changes and cancer	19 studies, 1966–2005	Association between marijuana smoking and increased tar exposure, alveolar macrophage dysfunction, increased oxidative stress, bronchial mucosa dysfunction	Although tissue changes seen, no significant association between marijuana use and cancer when adjusted for tobacco smoking
Nieder et al. (2006)	Case report and literature review	One case of TCBC	Heavy marijuana use was only risk factor in 45-year-old male with TCBC	TCBC associated with marijuana smoking in this patient
Rosenblatt et al. (2004)	Population-based case-control study	407 patients, aged 18 to 65 years with oral SCC; 615 controls recruited randomly by phone contact	OR adjusted for sex, education, age, alcohol, cigarette smoking is similar for cases and controls: OR 0.9 (95% CI 0.6–1.3)	OR showed no significant association between oral SCC and marijuana use
Taylor (1988)	Retrospective study; Respiratory tract cancer	Review of surgical pathology reports over 4 year period	7 of 10 patients under 40 years of age identified with respiratory cancer were marijuana users	Marijuana use may be an additional significant risk for developing respiratory cancer
Voirin et al. (2006)	Case-control study; Lung cancer and marijuana use	149 male cancer patients, 188 male controls	Increased risk for lung cancer with tobacco smoking: OR 3.9 for former smokers (95% CI 1.4–10.9); OR 17.1 for current smokers, 35+ year history of smoking (95% CI 6.3–46.3); OR 4.1 (95% CI 1.9–9.0) for past marijuana use and lung cancer when adjusted for age, tobacco use, occupational exposure	Linear relationship between risk of lung cancer and years of cigarette smoking; no clear dose–response relationship between lung cancer and intensity or duration of marijuana use; marijuana smoking may be a risk factor for developing lung cancer
Zhang et al. (1999)	Case-control study; Head and neck cancer and marijuana use	173 patients with SSC of the head and neck; 176 cancer-free controls	Increased risk with marijuana use, controlled for age, sex, race, passive smoke: OR (ever/never) 2.6 (95% CI 1.1–6.6)	Interaction effects of marijuana use with cigarette smoking, mutagen sensitivity, alcohol use; marijuana use may increase risk of head and neck cancer, suggested by strong dose–response pattern (marijuana use and day/years use)

AOR, adjusted odds ratio; CI, confidence interval; OR, odds ratio; RR, relative risk; SCC, squamous cell cancer; TCBC, transitional cell bladder cancer; THC, tetrahydrocannabinol.

study using 200 subjects or fewer. The possibility of selection bias and small sample size limit the generalizability of many of the studies.

Many of the studies used questionnaires to gain information about the subjects and the controls. Recall bias is a consideration in assessing the results and conclusions of these studies. Under-reporting of marijuana use or its frequency and duration may occur. Cigarette smoking as a confounder was considered in only a few of the studies, and in these studies, no increased risk of cancer could be determined when marijuana users were also cigarette smokers. Exposure to other confounders (e.g., alcohol, passive smoke) and carcinogens known to increase the risk of the cancer being investigated was generally not considered in these studies.

Since the development of cancer may evolve over many years, studies limited to young smokers may miss those who may go on to develop cancer. Cohort studies over long periods of time may be helpful in identifying the risk of smoking marijuana, especially if confounders can be identified and adjusted for in the statistical analyses.

Too few studies are reported that link marijuana use with a significant increased risk of developing head, neck, esophageal, lung, and bladder cancer. More studies are needed with larger sample sizes, controlled for confounders, and carried out for longer periods of time. More studies are also needed that consider other types of cancer seen in marijuana users. Studies also need to be replicated to enhance the reliability and validity of the results and generalizability of the studies.

Musculoskeletal system disease

Movement disorders

Only one epidemiological study was found in a review of the PubMed database that was published between 1988 and 2008 (Table 4.5). The study by Lozsadi et al. (2004) was a case report of a 25-year-old female who developed propriospinal myoclonus, confirmed by electromyography and frontal EEG, after a single exposure to inhaled marijuana smoke. No structural abnormalities of the spine were found.

Spinal cord function

Only one epidemiological study was found in the PubMed review related to marijuana use and spinal cord function. It reported on the use of alcohol and marijuana in young adults with spinal cord injury.

Young et al. (1995) used the Short Michigan Alcohol Screening Test to explore alcohol use in 123 patients with spinal cord injury. The test contains 13 questions designed to identify alcohol abuse. Patients were also questioned about marijuana use and other factors, including degree of physical impairment related to their spinal cord injury, health maintenance behaviors, depression, and social support. Compared with the alcohol users, the marijuana smokers (16% of respondents) tended to be younger at the time of their spinal cord injury, more depressed, and more stressed. The authors suggested that knowledge of alcohol and marijuana use would be useful information for rehabilitation treatment in spinal cord injured patients (Table 4.6).

Comments

No other reports of propriospinal myoclonus and marijuana use have been reported in the literature.

Table 4.5 Movement disorders

Study	Method	Sample	Incidence	Results
Lozsadi *et al.* (2004)	Case report	25-year-old female exposed to marijuana smoke	Development of propriospinal myoclonus confirmed by electromyography, frontal electroencephalography; no structural abnormality of the spine	

Table 4.6 Spinal cord injury

Study	Method	Sample	Incidence	Results
Young *et al.* (1995)	Convenience sample Alcohol and marijuana use Short Michigan Alcohol Screening Test and assessment of other demographics	123 community-based patients with spinal cord injuries	16% of the respondents smoked marijuana	Compared with alcohol users, marijuana users tended to be younger at the time of the injury, more depressed, more stressed

Too few studies have been published to generalize the characteristics of marijuana smokers with spinal cord injury. The descriptive study by Young *et al.* (1995) did not examine risk of spinal cord injury in persons who smoke marijuana; however, it does add to the body of knowledge about the demographic characteristics of users undergoing rehabilitation.

Digestive system disease

No relevant articles were found concerning marijuana and digestive disease.

Stomatognathic disease

Five articles were found in a review of PubMed literature from 1988 to 2008 that described epidemiological research on marijuana use and oral health. Two reviews, one prospective cohort study, and two case–control studies were found.

Darling & Arendorf (1992) reviewed various conditions found in the oral cavities of marijuana users, including xerostomia (dry mouth), caries, periodontitis, severe gingivitis, and mucosal abnormalities. They also described an untoward reaction to epinephrine-containing local anesthetics in some marijuana users.

Cho *et al.* (2005) also reviewed the oral health problems seen in marijuana users, including dental caries and periodontal disease associated with poor hygiene. Since the phytocannabinoids can interact with CB2 receptors on immune cells, marijuana users may be more likely to experience oral infections because of a depressed immune and inflammatory response. Marijuana smoke has also been found to contain carcinogenic materials, which can lead to mucosal dysplasia and premalignant changes in the mouth. The authors also described the hyperacute anxiety, dysphoria, tachycardia, and paranoia seen when a dental patient high on marijuana is given a local anesthetic containing epinephrine. The authors suggested that dental providers include questions about marijuana use prior to treating their patients.

Two case–control studies were described by Darling and coworkers. In the first study, Darling *et al.* (1990) compared the presence of *C. albicans* in 55 marijuana users, 58 tobacco users, and 50 non-smokers. The marijuana smokers also used tobacco and methaqualone. Compared with the tobacco smokers and non-smokers, the marijuana–tobacco–methaqualone users had an increase in the prevalence and density of oral *C. albicans*. No differences were found in the number of candidal infections found in the subjects and controls. (Also see review in the subsection on mycoses under Infections.)

In a later study, Darling & Arendorf (1993) used a larger sample to study the effect of marijuana use on oral health. Three hundred marijuana-methaqualone-tobacco users were compared with 152 tobacco smokers and 189 non-smokers. Leukoedema and precancerous leukoplakia lesions were found in all three groups; however, the leukoedema, xerostomia, and traumatic ulcers were the only lesions significantly different in the three groups.

A more recent prospective cohort study by Thomson *et al.* (2008) examined marijuana users from Dunedin, New Zealand starting at age 18 years, and then again periodically until age 32. A complete birth cohort (1972–1973) was studied and 903 (89%) of the original cohort of 1015 were followed through. In this study, the degree of combined periodontal attachment loss (CAL) was determined in the surviving cohort. (CAL refers to the detachment of the periodontal ligament from the alveolar bone and is often caused by periodontitis, other periodontal disease, or injury.) The subjects were categorized into three groups: those with no exposure to marijuana (293, 32.3%), those with some exposure to marijuana (428, 47.4%), and those with a high exposure to marijuana (182, 20.2%). Those with the highest exposure to marijuana had the highest number of incident attachment losses (23.6%) of all groups. Compared with the no exposure group, the users with the highest exposure to marijuana had the highest incidence of one or more CAL sites of ≥ 4 mm (RR 1.6; 95% CI 1.2–2.2); one or more CAL sites of ≥ 5 mm (RR 3.1; 95% CI 1.5–6.4, and incident attachment loss (RR 2.2; 95% CI 1.2–3.9). The variables controlled in this study included tobacco smoking (pack/years), sex, irregular use of dental services, and dental plaque. Although tobacco smokers had periodontal disease, no interaction between marijuana use and tobacco smoking was found in predicting periodontal disease. The authors suggested that marijuana use may be an independent predictor of periodontal disease.

These studies on oral health are summarized in Table 4.7.

Comments

Few studies have been reported and indexed in PubMed that look at the effects of marijuana use on oral health. Two of the case–control studies were carried out by some of the same researchers. Their subjects included marijuana users who also used methaqualone and tobacco, tobacco smokers, and non-smokers. It is not clear what the role of methaqualone had in affecting the risk for periodontal disease in the marijuana users. In the prospective cohort study, a group was followed for 14 years. Those with a high exposure to marijuana had a higher incidence of CAL than those in the other groups in the study and also more incident attachment loss. The measure used to determine what some and high exposure to marijuana entailed is not clear. The number of joints smoked and years of smoking were not delineated.

More epidemiological studies are needed to show the risk of periodontal disease in marijuana users. As in many studies reviewed in this chapter, self-report of marijuana use

Table 4.7 Stomatognathic disease

Study	Method	Sample	Incidence	Results
Cho et al. (2005)	Literature review			Marijuana users: poorer oral health, increased dental caries, increased periodontal disease Marijuana smoke carcinogenic, causing dysplasia, leukoplakia on oral mucosa; increased risk of infections through immunosuppression If "high", increased risk of anxiety, dysphoria, tachycardia, paranoia when administered local anesthetic with epinephrine
Thomson et al. (2008)	Prospective cohort study, 1972–1973 CAL	903 (89%) of cohort of 1015	After controlling for confounders (tobacco smoking, sex, irregular use of dental services, dental plaque) compared with non-smokers, those with heavy marijuana exposure: ≥ 1 CAL 4 mm, RR 1.6 (95% CI 1.2–2.2); ≥ 1 CAL 5 mm, RR 3.1 (95% CI 1.5–6.45); incident attachment loss, RR 2.2 (95% CI 1.2–3.9)	No interaction between marijuana exposure and tobacco use in predicting periodontal disease; marijuana smoking may be a risk factor independent of use of tobacco for periodontal disease including CAL and incident attachment loss
Darling et al. (1990)	Case–control study Marijuana and oral candidal carriage	58 marijuana users, 54 tobacco smokers, 50 non-smokers	Increased C. albicans in oral cavity of marijuana users: increased presence, density	No significant difference in candidal infections in the three groups
Darling & Arendorf (1992)				Marijuana use associated with xerostomia, caries periodontitis, severe gingivitis, oral mucosal disease; marijuana can cause abnormal stress response to local anesthetics containing epinephrine
Darling & Arendorf (1993)	Case–control study	300 marijuana–tobacco–methaqualone users, 152 tobacco smokers, 189 non-smokers	Leukoedema, leukoplakia found in all three groups	Marijuana users experienced more leukoedema, dry mouth, traumatic ulcers

CAL, combined attachment loss; CI, confidence interval; RR, relative risk.

may be under- or over-reported by the subjects. Controlling for other confounders (e.g., alcohol use, dose and duration of marijuana use) could offer greater reliability, validity, and generalizability to these studies.

Respiratory system disease

Twelve epidemiological studies examining marijuana use and the risk of respiratory disease were published between 1988 and 2008. The studies included five review articles and six case–control or prospective cohort studies.

Three reviews were written by Tashkin (1990, 2001, 2005) and summarized findings of pulmonary changes in individuals who smoked marijuana. In the first review, Tashkin (1990) described pulmonary changes found in smokers of marijuana and other smoked abused substances, including crack cocaine. Studies to this point suggested that marijuana smoking caused lung injury, including chronic respiratory tract symptoms such as acute bronchitis, disease of the respiratory mucous membrane, and alveolar macrophage dysfunction. The review also suggested that crack smoking may lead to respiratory tract dysfunction and acute lung injury.

In a second review, Tashkin (2001) expanded abused substances to include amyl and butyl nitrites, heroin, methamphetamine, and phencyclidine, in addition to marijuana and crack cocaine. Marijuana use was associated with lung injury, alveolar macrophage dysfunction, an increased risk of pulmonary infections, and respiratory cancer. Crack smoking was associated with an increase in asthma symptoms, and histological changes associated with acute lung injury syndrome. Heroin was found to exacerbate asthma symptoms, and nitrites, crystal methamphetamine, and phencyclidine studies showed pulmonary consequences.

In the most recent review, Tashkin (2005) stressed the respiratory effects of THC in marijuana. Although THC can cause modest short-term bronchodilation, chronic exposure to THC was associated with chronic cough and increased sputum production. Chronic airway inflammation and injury could lead to unregulated epithelial cell growth and lung cancer. Impaired alveolar macrophage activity, altered immune-related cytokine release, and decreased nitric oxide were also reported. These depressed inflammatory reactions may lead to increased pulmonary infections in chronic marijuana users. Tashkin suggested that, with the consideration of medicinal marijuana use, more studies are needed exploring long-term smoking risks in pulmonary health.

Van Hoozen & Cross (1997) reviewed marijuana smoking effects on pulmonary function. Since studying pulmonary function tests helps to predict chronic obstructive pulmonary disease, studies were reviewed to see whether this approach could also be used to predict chronic obstructive pulmonary disease in marijuana users. Similar to tobacco users, cough, wheezing, and increased sputum production are common findings in marijuana users. However, the authors concluded that the habitual marijuana user would need to smoke four to five joints per day for 30 years before developing chronic obstructive pulmonary disease. Other studies suggest that marijuana smoke is mutagenic and carcinogenic. Although epidemiological studies showed a potential for developing cancer of the larynx, oropharynx, and bronchial structures in marijuana smokers, the RR had not been substantiated by the reviewed research. The review also pointed out that respiratory changes in marijuana smokers are similar to those found in tobacco smokers. The authors suggested that more longitudinal studies are needed to show a relationship between upper airway bronchogenic cancers and marijuana smoking.

Tetrault *et al.* (2007) focused on the impact of marijuana smoking on pulmonary function and respiratory complications by reviewing 34 articles published between 1966 and 2005. The articles reviewed looked at results of airflow studies in short-term and long-term marijuana smokers. Eleven studies found an association between short-term marijuana use and bronchodilation, demonstrated by an increase in forced expiratory volume in 1 second (FEV_1) of 0.15 to 0.25 liters. In the studies looking at lung changes in long-term marijuana users, no consistent association was found between long-term use and measures of air flow obstruction. Fourteen studies that assessed respiratory complications found increased cough, sputum productivity, and wheezing in marijuana smokers. The OR for marijuana smoking and cough was 2.00 (95% CI 1.32–3.01). Some limitations were found in the quality of some of the studies reviewed, particularly in controlling for confounders such as concurrent tobacco smoking.

A prospective cohort study by Polen *et al.* (1993) explored the use of the healthcare system by 452 marijuana users who reported they did not smoke tobacco compared with a demographically similar control group of 450 non-smokers. The smoking status was assessed at health check-ups at a medical center between 1979 and 1985 and a review of medical records for a two-year follow-up. Comparative analyses were controlled for age, sex, race, education, marital status, and alcohol use. Marijuana users had a slight increased RR for respiratory-related outpatient visits (RR, 1.19; 95% CI 1.01–1.41). They also had an increased RR of 1.32 (95% CI 1.10–1.57) for injury, and an increased RR of 1.09 (95% CI 1.02–1.16) for office visits for other illnesses. Although not statistically significant, the marijuana users also had an increased risk of hospital admissions than their non-smoking counterparts (RR 1.51; 95% CI 0.93–2.46). While a strong RR was not found, the study found that marijuana smokers appeared to use the healthcare system slightly more than the non-smoking controls.

Roth *et al.* (1998) studied airway inflammation in 40 subjects who underwent videobronchoscopy, mucosal biopsy, and bronchial lavage. The subjects were non-smokers, marijuana-only smokers, tobacco-only smokers, or combined marijuana–tobacco smokers. The smokers (marijuana, tobacco, and marijuana–tobacco) showed more inflammatory changes than non-smokers, including vascular hyperplasia, submucosal edema, inflammatory cell infiltrates, and goblet cell hyperplasia. Bronchial lavage showed the highest percentage of neutrophils and interleukin-8 in the combined tobacco–marijuana smokers, and the lowest percentage of these inflammatory indicators in non-smokers. The authors suggested that smokers using only tobacco or only marijuana had fewer inflammatory changes than combined tobacco–marijuana smokers. However, all smokers had more inflammatory changes than non-smokers.

Stokes *et al.* (2000) studied whether cannabis might be a clinically important allergen in certain patients, particularly in areas where cannabis grows naturally. The subjects included 127 individuals undergoing multi-test routine skin testing. The Cannabis Skin Test was included in the battery of tests and 78/127 (61%) subjects tested positive for cannabis. Of these, 30 were randomly selected to determine a history of allergic rhinitis or asthma. Twenty-two had respiratory symptoms between July and September, the period of time when the cannabis pollen count was the highest (36% of the total pollen counted). All of the 22 subjects had positive skin tests for other weeds that pollinate at the same time as cannabis. Although more study is needed, the authors suggested that cannabis may be an aeroallergen for certain individuals.

Taylor and coworkers published two articles based on a cohort of young adults born in Dunedin, New Zealand in 1972–1973. The first study (Taylor *et al.* 2000) explored the respiratory effects of cannabis smoking and lung function using data from 943 of the initial cohort of 1037 subjects at age 21 years. A questionnaire was used to assess respiratory symptoms and all 943 underwent spirometry and methacholine challenge tests. The DSM-IIIR criteria were used to determine cannabis dependency. The three comparison groups in the study were cannabis dependent (91, 9.7%), tobacco smoking (264, 28.1%), and non-smoking. Adjusted odds ratios were determined for respiratory symptoms, lung function, and airway hyperresponsiveness (measured as the PC20, the provocative concentration of methacholine required to produce a 20% fall in the FEV_1). According to Taylor *et al.* (2000), compared with non-tobacco smokers, the cannabis-dependent group showed a significant ($p < 0.05$) increase in wheezing (61%), nocturnal wakening with chest tightness (72%), and a 144% increase in early morning sputum production ($p < 0.01$) after controlling for tobacco smoking. The respiratory findings in the cannabis-dependent group were similar to those who smoked 1 to 10 cigarettes per day. The ratio FEV_1/forced vital capacity (FVC) was also measured. An FEV_1/FVC ratio of < 80% was seen in 33 (36%) of the cannabis-dependent subjects compared with 20% for non-smokers ($p = 0.04$). Despite the young age of the cannabis smokers, significant respiratory function changes were evident.

The second study reported by Taylor *et al.* (2002) used the same subjects to compare respiratory changes in the group at ages 18, 21, and 26 years. Over 900 subjects remained in this prospective cohort study. When stratified for cumulative use of marijuana, the researchers found a significant linear relation between cannabis use (of > 900 joints) and FEV_1/vital capacity (VC) ($p < 0.05$). At age 18, 21, and 26 years, the mean percentage decrease in FEV_1/VC ratio was 7.2, 2.6, and 5.0%, respectively, with the major decrease in the cohort at age 21. The study showed a dose-dependent relationship between marijuana use and a decrease in pulmonary function. However, when controlled for age, weight, and tobacco smoking, there was no significant negative effect on the mean FEV_1/VC ratio ($p < 0.09$).

Moore *et al.* (2005) used the third National Health and Nutrition Examination Survey (1988–1992) to study respiratory effects of marijuana and tobacco smoking in a large US population ($n = 6728$). The responses of participants on the drug, tobacco, and health sections of the survey were analyzed in this study. Subjects also had a respiratory examination. Compared with non-marijuana users, the marijuana users had more symptoms of chronic bronchitis and chest sounds in the absence of a cold ($p = 0.02$), coughing most days ($p = 0.001$), increased mucus production ($p = 0.0005$), and wheezing ($p = 0.0001$). The study found that marijuana smokers and tobacco smokers had similar respiratory findings.

Table 4.8 summarizes these studies.

Comments

In a 20-year period, only six epidemiological studies were reported on the effects of marijuana smoking and respiratory disease. Five review articles were also published during this time period. Most of the case–control and prospective studies included a relatively large number of subjects (127 to 6728). Four of the studies controlled for tobacco use and other confounders in their analyses. Most of the results showed that there may be a slight increased in RR in marijuana users compared with non-smokers; however, marijuana and tobacco smokers both had similar respiratory findings, including evidence of inflammatory disease and abnormal pulmonary function tests. A fifth study provided evidence that cannabis may be an allergen.

While some of these studies controlled for confounders, not all of them controlled for the same confounders. The reliance on self-report may also introduce bias related to history

Table 4.8 Increased risk of respiratory disease with marijuana use

Study	Method	Sample	Incidence	Results
Moore et al. (2005)	Analysis of responses on NHANES III national survey Medical examination	6728 adults, aged 20 to 59 years	In analyses controlled for age, gender, asthma, marijuana users, compared with non-users, had more symptoms of chronic bronchitis ($p = 0.02$); cough, mucus production, wheezing (all $p = 0.001$ or less)	Marijuana smokers develop respiratory symptoms similar to tobacco smokers
Polen et al. (1993)	Prospective cohort study of outpatient visits for respiratory and other complaints, hospitalizations Check up and chart review 1979–1985	452 marijuana smokers, 450 non-smokers	In analyses controlled for age, sex, race, education, marital status, alcohol use, marijuana users, compared with non-smokers: outpatient visits, RR 1.19 (95% CI 1.01–1.41); injury, RR 1.32 (95% CI 1.10–1.57); other illnesses, RR 1.09 (95% CI 1.02–116); hospital admission, RR 1.51 (95% CI 0.93–2.46) (n.s.)	Marijuana smokers tended to have an increased risk for various health problems
Roth et al. (1998)	Cross-sectional study Marijuana smoking and airway inflammation Bronchoscopy (bronchial index), biopsy, and lavage	40 subjects, aged 20–49 years, divided into four groups: non-smokers, marijuana smokers, tobacco smokers, marijuana and tobacco smokers	Bronchial index higher in all smokers than non-smokers; biopsy showed more inflammatory changes in smokers: vascular hyperplasia, submucosal edema, inflammatory infiltrates, goblet cell hyperplasia Number of biopsy criteria present: smokers, 2 in 97%, 3 or more in 72%; none more than 1 in non-smokers Lavage showed correlation between percentage neutrophils and interleukin-8 levels; neutrophils > 20% in 1/9 marijuana smokers, 2/9 tobacco smokers, 5/10 marijuana–tobacco smokers, 0/10 non-smokers	Marijuana smoking associated with significant airway inflammation similar to that in tobacco smokers; all types of smokers showed more inflammatory changes than non-smokers
Stokes et al. (2000)	Convenience sample Cannabis as a clinically important allergen Pollen counts in US Midwest; skin testing	Convenience sample 127 total; 30 examined further for rhinitis during high pollen season	78 tested positive in skin test for cannabis and other weeds; 22/30 (73%) had respiratory signs and symptoms between July and September when pollen count elevated (36% cannabis pollen in pollen samples)	Cannabis is likely to be an allergen and affect some individuals, especially in areas where marijuana occurs naturally

Table 4.8 Cont.

Study	Method	Sample	Incidence	Results
Tashkin (1990)	Literature review Respiratory complications and marijuana, crack cocaine			Marijuana use associated with lung injury, chronic respiratory symptoms, acute bronchitis, tracheobronchial epithelial disease, alveolar macrophage dysfunction
Tashkin (2001)	Literature review Respiratory complications and marijuana, crack cocaine, amyl and butyl nitrites, heroin, methamphetamine, phencyclidine			Marijuana: airway injury; altered structure/ function of alveolar macrophages; predisposed to pulmonary infections and cancer Crack acute respiratory complications, exacerbation of asthma, acute lung injury syndrome Heroin: exacerbation of asthma Nitrites, crystal meth, phencyclidine: pulmonary dysfunction
Tashkin (2005)	Literature review Role of THC			Marijuana smokers: short-term effects include bronchodilation; long-term effects include chronic cough, sputum, airway infection and injury, altered epithelial cell growth (oxidative stress, mitochondrial dysfunction, inhibition of apoptosis) Increased susceptibility to infection from decreased macrophage phagocytic activity, altered cytokine function, altered nitric oxide
Taylor et al. (2000)	Prospective cohort study Lung changes in drug use (DSM-IIIR criteria for cannabis) Spirometry, methacholine challenge test	943 young adults, aged 21 years (born 1972–1973) divided into three groups: marijuana dependent (9.7%) tobacco smokers (28.1%), non-smokers (62.2%)	Analyses controlled for tobacco smoking: FEV_1/FVC < 80 in 36% marijuana smokers vs. 20% in non-smokers ($p = 0.04$); compared with non-smokers, marijuana smokers had increase of 61% wheezing, 65% exercise-induced shortness of breath, 72% nocturnal awakening, 144% early morning sputum production (all $p < 0.05$)	Respiratory symptoms and function decreased in marijuana smokers compared with non-smokers; respiratory symptoms of all smokers similar and more than seen in non-smokers
Taylor et al. (2002)	Prospective cohort Lung function in marijuana users Spirometry	900+ young adults, born 1972–1973; comparison of lung function at ages 18, 21, 26 years	Stratified for cumulative use of marijuana (≥ 900 or more), there was a linear relationship between marijuana use and percentage decreased mean FEV_1/VC ($p < 0.05$): 18 years, 7.2%; 21 years, 2.6%; 26 years, 5.0%	Compared with non-users, marijuana smokers had a decreased mean FEV_1/VC at ages 18, 21, and 26 years; however, when controlled for confounders (age, tobacco use, weight), there was no significant risk ($p = 0.09$)

Tetrault et al. (2007)	Literature review. Marijuana use and respiratory changes	34 publications, 1966–2005	Marijuana use and cough, OR 2.00 (95% CI 1.32–3.01)	Short-term marijuana smokers: bronchodilation Long-term marijuana smokers: inconsistent results for airflow obstruction, but associated with increased respiratory symptoms of obstructive lung disease
Van Hoozen & Cross (1997)	Literature review. Respiratory findings in marijuana and tobacco users			Respiratory findings in marijuana users similar to tobacco users; If α_1-antitrypsin normal, habitual marijuana users would have to smoke 4–5 joints/day for 30 years to develop chronic obstructive pulmonary disease; marijuana smoke is mutagenic and carcinogenic but relative risk for cancer not yet quantified for larynx, oropharynx, bronchi; upper airway cancer occurs more often than bronchogenic

CI, confidence interval; OR, odds ratio; RR, relative risk; DSM-IV, *Diagnostic and Statistical Manual of Mental Disorders*, 4th edition; FEV$_1$, forced expiratory volume in 1 second; FVC, forced vital capacity; NHANES, National Health and Nutrition Examination Survey; n.s., not significant; THC, tetrahydrocannabinol; VC, vital capacity.

of marijuana use. Some standardization terms and measurements might be helpful in comparing studies. For example, there seems to be different criteria for short term and long term when referring to length of smoking and defining moderate or heavy smokers. Some studies reported smoking habits in joints/day or cigarettes/day, while others used criteria such as one to five a day or 900/year. The DSM-IIIR criteria were used in one study for marijuana dependency. Two studies by Taylor *et al.* (2000, 2002) measuring pulmonary function used two different ratios – one, the FEV_1/FVC and the other FEV_1/VC. The lack of standardized criteria for categorizing groups or assessing smoking habits makes it difficult to compare studies and generalize the findings.

While there is some evidence that marijuana smoking is detrimental to respiratory health, more studies are needed to allow definitive conclusions. Longitudinal studies would be particularly helpful to assess cumulative affects of marijuana smoking.

Otorhinolaryngological disease

No relevant articles were found concerning marijuana and otorhinolaryngological disease.

Nervous system disease

Thirteen epidemiological articles were cited in the PubMed database between 1988 and 2008 on the association between marijuana and nervous system function. One review article and four case–control studies looked at development and brain mass. Two review articles, one meta-analysis, and five case–control studies addressed neuropsychological effects of marijuana use.

Neurodevelopment and neuropsychological studies

Neurodevelopment

Sundram (2006) reviewed the human and animal studies pertaining to brain development during perinatal exposure to marijuana. Animal studies have shown that the phyto-cannabinoids administered perinatally can affect offspring, particularly in the areas of motor control, neuroendocrine function, and nociception. Animal and human studies suggest that marijuana use is related to subtle changes in a variety of neurological functions, including cognitive defects – particularly visuospatial – and hyperactivity associated with impulsivity and inattention. Depressive symptoms, schizophrenia, and a tendency toward substance use disorders in adolescence have also been described in the literature. Some studies have shown that maternal use of marijuana during fetal development may influence the development of the dopamine and opioid neurotransmitter systems. Sundram (2006) suggested that, while marijuana use may affect neurodevelopment, other causes such as genetic and environmental factors may also have a role. Human and animal studies can increase knowledge of nervous system development and marijuana use that could expand information on the function of the EC system in human development.

A case–control study by Block *et al.* (2000) compared brain tissue volume and composition in 18 current young marijuana users with 13 non-marijuana-using controls. Using MRI, they measured brain volume – both global and regional – and gray and white matter. They found no evidence of cerebral atrophy in the frequent marijuana users and no changes in the volume of brain substance. Block *et al.* (2000) noted that other studies found an increase in volume of cerebrospinal fluid; however, their study found a lower volume.

Although there were some sex differences, there were no clinically significant MRI findings in their study.

Matochik *et al.* (2005) studied 11 heavy marijuana users and eight non-marijuana users in a case–control study to determine differences in brain tissue composition and gray and white matter tissue density. Based on MRI studies, they found that marijuana users, compared with non-users, had lower gray matter density in the right parahippocampal gyrus ($p = 0.0001$), bilaterally near the precentral gyrus and the right thalamus ($p < 0.04$), and lower white matter density in the left parietal lobe ($p = 0.03$). There was also higher white matter density around the left parahippocampal and fusiform gyri ($p = 0.002$). More structural differences were found in long-term heavy marijuana users than in others in the study, including a higher white matter density in the left precentral gyrus ($p = 0.045$). This preliminary report suggests that more studies are needed to confirm these findings.

Medina *et al.* (2007) studied hippocampal volume and symmetry in 16 alcohol users, 26 alcohol and marijuana users, and 21 controls who used neither alcohol nor marijuana. All subjects were aged 15 to 18 years. The 16 alcohol users had a significant difference in hippocampal symmetry ($p < 0.05$) compared with the other groups, including an increase in right to left asymmetry and a smaller left hippocampal volume; marijuana use was associated with left to right asymmetry and a larger hippocampal volume. The 26 marijuana–alcohol users were similar to the controls, but the controls, with greater right to left hippocampal volume, performed statistically better on verbal learning tests ($p < 0.05$). The authors concluded that alcohol and marijuana use is associated with hippocampal changes and verbal learning deficiencies.

A case–control study by Jager *et al.* (2007) used fMRI and voxel-based morphometry to study the effect of marijuana use on hippocampal-dependent associative memory in 20 frequent marijuana users and 20 controls (non-marijuana users), matched for age, gender, and intelligence quotient (IQ). They found that the marijuana users had lower activation of those areas of the brain known to be involved in associative learning (parahippocampus, right dorsolateral prefrontal cortex). There was no difference between subjects and controls in brain tissue composition and no relationship between the magnitude of brain activity and the composition of parahippocampal tissue. Jager *et al.* (2007) suggested that the lower brain activation may not reflect neurocognitive impairment but could be related to changes in cerebral perfusion or altered attention and alertness.

Neuropsychological studies

Gonzalez (2007) reviewed the scientific literature related to neurobehavioral function and marijuana use. He found that subjective mental status was altered in acute intoxication, but that the reporting of signs and symptoms of brain function and neuropsychological performance were not consistent in the literature. After a period of abstinence, the neuropsychological findings seen in marijuana users were mild and transient. Frequent heavy users of marijuana were more likely to have neuropsychological deficits. Neuroimaging studies show subtle differences in marijuana users and non-users, but significant findings are yet to be determined.

Pope *et al.* (1995) reviewed the literature for studies where subjects were given marijuana and then studied (drug-administration studies) and studies where heavy marijuana users abstained before participating in the study (naturalistic studies). While data supported that changes in attention, ability to perform psychomotor tasks, and short-term memory were consequences of marijuana use 12 to 24 hours prior to testing, the data do not support a prolonged residual effect on the CNS. They suggested that evidence for residual effects needs to be separate from (1) acute effects of the drug, (2) attributes of heavy marijuana users, and (3) the presence of a psychiatric disorder caused by or exacerbated by marijuana use. More studies are needed to support a "drug residue" effect 12 to 24 hours after acute intoxication and on the more lasting effects of marijuana on the CNS.

A meta-analytical study by Grant et al. (2003) reviewed 1014 studies on the residual neurocognitive effects of marijuana use. Only 11 studies met their criteria to be included in the meta-analysis. Two analyses were performed: the first included 623 marijuana users and 409 minimal and non-users; the second analysis involved 704 marijuana users and 484 non-users. Eight cognitive domains were studied. For six of the domains there was an effect size of zero; however, there was an increased effect size between marijuana use and learning and forgetting. Grant et al. (2003) concluded that, although few studies met research standards, the findings from these studies indicated that chronic users seem to have a decrease in the ability to learn and to remember information. They suggest the small effect size of the findings might indicate an acceptable margin of safety if marijuana is used therapeutically.

Jacobsen et al. (2004) reported on a case–control study on working memory in adolescent marijuana users. The controls in the study were tobacco users and non-smokers. Functional MRI was performed while subjects performed a working memory task. No results were reported in the abstract of this pilot study.

Chang et al. (2006b) used blood oxygen level dependent (BOLD) fMRI and neuro-psychological tests with 12 abstaining marijuana users and 12 active marijuana users. Nineteen controls, matched for age, sex, and education, also participated in this study. There were no significant differences in the use of marijuana or lifetime exposure to THC in the abstaining and active marijuana users. In both groups of marijuana users, there was a decrease in activity on the right prefrontal, parietal, and medial cerebellar areas during the psychological tests, except during the visual attention tasks, where greater activity was found in the frontal, parietal, and occipital areas of the brain ($p \leq 0.001$). Active users had more activation in the frontal and cerebellar regions than abstainers. Lower BOLD was found in users who started smoking early and had a greater cumulative THC than those who started smoking later in life and had lower THC levels. The lower BOLD fMRI was particularly found in the prefrontal and medial cerebellar areas. The changes seen in this study could be explained by a neuroadaptive process or altered brain development, especially in chronic users. Altered cerebral blood flow and volume or downregulation of CB1 receptors could also explain the results. The authors suggested that acute intoxication may be associated with neuroadaptive mechanisms, and in chronic users, the changes may be reversible.

Kanayama et al. (2004) used fMRI while participants worked on a spacial working memory task in their case–control study. Twelve long-term marijuana users who last smoked 6 to 36 hours earlier were matched with 10 control non-users. Brain activation was not correlated with selective demographic variables and length of marijuana use or levels of urine THC. There was increased brain activity in the spatial working memory areas (prefrontal cortex, anterior cingulate) of the long-term marijuana users. However, these subjects also had increased activity in the basal ganglia. The authors suggested that the marijuana users recruit additional areas of the brain (e.g., basal ganglia) to compensate for subtle neuropsychological deficits related to long-term use.

In a case–control study of response inhibition, Tapert et al. (2007) recruited 16 marijuana users and 17 non-using controls. None of the participants had neurological or other axis 1 diagnoses. A go/no-go task and BOLD fMRI were carried out on the controls and on the marijuana users 28 days after abstinence and showed no difference in task performance by the two groups. In the inhibition trials, the marijuana users did have an increased BOLD response in the prefrontal, frontal, and parietal lobes and the right occipital gyrus compared with non-users. In the "go" portion of the task, the marijuana users had an increase in BOLD in the prefrontal, insular, and parietal cortices ($p < 0.05$). This study showed that adolescent marijuana users had an increase in brain processing during inhibition tasks even 28 days after smoking. Questions raised by this study include whether the increased brain processing occurred before or as a result of regular use of marijuana, and whether there is a risk associated with increased brain processing.

A case–control study by Pillay *et al.* (2008) involved 11 marijuana users and 16 controls. Right and left finger tapping tasks during fMRI at Brodmann's area were carried out 4 to 36 hours after last use of marijuana and 7 and 28 days after abstinence (Table 4.9). The authors suggest that there was residual diminished brain activity in the motor cortex even 28 days after discontinuation of marijuana use.

Table 4.10 summarizes the studies on neurodevelopment and neuropsychology. The section below, Neurological manifestations, also contains relevant information.

Comments

The two recent review articles provide information about what is known about marijuana use and the effect on nervous system development prenatally (Sundram 2006), and also the effect of marijuana use on neurobehavioral function (Gonzalez 2007). The majority of studies in this section were case–control studies, with small subject size (11 to 20 marijuana users). Most of the studies used fMRI and a variety of psychological tests to assess a variety of marijuana users. Some of the users were described as "heavy users," "long-term users," or "occasional users." The length of abstinence varied from study to study. The small number of studies indicates that more are needed, using larger sample size and the same or similar psychological tests to enhance confidence in the findings.

The meta-analysis by Grant (2003) points out the difficulty in comparing results of these studies. Only 11 studies out of 1014 could be used in their analysis of research on the residual CNS effects of marijuana use. Meta-analytical studies could be useful in synthesizing the information from various research articles, and with a larger sample size, the meta-analyses could potentially be useful in generalizing the data.

Central nervous system disease

Eleven epidemiological articles relating to marijuana use and CNS diseases published between 1988 and 2008 were found in a review of PubMed. Two of the articles were reviews; the other nine were case series and reports (seven), case–control (one), or cross-sectional (one) studies.

One review by Gordon & Devinsky (2001) looked at the safety of marijuana and alcohol use in patients taking antiepileptic drugs for seizure activity. While alcohol withdrawal seemed to lower the threshold and increase the risk for seizures, marijuana may have an antiepileptic effect, particularly in the control of tonic–clonic and partial seizures. However, the role of marijuana and seizures in epilepsy is not as well researched as the role of alcohol in epilepsy. According to the authors, the marijuana–epilepsy studies reviewed were inconclusive. Compliance in taking antiepileptic drugs could be a problem in marijuana

Table 4.9 Changes in fMRI at Brodmann's area with motor tests

Brodmann's area[a]	Left finger tapping						Right finger tapping					
	Day 0		Day 7		Day 28		Day 0		Day 7		Day 28	
	⇑	⇓	⇑	⇓	⇑	⇓	⇑	⇓	⇑	⇓	⇑	⇓
6		C		C, I	C			I	I			I
24												
32		C, I			C		C, I		C, I			C
4					C							

C, contralateral side; I, ipsilateral side.
[a] 6, supplemental motor cortex; 4, primary motor cortex; 24, in cingulate cortex; 32 in cingulate cortex.

users since poor short-term memory is often a consequence of marijuana use. Failure to take the antiepileptic drugs could result in increased seizure activity.

Moussouttas (2004) reviewed all reported cases of marijuana-related cerebral ischemic events as well as selective human and animal studies. He concluded that the exact relationship between marijuana smoking and cardiovascular events could not be determined but cerebral vasospasm appeared to be a likely cause of the ischemic events. Other possibilities include emboli of cardiac origin and systemic hypotension.

Seven case reports were found that described patients with ischemic strokes after smoking marijuana. Zachariah (1991) reported on two young men who developed cerebral infarcts after a heavy episode of marijuana smoking. No other confounders (alcohol, other illicit drugs) were evident, and neurodiagnostic tests found no evidence of atherosclerosis. Vasospasm related to changes in systemic blood pressure was thought to be the cause of the strokes.

Geller et al. (2004) described three male adolescents who developed cerebellar infarcts soon after smoking marijuana. This retrospective case and chart review followed the three subjects for five years. Neurodiagnostic testing with CT, MRI, arteriography, cerebellar biopsy, and necropsy confirmed posterior cerebral circulation ischemic strokes. Symptoms at the time of the infarct included headache, visual disturbances, ataxia, and varying levels of unconsciousness and lethargy.

Finsterer et al. (2004) described a 37-year-old male who developed temporary left hemiparesis, hemihypesthesia, and visual impairment 15 minutes after smoking marijuana, which completely resolved three days later. The subject was a long-term marijuana user (10 years) who reportedly smoked two to three joints a week for six months prior to the episode. He had no significant risk factors for cerebrovascular disease. Other than potential mild hyperlipidemia associated with tobacco use, the authors suggested that marijuana use contributed to the stroke onset.

Mateo (2005, 2006) described three patients with cerebral strokes after smoking marijuana. In the first case (Mateo et al. 2005), neuroimaging performed on one patient showed three infarcts in three different arterial areas of the brain and areas that suggested lesions of toxic or inflammatory etiology. The later article (Mateo et al. 2006) described two other patients (aged 26 and 29 years) who had temporal lobe infarcts after smoking marijuana. None of the three patients had risk factors for cerebrovascular disease.

Table 4.10 Neurodevelopment and neuropsychological studies

Study	Method	Sample	Incidence	Results
Block et al. (2000)	Case–control study Volume and composition brain tissue MRI	18 current, frequent marijuana users, 13 non-using controls	Measured global, regional brain volume, gray/white matter	Marijuana users: no evidence of atrophy, global or regional changes in volume, CSF volume lower than controls, some sex differences No abnormal clinical signs in any subjects
Chang et al. (2006b)	Case–control study Visual attention and cerebellar function BOLD fMRI, neuropsychological tests	12 abstaining marijuana users, 12 active marijuana users, 19 controls matched for age, sex, education	Marijuana users (all): decreased activity right prefrontal lobe, parietal, cerebellar region; greater activity frontal, parietal, occipital areas ($p \leq 0.001$); BOLD signals normalized in abstainers Active users: greater frontal, cerebellar activity than non-users; lower BOLD in prefrontal, cerebellum in users smoking at earlier age, greater THC exposure	Neuroadaptive processes may be functioning or there is altered brain development in chronic users; changes could be related to altered cerebral blood flow, downregulation of CB1 receptors
Gonzalez (2007)	Literature review Neurobehavioral function, cannabis use		Acute intoxication: change in subjective mental status; neuropsychological function After abstinence: mild, transient deficits in neuropsychological performance	Subtle changes in brain function of unknown significance; changes mostly in heavy users
Grant et al. (2003)	Meta-analysis of 11 of 1014 studies Residual effects of marijuana use	Study 1: 623 marijuana users, 409 non-users Study 2: 704 marijuana users, 484 non-users	8 cognitive domains examined: 6 domains, no effect size; 2 domains (learning, forgetting) with slight increased effect size	Few studies met current research standards; chronic users had decrease in ability to learn, remember; therapeutic marijuana may fall within "acceptable margin of safety"
Jacobsen et al. (2004)	Case–control study Working memory tasks fMRI pilot study	Adolescent marijuana users, 2 control groups matched for tobacco, non-smoking		

Table 4.10 Cont.

Study	Method	Sample	Incidence	Results
Jager et al. (2007)	Case–control study Marijuana use and hippocampal-associated memory fMRI, voxel-based morphometry	20 frequent marijuana users, 20 controls (non-users) matched for age, gender, IQ	Marijuana users: lower activity in associative learning brain areas (parahippocampus, right dorsal lateral prefrontal cortex); no difference in brain tissue composition	No association between parahippocampal tissue and magnitude of brain activity; lower brain activity may represent change in cerebral perfusion, differences in attention rather than neurological impairment
Kanayama et al. (2004)	Case–control study SWM task fMRI	12 long-term marijuana users, 6–36 h after last smoke, 10 controls (non-users)	Marijuana users: increased activity in SWM areas (prefrontal cortex, anterior cingulate) in long-time users; recruited non-SWM areas (basal ganglia)	Results not affected by age, education, verbal IQ, lifetime marijuana use, urine THC levels; marijuana users had more widespread brain activity, suggesting subtle neurophysiological deficits or compensation using other areas of brain
Matochik et al. (2005)	Case–control study Brain composition, particularly gray/white brain density Voxel-based morphometry, T_1-weighted MRI	11 heavy marijuana users, 8 non-users	Marijuana users: lower gray matter density in parahippocampal gyrus ($p = 0.0001$); greater density bilaterally near precentral gyrus, right thalamus ($p < 0.04$); lower white matter density parietal lobe ($p = 0.03$); higher white matter density left parahippocampal and fusiform gyri ($p = 0.002$); also precentral gyrus in long-term users	Evidence of possible structural differences in marijuana users, particularly long-term users
Medina et al. (2007)	Case–control study Alcohol/marijuana use and hippocampal volume and symmetry	15–18 year olds after 2 days abstinence: 16 alcohol users, 26 marijuana and alcohol users, 21 controls Excluded: those with prenatal exposure, left handers, those with psychiatric or neurological disorders	Alcohol users had significant differences from others: increased use; increased asymmetry (right > left); smaller hippocampal volume Marijuana: increased left > right asymmetry; larger left hippocampal volume Marijuana/alcohol users: no difference from controls Controls: functionally better than others on verbal learning test ($p = 0.05$)	Alcohol and marijuana affect hippocampal symmetry in opposite manners; verbal learning decreased in alcohol and marijuana users compared with controls

Reference	Study type	Sample	Results	Conclusions
Pillay et al. (2008)	Case–control study Motor function in marijuana users fMRI of BA, finger tapping	11 marijuana users, 16 controls Testing 4 to 36 h after marijuana use and after 7 and 28 days of abstinence	Overall: decreased contralateral SMA activity from day 0 to day 28 Left finger tapping: decreased fMRI signals from SMA contralateral side day 7, ipsilateral side day 7 only; BA 32 contralateral and ipsilateral sides day 0; contralateral PMC, day 28 Right finger tapping: decreased fMRI BA 32 ipsilateral side on days 0 and 7, contralateral side on day 0, 7, and 28; BA 6 ipsilateral side on days 0, 7, and 28	BA 24 unaffected; diminished brain activity persists even after 28 days of abstinence
Pope et al. (1995)	Literature review Residual neuropsychological effects	Drug-administered studies vs. naturalistic studies (drug abusers after abstinence)		Data supports drug effect lasting 12–24 h with changes in attention, psychomotor tasks, short-term memory; prolong drug residual effect on CNS inconclusive
Sundram (2006)	Literature review	Human, animal perinatal marijuana exposure studies		Phytocannabinoid effect seen perinatally through adolescence Human and animal studies show subtle effect on later function: cognitive defects, particularly visuospatial, impulsivity, inattention, hyperactivity, depression, substance use disorders; gender differences in effects on sex hormones Animal studies show deficits in motor control, neuroendocrine function, nociception Fetal studies indicate influence on development of opioid, dopaminergic receptors
Tapert et al. (2007)	Case–control study Response inhibition BOLD fMRI, go/no-go test	Subjects with no neurological deficits or axis 1 diagnoses: 16 marijuana users (by history), 28-day abstinence, 17 controls (non-users)	No difference in task performance Inhibition trials: marijuana users had more BOLD response in prefrontal, frontal, parietal lobes; right occipital gyrus; Go trials: marijuana users had more BOLD response in prefrontal, insular, parietal cortex ($p < 0.05$)	Even after 28 days abstinence, marijuana users had increased brain processing during inhibition tests Questions: did brain processing change occur before marijuana use or caused by marijuana use? Is there a risk associated with increased brain processing?

BA, Brodmann's area; BOLD, blood oxygen level dependent; CB1 and CB2, cannabinoid receptors; CSF, cerebrospinal fluid; EC, endocannabinoids; fMRI, functional magnetic resonance imaging; IQ, intelligence quotient; MRI, magnetic resonance imaging; PMC, primary motor cortex; SMA, supplemental motor cortex; SWM, spatial working memory; THC, tetrahydrocannabinol.

Mateo *et al.* (2006) also reported on 18 other patients who experienced cerebrovascular ischemia after using marijuana.

A case–control study was described by Herning *et al.* (2001). Vascular studies were used to compare cerebral vascular characteristics of 16 abstinent marijuana smokers with 19 controls, ages 18 to 30 years. Cerebrovascular perfusion data and transcranial Doppler sonography showed that the marijuana smokers had vascular findings similar to healthy 60 year olds. Cerebrovascular resistance and systolic velocity in the anterior and middle cerebral arteries was significantly increased ($p < 0.005$) in the marijuana users compared with controls. Based on their findings, the authors suggested that chronic marijuana smoking may be a risk factor for stroke.

A cross-sectional study of 51 chronic schizophrenics receiving neuroleptic drugs was carried out to assess the risk of tardive dyskinesia in marijuana smokers (Zaretsky *et al.* 1993). (Tardive dyskinesia is often a consequence of long-term use of neuroleptic drugs. Symptoms include repetitive and involuntary movements of the facial muscles, arms, and legs.) A clinical researcher administered a questionnaire and obtained information on drug and alcohol use, and smoking habits. An assessment of involuntary movement was carried out by a trained rater. The study showed that women and older patients with a long duration of schizophrenia tended to have elevated scores on the Abnormal Involuntary Movement Scale. Multiple regression analysis showed a strong correlation between marijuana smoking and tardive dyskinesia, more so than other possible factors.

Two other case reports described sequelae occurring after smoking marijuana. Stracciari *et al.* (1999) reported transient amnesia occurring in an individual after smoking marijuana. Bonkowsky *et al.* (2005) described a two-year-old girl with acute marijuana intoxication who experienced ataxia and shaking in a seizure-like episode.

These studies are summarized in Table 4.11.

Comments

Most of the support for an increased risk of cerebral ischemia in marijuana users comes from seven case reports. Only one study evaluating cerebral vascular flow was found and, in this study, the marijuana users were abstaining from marijuana use. However, this small study did show some significant differences in cerebral blood flow in marijuana users compared with the controls.

None of the studies reported statistical evidence that marijuana use is a risk for CNS disease. Further research is needed to clarify the role of marijuana in ischemic cerebral episodes, the relationship between marijuana and tardive dyskinesia, and the interaction between marijuana and drugs used to treat seizures and neurological disorders. More studies are needed showing the effect of marijuana use and cardiovascular responses, particularly since some laboratory studies have found that ECs and marijuana binding to cannabinoid receptors in the heart and blood vessels can lead to vasodilatation and endothelial growth and proliferation.

Chronobiology and sleep disorders

One article (Leon-Carrion & Vela-Bueno 1991) was found in a review of PubMed citations from 1988 to 2008. The results of this study on the effect of cannabinoids on cognitive styles and communication between the two cerebral hemispheres found that there was a difference between hashish users and controls. The Basic Rest–Activity Cycle (BRAC) test was

Table 4.11 Central nervous system disease

Study	Method	Sample	Incidence	Results
Zacharia (1991)	Case report	2 young men who developed cerebral infarcts after heavy use of marijuana; no evidence of alcohol or use of other illicit drugs		No atherosclerotic causes; vasospasm suspected
Herning et al. (2001)	Case–control study Cerebrovascular blood flow velocity Transcranial Doppler sonography in cerebrovascular perfusion	Subjects aged 18–30 years: 16 abstaining marijuana users, 19 controls	Increased pulsatility index (measure of cardiovascular resistance) and systolic velocity in marijuana users ($p < 0.005$)	Findings in marijuana users similar to 60 year olds; stroke may be a risk factor in marijuana smokers
Geller et al. (2004)	Retrospective case and chart review	3 male adolescents with onset of stroke after smoking marijuana	Cerebellar infarct within days of smoking marijuana: symptoms of headache, visual disturbance, ataxia, varying lethargy, unconsciousness; confirmed by CT, MRI, cerebral arteriography, cerebellar biopsy, necropsy	Episodic marijuana smokers (adolescents) are at risk for developing cerebellar infarction
Gordon & Devinsky (2001)	Literature review Safety of alcohol and marijuana use in epileptics			Alcohol (1–2 drinks) had no effect on increased seizure activity or level of antiepileptic drugs; withdrawal increased risk of seizures Marijuana studies inconclusive, insufficient data in users and seizure activity Cannabinoids may have antiepileptic effect, particularly for partial and tonic–clonic seizures; animal models show lower threshold for seizure activity
Moussouttas (2004)	Literature review Marijuana use and cerebral ischemia	All reported cases of marijuana-related cerebral ischemia; selected human, animal experimental studies		Marijuana use related to cerebral ischemia, infarction; etiology: likely to be cerebral vasospasm; other possible causes include cardioembolism; systemic hypotension; exact association between marijuana use and cerebral ischemia undetermined

187

Table 4.11 Cont.

Study	Method	Sample	Incidence	Results
Finsterer et al. (2004)	Case report Marijuana use and stroke	37-year-old male, smoker for 10 years; 2–3 joints/week for 6 months; mild cigarette smoker; dyslipidemia; no classic risks for cerebrovascular disease; with stroke	Right occipital ischemic stroke; onset 15 min after smoking joint with 250 mg marijuana; laboratory and radiography studies normal	Stroke likely caused by marijuana smoking
Mateo et al. (2005)	Case report Marijuana use and stroke Neuroimaging	One patient with 2 recurring strokes immediately after smoking marijuana	Neuroimaging: 3 infarcts in different cerebral arteries; non-atherosclerotic arterial disease (toxic or inflammatory origin)	Mechanism of stroke etiology unclear
Mateo et al. (2006)	Case series Marijuana use and stroke	Two patients (26 and 29 years) with temporal strokes after marijuana use	Described 18 other patients with ischemic stroke after marijuana use	Etiology unclear
Zaretsky et al. (1993)	Cross-sectional study Marijuana use and tardive dyskinesia Questionnaire and abnormal movement assessment (AIMS)	51 chronic schizophrenics taking neuroleptic drugs	Trend for females and older patients with long-term schizophrenia to have increased scores on AIMS	Multiple regression analysis: marijuana smoking correlated best with tardive dyskinesia
Stracciari et al. (1999)	Case report Marijuana use and amnesia	Individual with sudden transient amnesia with acute marijuana use	Amnesia of long duration, characteristic of global amnesia-like episode	Marijuana use may trigger transient amnesia
Bonkowsky et al. (2005)	Case report Marijuana use and seizures	2-year-old girl with acute marijuana intoxication	Seizure-like activity, ataxia, shaking	Marijuana exposure may trigger seizure activity

AIMS, Abnormal Involuntary Movement Scale; CT, computed tomography; MRI, magnetic resonance imaging.

Table 4.12 Chronobiology and sleep disorders

Study	Method	Sample	Incidence	Results
Bolla *et al.* (2008)	Case–control study Sleep patterns in marijuana users Polysomnography	Men and women aged 18–39 years: 17 heavy marijuana users tested 2 days after drug abstinence, 14 matched drug-free controls	Heavy marijuana users: lower sleep times, longer sleep onset; less slow wave sleep, shorter REM latency; worse sleep efficiency; no improvement after night of adaptation	Abstaining heavy marijuana users experience greater sleep disturbances than drug-free controls; suggests poor sleep quality may influence success of drug treatment
Leon-Carrion & Vela-Bueno (1991)	Case–control study Cannibis use and cognitive styles and cerebral hemispheric communication BRAC assessment		BRAC was altered in cannabis users	There was a difference between cannabis users and controls on the BRAC, suggesting an altered biological rhythm

BRAC, Basic Rest–Activity Cycle; REM, rapid eye movement.

used to assess the effect of hashish. This test can be used to assess control of the biological clock on rest–activity cycles and effects on various stages of sleep.

A second case–control study by Bolla *et al.* (2008) looked at sleep disturbances in marijuana users. All of the subjects in the study were aged 18–30 years and included men and women. Polysomnographic results were recorded for two nights after marijuana users abstained from drug use. The 17 heavy marijuana users differed from the 14 drug-free controls in the following areas: the marijuana users experienced less slow wave sleep, shorter rapid eye movement (REM) latency, lower sleep times, worse sleep efficiency, longer sleep onset, and experienced worse sleep continuity than the controls. After a night of adaptation, the marijuana users showed no improvement in the sleep parameters. The authors suggest that poor sleep quality after discontinuing marijuana use may influence marijuana treatment failure.

These two studies are summarized in Table 4.12.

Comments
The first abstract provided little information about the study, including what the sample size was, the methods of measuring BRAC, and the results of the findings. Further study on the effect of illicit drugs, and particularly marijuana, on biological rhythms would be helpful in identifying those at risk for injury owing to altered alertness. The second study found differences between heavy marijuana users and drug-free controls. The study was limited in the number of subjects. Replication of both of these studies with larger sample sizes may help to determine the relationship between marijuana use and altered sleep.

Neurological manifestations
Five epidemiological studies and reviews on the association between neurological manifestations and marijuana use were found in a 1988–2008 PubMed search. They related to cognition and psychomotor tasks.

A study by Schwartz *et al.* (1989b) examined short-term memory changes in marijuana users in a study of 27 adolescents; 10 marijuana dependent, 8 short-term marijuana abusers, and 9 who never used any illicit drugs. Subjects were matched for age, IQ, and screened for learning disabilities. Phencyclidine and alcohol users were excluded from the study. Seven neuropsychological tests were administered at the beginning of the study and again six weeks later. A significant difference was found between marijuana-dependent users and the two other groups on two tests at the beginning of the study: Benton Visual Retention Test ($F_{2,24} = 6.07$) and the Weschler Memory Scale Prose Passages ($F_{2,23} = 7.04$). Six weeks later, after a supervised abstinence of marijuana, the marijuana-dependent group's scores improved, but not significantly, on both tests. The researchers concluded that short-term memory deficits were found in marijuana-dependent adolescents as long as six weeks after commencing abstinence.

Wilson *et al.* (1994) studied the performance of 10 experienced marijuana smokers on five cognitive neuromotor tests. Each subject was tested on three separate days after smoking a cigarette with 1.75% THC, 3.55% THC, or a placebo. This randomized double-blind repeated-measures study tested smokers before and 30, 90, and 150 minutes after smoking the cigarettes. The authors reported that, of the five tests, the digit-symbol substitution test with memory (a test of speed of information processing) and the reaction time task (a measure of response time to visual and auditory cues) were most affected by marijuana use.

Rizzo *et al.* (2005) studied the effects of MDMA and THC on cognition. Cognitive processing was compared in two groups: dual MDMA/THC users and THC users only. Subjects were asked to report the detection of travel (left/right) of a visual stimulus. While both groups performed poorly, the MDMA/THC group performed worse. The authors suggested that marijuana and MDMA use has a negative effect on driving ability and users had an increased risk of crashing a vehicle.

Messinis *et al.* (2006) studied verbal and psychomotor functioning 24 hours after drug abstinence in 20 long-term and 20 short-term heavy, frequent marijuana users and compared these with 24 controls. While long-term users performed significantly worse on verbal memory and psychomotor speed tests, both long-term and short-term users scored poorly on verbal fluency, verbal memory, attention, and psychomotor speed tests. The authors suggested that those individuals with longer years of frequent marijuana use have greater cognitive impairment than their counterparts who smoked marijuana for a shorter period of time.

Ramaekers *et al.* (2006) studied the effect of smoking high-potency marijuana (THC 13%) on performance in cognitive and motor function tests by 20 recreational marijuana users. In this double-blind, placebo-controlled, three-way crossover study, three different doses of marijuana were used: 0 (placebo), 250, and 500 μg/kg body weight. Tested at intervals from 15 minutes to six hours after smoking, the performance of the smokers showed that the high-potency marijuana cigarettes had the greatest effect on several performance tests. The 500 μg/kg THC significantly impaired motor control, executive function, and motor impulsivity, and increased risk taking. The effect of the THC lasted at least six hours after smoking. The authors suggested that the higher dose of THC should be used in performance studies rather than the lower (4% THC) dose typically used.

Theses studies are summarized in Table 4.13. The section above on Neuropsychological manifestations also contains relevant articles.

Table 4.13 Neurological manifestations

Study	Method	Sample	Incidence	Results
Messinis et al. (2006)	Case–control study Verbal and psychomotor function in marijuana users	20 long-term marijuana users, 20 short-term heavy, frequent marijuana users, 24 non-users; 24 h abstinence prior to testing	Long-term users performed significantly worse than others; both short- and long-term users performed poorly on verbal fluency, verbal memory, attention, and psychomotor speed tests	Long-term marijuana users had greater cognitive impairment than short-term users
Ramaekers et al. (2006)	Convenience sample; double-blind, placebo-controlled, three-way crossover study Performance on cognitive, psychomotor tests in users of high-potency marijuana	20 recreational marijuana users, receiving one of three marijuana doses: 0, 250, 500 µg/kg THC; tested at intervals after smoking: 15 min to 6 h	High-dose THC (13%) significantly impaired motor control, executive function, motor impulsivity; increased risk taking	Greater impairment of cognitive and motor function with high dose (THC 13%) than in normal dose (THC 4%) in recreational marijuana users; effect of high dose THC lasted at least 6 h
Rizzo et al. (2005)	Case–control study Cognitive processing (heading) in marijuana and ecstasy users Optical flow test	Marijuana users, marijuana + MDMA users	Both groups performed poorly on optical flow test; the marijuana–MDMA users were most impaired	Marijuana/MDMA users at risk for motor vehicle crashes because of heading impairment
Schwartz et al. (1989b)	Case–control study Marijuana use and memory Auditory/verbal neuropsychological tests (7)	27 adolescents: 10 marijuana dependent, 8 short-term marijuana users, 9 never used illicit drugs	At start of study, significant differences in marijuana-dependent users: Benton Visual Retention Test ($F_{2,24} = 6.07$); Weschler Memory Scale Prose Passages ($F_{2,23} = 7.04$); 6 weeks later, scores improved but not significant	Short-term memory deficits found in marijuana-dependent users compared with two other groups; impairment improved but still present 6 weeks later
Wilson et al. (1994)	Randomized double-blind repeated-measures study Cognitive and neuromotor function in marijuana users Cognitive, neuromotor tests (5)	10 male volunteers, experienced marijuana users	Tests given 30, 90, 150 min after smoking three types of cigarettes (placebo, 1.75% THC, 3.55% THC): of the 5 tests, the digit–symbol substitution test with memory and reaction time task most affected by marijuana use	Tests vary in their ability to measure cognitive and neuromotor function

MDMA, 3,4-methylenedioxymethamphetamine (ecstasy); THC, tetrahydrocannabinol

Comments

Only five studies looking at the performance of marijuana users on cognitive and psychomotor tests were found in the PubMed database. In the four studies reporting sample size, the combined subjects and controls numbered 10, 20, 27, and 64. The tests reported ranged from one to seven and varied from study to study. The small sample size and lack of similarity of tests used to assess cognitive and psychomotor function make it difficult to generalize the findings of these studies. Another limitation of the group as a whole is the varying dose of marijuana reported in two studies: 1.75 and 3.55% THC in one, 13% THC in the other. One study reported subjects abstained from using marijuana for 24 hours, while another indicated subjects abstained for six weeks. One study indicated various confounders were controlled (age, alcohol, IQ, learning disabilities, phencyclidine use), while the other studies did not report any confounders considered in their analyses. Terms varied in their description of marijuana use in the subjects. For example, short-term and long-term users, recreational users, and experienced marijuana users were terms used to describe the subjects, which also make it difficult to compare results of these studies. Few of the abstracts reviewed provided statistics for their findings, instead suggesting "significant differences" or "a higher proportion" to describe the results. Because of these limitations, making confident conclusions on the effect of marijuana on cognition and psychomotor activity is difficult.

Ocular disease

Two reviews and two descriptive reports were found on a PubMed review of articles on marijuana use and eye diseases published between 1988 and 2008 (Table 4.14). Both reviews were similar and explored the pharmacological effects of several illicit drugs including marijuana, and discussed various eye conditions. The review by McLane & Carroll (1986) and the review by Urey (1991) both described infectious eye conditions, toxic effects of the illicit drugs, and other conditions seen in drug abusers.

Levi & Miller (1990) described five individuals who used marijuana or hallucinogens or both marijuana and hallucinogens. The individuals had persistent or recurring visual disturbances, including image alteration (including shimmering, movement, and streaking). No neurological cause of the illusions could be found, including migraine, epilepsy, or cerebral lesions. The authors suggested that detailed drug histories be obtained on individuals describing visual illusions.

Laffi & Safran (1993) described a patient who developed visual changes after using hashish for five years. The 23-year-old male experienced random, flickering black and white visual spots one day after discontinuing use of hashish. He also reported difficulty with depth perception. These visual changes lasted for several months.

Comments

The last review of the literature related to eye diseases and marijuana use was over 15 years ago (1991). It would seem appropriate to repeat a review of the in vitro and in vivo laboratory studies and the clinical research findings on this topic. The reports by Levi & Miller (1990) and Laffi & Safran (1993) provide some support that visual illusions may be drug related and not caused by other cerebral events.

Table 4.14 Eye diseases

Study	Method	Sample	Incidence	Results
Laffi & Safran (1993)	Case report Visual distortion with marijuana use	23 year old with 5-year history of hashish consumption	Developed visual changes 1 day after discontinuing hashish use: small, randomly flickering black and white spots; increased with physical activity, reading; experienced problems with depth perception	Visual distortion can occur after stopping hashish use; symptoms lasts for months
Levi & Miller (1990)	Descriptive study, case series Drug use and illusions	5 users of marijuana, hallucinogens, or both marijuana and hallucinogens	Despite absence of neurological findings of ophthalmic disease, 5 drug abusers had persistent symptoms: image distortion (shimmering, movement, streaking)	Illusions in these 5 users persisted or recurred even after months or years of abstinence and were not related to migraine, epilepsy, or intracranial lesions; patients with illusions should be questioned about drug use
McLane & Carroll (1986)	Literature review			Ocular damage can occur by drug toxicity, route of drug administration, injury while under the influence of the drug; reviewed four other groups of drugs besides marijuana and discussed effects of the drugs
Urey (1991)	Literature review			Review of pharmacological effects of various illicit drugs on the eye, including marijuana; diseases discussed: acquired immunodeficiency syndrome, cytomegalovirus retinitis, bacterial and fungal endoohthalmitis, quinine poisoning, talc retinopathy

Male urological disease

Renal disease

One review and two case–control epidemiological studies were found in a search of PubMed articles on renal disease and marijuana use. The review by Crowe *et al.* (2000) reviewed the glomerular, interstitial, and vascular renal complications commonly found in individuals using illicit drugs. Besides reviewing the effect of the drugs on the kidney, other mechanisms for renal damage were also explored.

Vupputuri *et al.* (2004) studied the association between marijuana use in hypertensive patients and the risk for developing mild renal disease. A median seven-year follow-up of 647 patients with hypertension found that patients on any illicit drug had an RR of declining renal functions (measured by an elevated creatinine level of 6.0 mg/L or more) (RR 2.3; 95% CI 1.0–5.1). The patients who used marijuana (22.7%) also had an increased creatinine level, but this was not statistically significant. Patients with cocaine use (6.7%) had an RR of 3.0 (95% CI 1.1–8.0), and those using psychedelics (3.1%) had an RR of 3.9 (95% CI 1.1–14.4). Various confounders were controlled in this study: age, race, education, income, smoking, and alcohol use. Systolic blood pressure, use of hypertensive drugs, BMI, diabetic history, and hyperlipidemia were also considered in the analyses.

Neoplastic disorders

A case–control study by Chacko *et al.* (2006) examined a convenience sample of 52 men aged 59 years or younger who were diagnosed with TCBC and 104 age-matched controls with no history or signs and symptoms of TCBC. The subjects completed a questionnaire assessing past exposure to known TCBC carcinogens and marijuana use. Forty-six (88.5%) of the men with TCBC acknowledged habitual marijuana use, and 72 (69.2%) of the controls habitually used marijuana. The researchers noted there was a statistically significant difference ($p = 0.0008$) between the number of habitual marijuana users with TCBC and the habitual marijuana-using controls. They also found a significant correlation between marijuana use and the stage, grade, and recurrence of the cancer. Although a large number of both the TCBC group and the controls were habitual marijuana users, the authors suggested that marijuana smoking increased the risk of TCBC. No risk data were provided, and it is not clear whether confounders such as cigarette smoking were considered in this study.

Male genitalia

One review, one case–control study, and one review of a database were found in the PubMed review of epidemiological studies reported in 1988 to 2008. The review by Thompson (1993) looked at the causes of male infertility and included marijuana as one of the potential causes. The case–control study by Close *et al.* (1990) explored pyospermia in infertile males and the relationship to marijuana smoking. Seminal fluid analysis, sperm penetration assay, and testing for sperm autoimmune antibodies were carried out in 164 males in infertile relationships. Compared with non-users, significant increases in leukocytes in seminal fluid were found in marijuana users ($p < 0.007$), cigarette smokers ($p < 0.02$), and heavy alcohol users ($p < 0.01$). There were no differences between the non-users and the marijuana, cigarette, and alcohol users in decreased sperm count, sperm motility, percentage of oval sperm, or antisperm antibodies. When controlled for STD and multiple substance exposures, multivariate analyses found a non-significant association between marijuana use and an increase in seminal fluid leukocytes ($p = 0.12$). However, there was a significant association found with cigarette use ($p = 0.006$).

Johnson *et al.* (2004) reviewed the data from the 1981–1983 Epidemiologic Catchment Area Project to study the association between sexual dysfunction and drug and alcohol use. Only the 3004 participants who were asked about sexual dysfunction were included in the analysis. Controlling for confounders, inhibited orgasm and painful sex were associated with marijuana and alcohol use. Illicit drug abusers were also more likely to have inhibited sexual excitement (but not inhibited sexual desire) compared with non-drug users.

These studies are summarized in Table 4.15.

Comments

With only one study suggesting marijuana might increase the risk of bladder cancer and another finding no significant decrease in renal function in marijuana users, further study is needed to explore the relationship between marijuana use and urological disease. Since TCBC is associated with cigarette smoking, studies comparing smokers who use marijuana, cigarettes, or both would be helpful in assessing risk in each group of smokers.

Limited information is available in the one review related to causes of infertility. The two studies on pyospermia and sexual dysfunction suggest some association with marijuana use; however, more studies are needed to clarify the risks associated with marijuana use.

Female genital and neonatal/congenital disorders

Genital and pregnancy disorders

Five articles related to marijuana use and female genital diseases were found in a PubMed search from 1988 to 2008. Eleven articles on pregnancy complications in marijuana users were also found.

Female genital disorders

One review article by Buck *et al.* (1997) reviewed Medline, Index Medicus, and reference lists for articles on factors that might influence female infertility, including cigarette smoking, alcohol, caffeine, drug use, physical exercise, and BMI. The authors suggested that several types of primary infertility in women could possibly be related to use of cocaine, marijuana, and alcohol, as well as use of thyroid medicine and exercise. Extremes in body size were also identified as a risk factor. At least two studies reviewed found that cigarette smoking and use of intrauterine devices were risk factors for primary tubal infertility.

A case–control study by Mueller *et al.* (1990) studied the risk of infertility in a sample of infertile women who used marijuana, lysergic acid diethylamide (LSD), amphetamines, cocaine, or other abused drugs. These women were matched with controls with proven fertility. They found that marijuana use in their study was consistent with animal studies demonstrating that ovulation was transiently disrupted with marijuana use. There was an RR of marijuana interference with ovulation of 1.7 (95% CI 1.0–3.0). In women who used marijuana within one year of trying to become pregnant, there was an RR of 2.1 (95% CI 1.1–4.0) of interference with ovulation. The study found no increased risk of infertility related to frequency or duration of marijuana use. No other drug use showed significant risk of infertility, except for cocaine use, which was associated with a tubal abnormality (RR 11.1; 95% CI 1.7–70.8).

Table 4.15 Male urological disorders

Study	Method	Sample	Incidence	Results
Chacko et al. (2006)	Case–control study Marijuana use and TCBC Questionnaire	52 males with TCBC, under 60 years of age; 104 age-matched controls	Significant difference in habitual marijuana smoking: 46 (88.5%) in TCBC group and 72 (69.2%) in controls ($p = 0.0008$) Marijuana use also significantly correlated with stage, grade of cancer, and number of recurrences Confounders: potential carcinogens, radiation, agent orange, tobacco and marijuana use, smoked and processed meats	Marijuana smoking might increase the risk of TCBC
Close et al. (1990)	Case–control study Pyospermia in infertile men Analysis of seminal fluid, sperm penetration assay, sperm autoantibodies	164 males: marijuana users, cigarette smokers, heavy alcohol users; non-users	Compared with non-users, increase in number of leukocytes in seminal fluid of cigarette smokers ($p < 0.02$), marijuana users ($p < 0.007$), and alcohol users ($p < 0.01$) Controlled for STDs and multiple substance exposure, marijuana use not associated with trend toward seminal fluid leukocytes ($p = 0.12$) Compared with non-users, no significant differences in sperm count, motility, percent oval sperm, sperm autoantibodies	Cigarette smokers had more statistical significant findings than marijuana smokers, alcohol users, or controls
Crowe et al. (2000)	Literature review Substance abuse and renal function			Renal complications more common with use of illicit drugs; some substances nephrotoxic; dysfunction may be chronic and irreversible; acute dysfunction may be reversible
Johnson et al. (2004)	Descriptive analysis of database: Epidemiological Catchment Area Project 1981–1983	3004 responses to sexual dysfunction questions	Controlling for confounders, inhibited orgasm associated with marijuana use and alcohol use; illicit drug abusers more likely to have inhibited sexual excitement but not inhibited sexual desire	Sexual dysfunction can occur in illicit drug users

Thompson (1993)	Review Male infertility causes			Some causes of male infertility can be identified
Vupputuri et al. (2004)	Longitudinal study at Veteran's Association clinic for high blood pressure Effect of illicit drug use and kidney function Interview for drug use with 7-year follow-up of creatinine level	647 hypertensive patients (1977–1999): 147 (22.7%) marijuana users	Mild kidney decline, any illicit drug, RR 2.3 (95% CI 1.0–5.1); marijuana users, RR not significant although creatinine level did increase Analyses adjusted for confounders	Users of cocaine and psychedelic drugs had higher RR: cocaine, RR, 3.0 (95% CI 1.1–8.0); psychedelics, RR 3.9 (95% CI 1.1–14.4)

STD, sexually transmitted disease; TCBC, transitional cell bladder cancer.

Two studies looked at the risk of vaginal infections and marijuana use. Crosby *et al.* (2002) looked at predictors of *Trichomonas vaginalis* in marijuana users. The subjects included 522 low-income African American adolescents, aged 14–18 years, who were part of an HIV prevention intervention study with baseline assessement and follow-up at 6 and 12 months. The subjects performed self-administered vaginal swabs, completed a survey, and had personal interviews. At baseline, 12.9% of the girls were infected with *T. vaginalis*. At six months, 8.9% were infected, and at 12 months, 10.2 % were infected. Marijuana use was the strongest predictor of *T. vaginalis* infection. Marijuana users were six times more likely to have the infection than non-marijuana users (AOR 6.2; $p = 0.0003$). Three other significant factors were identified: having sex partners five years older than the subject (AOR 2.6; $p = 0.005$), having sex with non-steady partners (AOR 1.9; $p = 0.02$), and a history of delinquency (AOR 1.3; $p = 0.02$).

Beigi *et al.* (2004) conducted a one-year longitudinal study of 1248 women to determine the risk of vaginal yeast infections in marijuana users. The women were tested at baseline, and at 4, 8, and 12 month intervals. Vaginal yeast was detected in 873 (70%) women at one or more visits. Only 4% had yeast infections on all four visits. Marijuana use in the last four months was associated with the presence of vaginal yeast. Other main risk factors included use of depomedroxyprogesterone acetate in the previous four months and sexual intercourse in the previous five days.

The fifth study (Holt *et al.* 2005) looked at the level of risk of ovarian cysts by marijuana users whose BMI was < 20, 20–25, or > 25. Marijuana use was of interest since cigarette smoking had been identified as a risk factor for functional ovarian cysts. The BMI was used as a variable since one previously published study found that the BMI could modify the risk of functional ovarian cysts in cigarette smokers. The data were collected over a five-year period in a case–control study of 586 women with functional ovarian cysts and 757 age-matched controls. The researchers found that when the BMI increased, the risk of ovarian dysfunction decreased. The OR in marijuana users was 2.05 (95% CI 0.85–4.75) for BMI < 20, 1.78 (95% CI 1.00–3.17) for BMI 20–25, and 0.72 (95% CI 0.36–1.42) for BMI > 25. Cigarette smokers also had a similar decline in risk for ovarian dysfunction as their BMI increased, despite evidence that cigarette smoking increases the risk for functional ovarian disease. The authors suggested that the increase in BMI in some way modifies the adverse effect of smoking on ovarian cyst development.

Table 4.16 summarizes these studies on female infertility and genital disease.

Pregnancy complications

Three reviews and eight studies described pregnancy complications associated with drug abuse, particularly marijuana. A review by Lee (1998) found conflicting information in studies involving pregnant women who smoked marijuana. Since many pregnant women were both cigarette and marijuana users, the effect of the chemicals in cigarettes and in marijuana were difficult to differentiate. However, there was greater evidence that cigarette smoke was more harmful than marijuana use during pregnancy.

Concerned about anesthesia interactions in pregnant marijuana users, Kuczkowski (2004) carried out a Medline search for articles on drug abuse – particularly marijuana – and fetal outcomes. The peripartum marijuana user presents challenges to the anesthesia provider because of the unpredictable clinical presentation, the difficulty in accurately predicting drug use, and the complex interactions of THC and other marijuana chemicals. Without any guidelines for anesthesia administration or analgesia use, Kuczkowski (2004)

Table 4.16 Female genital diseases

Study	Method	Sample	Incidence	Results
Beigi et al. (2004)	Longitudinal study, 1 year Vaginal yeast colonization	1248 women tested at baseline, 4, 8, and 12 months	70% had vaginal yeast on one or more visits; only 4% had yeast on all 4 visits	Marijuana use in previous 4 months is one of several factors associated with vaginal yeast colonization
Buck et al. (1997)	Literature review Lifestyle factors and female infertility	Medline, *Index Medicus*, reference lists		Possible risk factors for several subtypes of primary infertility: cocaine, marijuana use; thyroid medication; exercise; caffeine use
Crosby et al. (2002)	Case-control study Predictors of *Trichomonas vaginalis* infection Self-administered vaginal swabs; personal interview and survey	522 low-income African Americans, aged 14–18 years, enrolled in an HIV prevention intervention study	Tests at baseline, 6, 12 months: infection 12.9% at baseline, 8.9% at 6 months, 10.2% at 12 months; strongest predictor of infection: marijuana use (biologically confirmed), AOR 6.2 ($p = 0.0003$)	Other factors: sex partners 5 years older (AOR 2.6; $p = 0.0003$), sex with non-steady partners (AOR 1.9; $p = 0.005$), history of delinquency (AOR 1.3; $p = 0.02$)
Holt et al. (2005)	Case-control study, data from 1990–1995 Ovarian cysts, BMI, and marijuana use	586 women with functional ovarian cysts, 757 age-matched controls	Multivariate analyses, controlled for age, education, reference year: risk for functional ovarian cyst in marijuana users: BMI < 20, OR 2.05 (95% CI 0.89–4.75); BMI 20–25, OR 1.78 (95% CI 1.00–3.17); BMI > 25, OR 0.72 (95% CI 0.36–1.42)	As BMI increased, risk of functional ovarian cyst decreased; lower BMI associated with increased risk of ovarian cyst; similar decline in risk with increased BMI in cigarette smokers
Mueller et al. (1990)	Case-control study Primary infertility and drug use	Infertile women users of illicit drugs, matched fertile women controls	Low-frequency marijuana users slight increased risk for infertility through ovulation abnormality (RR 1.7; 95% CI 1.0–3.0); risk increased in marijuana use within 1 year trying to get pregnant (RR 2.1; 95% CI 1.1–4.0)	Marijuana use consistent with animal studies, transient disruption of ovarian function; no consistent effects of frequency or duration of marijuana use; no risks associated with other drug use

AOR, adjusted odds ratio; BMI, body mass index; CI, confidence interval; HIV, human immunodeficiency virus; OR, odds ratio; RR, relative risk.

suggested that the anesthesiologist needs to individualize treatment on a case-by-case basis in the peripartum period.

A study by von Mandach (2005) reviewed the reports of complications of pregnancy in marijuana users, including placenta abruptio, preterm labor, spontaneous abortion, and fetal stillbirth. Since marijuana has been found to cause vasoconstriction, these complications are a possibility in marijuana-using pregnant females. However, since many marijuana users are also polydrug users, the effects of comorbid use of MDMA, LSD, and other drugs make it difficult to differentiate causes of or risks for pregnancy complications.

Witter & Niebyl (1990) carried out a retrospective analysis from a database of 8350 women during their pregnancies looking at marijuana use and pregnancy outcomes. A history of only marijuana use during pregnancy was seen in 417 women (5%). The findings showed no association between marijuana use and prematurity or congenital anomalies. Because many marijuana users also smoked cigarettes and drank alcohol during their pregnancy, it was difficult to isolate the effect of marijuana on adverse pregnancy outcomes.

Czeizel et al. (2004) carried out a retrospective study of 81 patients with orofacial cleft with matched controls, and 537 with congenital limb deficiencies, also with matched controls using the Hungarian Congenital Abnormality Registry. The purpose of the study was to determine the reliability of self-report of smoking and alcohol use during pregnancy. Mothers were mailed a structured questionnaire, while fathers and other family members were personally interviewed using the same questionnaire. The researchers found that there was low reliability in the correlation between self-reported information given by the mothers regarding marijuana use during pregnancy and the information from fathers and family members. Conversely, in the control group, there was a good correlation between self-report and family information. Regarding the use of alcohol, there was a low reliability for both the affected mothers and the controls. As a result of this study, data on smoking and alcohol use during pregnancy were not used in analysis of the dataset on congenital abnormalities.

Two studies explored the risk of placenta abruptio in pregnant women. Williams et al. (1991) used a large cross-sectional database collected from 1977 to 1980 to identify 143 cases of placenta abruptio; 1257 random controls were used. Odds ratios were significant for the following conditions and the risk of placenta abruptio: chronic hypertension (OR 3.1; 95% CI 1.1–8.4), but for pregnancy-induced hypertension, there was no association with abruption; advanced maternal age (OR 2.3; 95% CI 1.3–3.9); low pregnancy BMI (OR 2.3; 95% CI 1.3–4.1; 4); history of prior stillbirth (OR 3.5; 95% CI 1.8–7.0); and weekly marijuana use during pregnancy (OR 2.8; 95% CI 1.2–6.6). There was a borderline significant association between the number of cigarettes smoked and risk of placenta abruptio (OR 1.5; 95% CI 1.0–2.2).

Budde et al. (2007) carried out a retrospective case–control study of placenta abruptio in all singleton pregnancies between 2001 and 2005. Univariate analyses found that the incidence of placenta abruptio in an economically disadvantaged population was 1.0%, and the overall perinatal mortality of abruptio was 13%. Three conditions showed an increased risk for placenta abruptio: preterm membrane rupture (OR 4.79; 95% CI 1.52–15.08), noncompliance with antenatal care (OR 2.93; 95% CI 1.06–8.90), and severe IUGR and elevated homocysteine levels (OR 45.55; 95% CI 7.06–458.93). The placenta abruptio group had significantly more incidents of IUGR than the control group ($p = 0.032$). Preterm rupture and an elevated homocysteine level were the major risk factors for placenta abruptio, but there was no association between smoking or pre-eclampsia and placenta abruptio. In multivariate analyses, preterm rupture of the membranes and elevated homocysteine levels were more commonly found in the abruptio group and were identified as a significant risk for placenta abruptio. This group also had a higher incidence of marijuana use, domestic violence, and mental health problems.

The relationship between marijuana use and chromosomal abnormalities was studied by Kline *et al.* (1991), who reviewed 567 cases of spontaneous abortion with normal karyotypes and 393 cases of spontaneous abortion with chromosomal aberrations. In the group with chromosomal aberrations, there were 212 cases of trisomy, 71 of monosomy X, 49 triploidies, and 61 other chromosomal abnormalities. The OR was 1.1 (95% CI 0.7–1.5) for reported marijuana use comparing with controls (n = 2042) and those with normal chromosomes; for those with abnormal chromosomes the OR was 1.2 (95% CI 0.7–1.9). There were no differences between marijuana users and controls for trisomy (AOR 0.8; 95% CI 0.4–1.8), monosomy (AOR 1.8 95% CI 0.7–4.3), or triploidy (AOR 1.3; 95% CI 0.4–4.5). Overall, there was no association between marijuana use during the perifertilization period and trisomy abnormalities, nor between marijuana use and normal chromosome spontaneous abortions. Small numbers made it difficult to determine the effect in other aneuploid cases.

Zhang & Bracken (1996) used a tree-based analysis, logistic regression, and Mantel–Haenszel test to assess potential risk confounders for spontaneous abortion. Data from 1988 to 1991 were used to identify 11 putative risk factors for spontaneous abortion and 19 potential confounders, including marijuana use and passive exposure to marijuana. The three major risks were carrying loads greater than 9 kg at least once a day (RR 1.71; 95% CI 1.25–2.32; 2), drinking three or more cups of coffee per day (RR 2.34; 95% CI 1.45–3.77), and reaching over the shoulders (marginally significant; RR 1.35; 95% CI 1.02–1.78). The authors found that analyzing the data using the tree analysis and Mantel–Haenszel test was a good method to explore risk for spontaneous abortion when many confounders exist.

A study by Shiono *et al.* (1995) used an interview method and serum tests from 7470 pregnant women to study cocaine and marijuana use and pregnancy outcomes. They were particularly interested in LBW (under 2500 g), preterm birth (prior to 37 weeks), and placenta abruptio. Of the 7470 women studied from seven prenatal clinics from 1984 to 1989, 172 (2.3%) used cocaine and 821 (11.0%) used marijuana during the pregnancy. Drug use was assessed by interview and laboratory testing. While cocaine use was strongly associated with placenta abruptio (AOR 4.2; 95% CI 1.9–9.5), marijuana use was not associated with any of the three outcomes (LBW, AOR 1.1; preterm labor, AOR 1.1; placenta abruptio, AOR 1.3). However, cigarette smoking was associated with a slightly increased risk of having LBW babies (AOR 1.5; 95% CI 1.2–1.8).

Holland *et al.* (1997) studied preterm delivery in women who abused drugs during and experienced physical trauma during their pregnancies. In this prospective study, 157 (2.3%) of 6828 live births were associated with physical trauma. Most of the incidents of trauma were insignificant (153) or minor (2), but two women experienced severe trauma. Fifty-four percent of the women agreed to be screened for alcohol, marijuana, and cocaine; 11% tested positive for one or more substance. Preterm labor and delivery occurred in 32 (21%) of the 153 patients experiencing insignificant trauma, with a morbidity rate of 50:1000 and a mortality rate of 20:1000.

Table 4.17 summarizes these studies.

Table 4.17 Pregnancy complications

Study	Method	Sample	Incidence	Results
Lee (1998)	Literature review Marijuana use in pregnancy			Many pregnant marijuana users are polydrug and alcohol users so difficult to pin-point chemical cause; conflicting information on reports of marijuana use; more evidence for effects of smoking reversed with smoking cessation
Kuczkowski (2004)	Literature review Drug abuse, pregnancy, fetal outcomes, anesthesia concerns	Medline search		No guidelines for anesthesia, analgesia administration in peripartum period; individualize care on case to case basis
von Mandach (2005)	Literature review Drug abuse in pregnancy			Marijuana can cause vasoconstriction, may affect placental vessels (placenta abruptio, preterm labor, spontaneous abortion, stillbirth); pregnant drug users often polydrug users, so difficult to determine risk for one drug
Witter & Niebyl (1990)	Retrospective analysis Marijuana use, pregnancy outcomes	8350 women, 417 (5%) history of only marijuana use	No association between marijuana use and prematurity, congenital anomalies; many women smoking marijuana also used cigarettes and alcohol	Prematurity, congenital anomalies could also be caused by cigarettes, alcohol
Czeizel et al. (2004)	Retrospective study of data from Hungarian Congenital Abnormality Registry Reliability of self-report of smoking, alcohol use during pregnancy Structured questionnaire for mothers, fathers, family	81 offspring with orofacial cleft and matched controls, 537 offspring with congenital limb deformity and matched controls	Mothers mailed structured questionnaire; Fathers, family interviewed with same questionnaire Low reliability in self-report of information on smoking by case mothers but not control mothers; low reliability of self-report of information on alcohol use in both case and control mothers	Self-report of smoking and alcohol use is unreliable

Study	Design	Sample	Results	Conclusion
Williams et al. (1991)	Retrospective study, large cross-sectional database, 1977–1980 Risk of placenta abruptio	143 with placenta abruptio, 1257 random controls	Major risk factors for placenta abruptio: Chronic high BP (OR 3.1; 95% CI 1.1–8.4); advanced maternal age (OR 2.3; 95% CI 1.3–3.9); low BMI (OR 2.3; 95% CI 1.3–4.1); history of prior stillbirth (OR 3.5; 95% CI 1.8–7.0); weekly marijuana use during pregnancy (OR 2.8; 95% CI 1.2–6.6); cigarette smoking (OR 1.5; 95% CI 1.0–2.2; borderline significant)	Marijuana use is is a risk factor for placenta abruptio
Budde et al. (2007)	Retrospective case–control study, 2001–2005 data Risk for placental abruptio		Incidence of placental abruptio 1.0%; mortality with births 13% Risk factors for placental abruptio: preterm membrane rupture (OR 4.79; 95% CI 1.52–15.08); non-compliant prenatal care (OR 2.93; 95% CI 1.06–8.90); severe IUGR, elevated plasma homocysteine (OR 45.55; 95% CI 7.06–458.93)	Severe IUGR more common in abruption group vs. controls ($p = 0.032$); preterm rupture of membranes, increased homocysteine level both significant dependent risk factors for abruption; abruption group had more marijuana use, domestic violence, mental health problems
Kline et al. (1991)	Analysis of spontaneous abortions of known karyotype	Normal karyotype and spontaneous abortion, abnormal karyotype and spontaneous abortion (212 trisomies, 71 monosomy X, 49 triploidies, 61 other), 2042 controls	Marijuana use and spontaneous abortion, normal karyotype, OR 1.1 (95% CI 0.07–1.5); spontaneous abortion, aneuploidy, OR 1.2 (95% CI 0.7–1.9); trisomies, OR 0.8 (95% CI 0.4–1.8; n.s.); monosomy X, AOR 1.8 (95% CI 0.7–4.3); triploidy, AOR 1.3 (95% CI 0.4–4.5)	No association with marijuana use and normal or abnormal karyotype and spontaneous abortion
Zhang & Bracken (1996)	Tree-based analysis, logistic regression, Mantel-Haenszel test of 1988–1991 dataset Risk factors and potential confounders for spontaneous abortion	Assessed 11 putative risk factors, 19 potential confounders (including marijuana)	Risks: carrying loads > 9 kg at least once a day (RR 1.71; 95% CI 1.25–2.32); drinking 3 or more cups coffee/day in first months of pregnancy (RR 2.34; 95% CI 1.45–3.77); reaching over shoulders (RR 1.35; 95% CI 1.02–1.78)	Tree-based analysis a good method to explore risk when many confounders exist; in this analysis, marijuana use was a confounder and not a risk factor

Table 4.17 *Cont.*

Study	Method	Sample	Incidence	Results
Shiono *et al.* (1995)	Retrospective study Risk of LBW, preterm birth, placenta abruptio with cocaine, marijuana use Interview, serum test	7470 pregnant women from seven clinics: 172 (2.3%) used cocaine during pregnancy; 822 (11.0 %) used marijuana	Cocaine strongly associated with placenta abruptio (AOR 4.2; 95% CI 1.9–9.5); marijuana not associated with any outcomes (LBW, AOR 1.1; preterm labor, AOR 1.1; placenta abruptio, AOR 1.3); cigarette smoking associated with LBW (AOR 1.5; 95% CI 1.2–1.8)	Cocaine associated with placenta abruptio; cigarette smoking associated with LBW; marijuana not associated with any of three outcomes
Holland *et al.* (1997)	Prospective study Preterm delivery, drug abuse, trauma	Pregnant patients with physical trauma: 6828 live births (157 [2.3%] associated with trauma); 85 (54%) screened for drugs and 9 (11%) positive for one or more drug	Morbidity/mortality in 153 trauma patients: morbidity 50:1000; mortality 20:1000; 21% of patients with insignificant trauma had preterm labor and delivery	Trauma and drug use can be risk factors for preterm delivery

AOR, adjusted odds ratio; BMI, body mass index; BP, blood pressure; CI, confidence interval; HIV, human immunodeficiency virus; IUGR, intrauterine growth retardation; n.s, not significant; OR, odds ratio; RR, relative risk.

Comments

This diverse subsection on marijuana and female genital disease and pregnancy complications provides some insight to risks of marijuana use in pregnant women. While the literature review on infertility in marijuana users was inconclusive, the fairly large case–control study found marijuana users were at risk for primary infertility. The two studies on vaginal infections indicate that marijuana use is associated with trichomoniasis and yeast infections. Since the ECs can bind to CB2 receptors on immune cells, an increased risk of infection might be expected with marijuana use. There was a single study on the increased risk for functional ovarian cysts in marijuana users with a low BMI. These five studies provide some input into the relationship of marijuana and female genital disease; however, although several studies had large sample sizes, more studies are needed to confirm the results before the information can be used more generally to guide practice or show evidence of risk association.

A difficulty in the pregnancy-complication studies was the polysubstance use by pregnant women. Concurrent cigarette smoking and drug abuse in undesirable pregnancy outcomes provide challenges in parsing the effects of the chemicals in these substances on specific outcomes. Some of the studies did find that marijuana use was associated with placenta abruptio; however, other studies found no relationship between marijuana use and prematurity or congenital abnormalities, LBW, or placenta abruptio. One study looked at chromosomal abnormalities in spontaneously aborted fetuses in marijuana users. Use of marijuana did not appear to significantly increase the risk of aneuploidy when smoking occurred in the first trimester. Further studies on these topics could provide greater insight into the role of marijuana use and pregnancy risk outcomes.

Two studies provided information related to research methodology. One study confirmed the findings of others in this chapter that self-report of drug use can be unreliable. Obtaining information from spouses and family members could provide additional information about drug use in the patients being studied. Use of a tree-based methodology and tests to examine association among possible confounders provides additional statistical tools to analyze research data.

Congenital, hereditary, and neonatal diseases and abnormalities

In the review of PubMed literature published between 1988 and 2008 related to marijuana use, there were 10 articles on congenital diseases, including two reviews and eight research studies; two articles on neonatal diseases, including one review and one research study; and six articles on congenital abnormalities, including one review and five research studies. These articles are reviewed in three sections.

Congenital disorders

Behnke & Eyler (1993) reviewed the effects on the fetus and neonate of alcohol, marijuana, nicotine, opiates, and cocaine use by pregnant women. The review included information on the possible long-term effects of these drugs on the developing infant. Schempf (2007) reviewed adverse birth outcomes associated with marijuana, opiate, and cocaine use. While cocaine use was associated with decreased fetal growth, studies of cocaine and other illicit drug use often did not control for social, psychosocial, and contextual factors that might affect fetal outcomes. The authors suggested further research to study the effects of these factors on the developing neonate.

Frank et al. (1990) studied body proportionality and composition in a multiethnic sample of 1082 newborns. Self-report of marijuana and cocaine use by the mothers and urine samples for drug use were obtained. Infants of marijuana users tended to have a depressed mean arm circumference (non-fat areas) ($p < 0.05$) when the data were analyzed controlling for other drugs and confounders. Infants of cocaine users had decreased subscapular fat folds, and decreased fat and non-fat arm areas ($p < 0.05$). Infants of both marijuana users and cocaine users had LBW. The authors suggested that the mechanism for the IUGR in marijuana-using mothers may be related to maternal–fetal hypoxia, while the decreased body weight in infants of cocaine-using mothers was related to altered nutrient transfer and fetal metabolism.

Day and coworkers conducted two longitudinal studies on women beginning with their pregnancies. In the first study (Day *et al.* 1991), they interviewed mothers of 519 newborns during each trimester and assessed growth parameters, external features, and gestational age. They found a small, significant negative effect of marijuana use during the first trimester – especially the first two months – on birth length, and a positive effect of marijuana use during the third trimester on birthweight. Once controlling for various confounders, all other effects were non-significant.

In the second study (Day *et al.* (1994), they also interviewed pregnant women during their fourth and seventh months of pregnancy and evaluated the mothers and their offspring at delivery, at 8 and 18 months, and at three and six years of age. The study comprised 668 children. They found that at age six, children of alcohol-using mothers had smaller weight and height, smaller head circumference, and a narrower palpebral fissure width than other children. Appetite differences were also found. At age six, children of mothers who smoked cigarettes and marijuana during their pregnancy had no significant growth and development changes or morphological abnormalities.

In another longitudinal study, Cornelius *et al.* (1995) looked at the effect of tobacco and marijuana use during pregnancy on the growth and development of infants. Adolescent mothers of 310 offspring were interviewed in the middle of their pregnancy and at delivery. The infants were examined 24 to 36 hours after birth. The average age of the mothers was 16.1 years (range, 12–18); 70% were African American. While marijuana use was only associated with a decrease in gestational age and an increased rate of minor morphological changes in infants of white women, tobacco use was associated with a decreased birthweight and length, and a decrease in head and chest circumference. There was no increase in the morphological abnormalities in infants of women who smoked tobacco. The authors suggested that the young age of the tobacco- and marijuana-using mothers could increase the risks of negative outcomes in the infants.

In 2002, Cornelius *et al.* published another study on 345 live births surviving to six years of age. The focus of this prospective study was to assess child growth for mothers who used alcohol, tobacco, or marijuana during pregnancy. The mothers were recruited for the study between 1990 and 1995. After controlling for confounders, the authors found that fetal exposure to alcohol and marijuana was significantly associated with growth defects but at specific exposure times. Exposure to alcohol during the second and third trimesters was associated with decreased height, and third trimester use led to infants with decreased skinfold thickness. Exposure to marijuana during the second trimester was associated with decreased stature. Tobacco use during the first trimester was significantly associated with increased skinfold thickness in children at age six. Their study suggests there are long-lasting effects, at least to six years of age, in children of mothers who used alcohol, tobacco, or marijuana during their pregnancy.

In a population-based case–control study, Williams *et al.* (2004) studied maternal lifestyle effects on the development of simple ventricular septal defects in infants. Maternal self-reports and paternal proxy reports of mothers' drug use were conducted to determine intrauterine exposure to alcohol, cigarette smoke, and illicit drugs. During the period 1968 to 1980, 122 children with simple ventricular septal defects were identified from the Atlanta Birth Defects Case–Control Study; 3029 controls were recruited. Alcohol use in mothers was associated with simple ventricular septal defects with heavy use self-report and moderate use proxy report. In marijuana users, there was a two-fold increased risk of simple ventricular septal defect, and an increased risk with regular use (three or more days/week).

Steinberger *et al.* (2002) reported on a population-based case–control study in infants with a single ventricle. Data from the Baltimore–Washington Infant Study (1981–1989) were used. Controls were 3572 normal infants with no cardiac abnormalities. Of the children with congenital cardiovascular defects, 55 (1.25%) had a single ventricle, however only 48 (87.3%) of the parents were interviewed for the study. Maternal and paternal alcohol and marijuana use were explored. Paternal use of alcohol and marijuana was associated with all cases of single ventricle. The ORs were 2.0 (95% CI 1.1–3.9) for paternal alcohol use, 2.4 (95% CI 1.1–5.1) for paternal cigarette use, and 2.2 (95% CI 1.0–5.2) for paternal marijuana use., The only significant risk associated with the mothers with an abnormal ultrasound was a previously induced abortion (OR 2.2; 95% CI 1.1–11.5). The authors concluded that paternal smoking and alcohol use were major risk factors for a single ventricle.

Wilson *et al.* (1998) reported on potential causes for eight cardiac malformations using the Baltimore–Washington Infant Study database. The only illicit drug associated with one of the eight cardiac malformations was marijuana. They found that there was a relationship between paternal use of marijuana and transposition of the great arteries with an intact ventricular septum.

These studies on congenital disorders are summarized in Table 4.18.

Congenital abnormalities

One review article and five studies reported on congenital abnormalities associated with marijuana use. In a review, Day & Richardson (1991) reported on the characteristics of maternal users and the result of studies on neonatal outcomes. Female marijuana users who smoked during their pregnancy tended to be less educated and of a lower social class than non-users; they were also more likely to be African American and to abuse other substances during their pregnancy. The researchers found contradictory or equivocal results in the studies on prenatal drug use and birth outcomes. In prospective studies, relationships between marijuana use and birthweight were not found. There was some suggestion of decreased birth length in the infants. Some studies suggested that marijuana use was associated with small birth size, but in many of the studies, there were no controls for other illicit drug use. Infant growth outside the neonatal period did not appear to be affected by marijuana used during the prenatal period. Conflicting results were found in studies looking at marijuana use and gestational age and neurobehavior in infants. The two morphological studies reviewed tended to report no association between marijuana use and infant outcomes. Overall, there were conflicting results and too few studies to make definitive associations between marijuana use and untoward birth outcomes.

Forrester & Merz (2007) reported on a study of 52 children in the Hawaiian Adverse Pregnancy Outcome Registry who were born with selected birth defects between 1986 and

Table 4.18 Congenital disorders

Study	Method	Sample	Incidence	Results
Behnke & Eyler (1993)	Literature review Effects of commonly used drugs on fetus			Long-term use of illicit drugs can increase risk for congenital disease
Schempf (2007)	Literature review Adverse birth outcomes	Recent research in epidemiological literature on marijuana, opiates, cocaine		Many studies did not control for use of other drugs or socioeconomic-contextual factors; cocaine was associated with decreased fetal growth
Frank et al. (1990)	Multiethnic sample Body proportionality and composition Self-report of marijuana, cocaine use, drug urine samples	1082 newborns and mothers	Controlled for use of other drugs, confounders, infants of marijuana users had decreased arm muscle circumference (non-fat) ($p < 0.05$); infants of cocaine users had decreased subscapular fat folds, fat and non-fat arm areas ($p < 0.05$); Infants of users of both had decreased birthweight	Marijuana may affect fetal oxygenation while cocaine may affect nutrient transfer to fetus
Day et al. (1991)	Longitudinal study Interview pregnant women every trimester	519 newborns	Small significant negative effect of marijuana use during first 2 months of pregnancy on birth length; positive effect of marijuana use in third trimester on birthweight	After controlling for confounders, few marijuana effects on growth and development
Day et al. (1994)	Cohort study, 6-year follow-up Interviews and infant assessments	668 children and their mothers	Mothers evaluated during 4th, 7th months of pregnancy; mothers/newborns evaluated at delivery; infants evaluated at 8 and 18 months, 3 and 6 years Infants of marijuana-using mothers had no significant changes in growth and development at age 6; infants of alcohol-using mothers had smaller weight, height, head circumference, palpebral fissure width at age 6; also appetite changes	Long-term consequences of marijuana use during pregnancy inconclusive No relationship between prenatal alcohol, marijuana, tobacco use and rate of morphological abnormalities

Cornelius et al. (1995)	Longitudinal study Marijuana and tobacco use during pregnancy and infant growth and development Interviews and infant assessments	Adolescent mothers of 310 offspring, average maternal age 16.1 years (range, 12–18), 70% African American	Interview mid-pregnancy, delivery; infants assessed 24–36 h after birth Prenatal marijuana use: reduced gestational age at birth; increase in minor physical abnormalities in whites; no abnormal growth outcomes Tobacco use: decreased birthweight, length, head–chest circumference	Reduced gestational age more likely in marijuana users; decreased infant birthweight, length more common in tobacco users
Cornelius et al. (2002)	Prospective study from 1990–1995 Long-term effects of substance abuse on child growth	443 cases recruited, 345 survived to age 6	After controlling for confounders, alcohol, marijuana exposure significantly associated with growth defects seen at age 6 Alcohol second, third trimester exposure, decreased height; marijuana second trimester exposure, shorter stature; tobacco: first trimester exposure, increased skinfold thickness	Long-lasting consequences may be present in children whose mothers used alcohol, tobacco, and marijuana during pregnancy
Williams et al. (2004)	Population-based case–control study (1968–1980 data) VSD and maternal lifestyle Maternal reports, paternal proxy reports	122 with simple VSD, 3029 controls	Alcohol use: heavy (self-report) or moderate (proxy) associated with simple VSD; marijuana use gave two-fold increase of simple VSD; increased risk with regular use (3 or more times/week)	Marijuana use associated with increased incidence of simple VSD
Steinberger et al. (2002)	Population-based case–control study using data from the Baltimore–Washington Infant Study Database (1981–1989) Incidence of single ventricle Interviews, maternal and paternal	55 infants, single ventricle (1.25% of all cardiovascular defects), 48 interviews (maternal and paternal); 3572 controls	Paternal association with infant single ventricle: alcohol (OR 2.0 (95% CI 1.1–3.9); cigarettes (OR 2.4; 95% CI 1.1–5.1); marijuana (OR 2.2; 95% CI 1.0–5.2) Maternal marijuana use only associated with abnormal ultrasound with previous induced abortion (OR 3.2; 95% CI1.1–11.5)	Paternal use of abused substances associated with cases of single ventricle
Wilson et al. (1998)	Descriptive study, Baltimore–Washington Infant Study Database (1981–1989) Cardiac malformations		8 attributable factors associated with cardiac malformations	Only marijuana use in fathers associated with transposition of great arteries with intact ventricular septum (7.8%)

CI, confidence interval; OR, odds ratio; VSD, ventricular septal defect.

2002. The birth defects included CNS, cardiovascular, oral clefts, and limb abnormalities. Forrester studied the maternal use rates for methamphetamine (0.52%), cocaine (0.18%), and marijuana (0.26%). The methamphetamine rates were significantly higher than expected for 14 (26%) of the birth defects; the cocaine use rates were significantly higher than expected for 13 (24%) of the birth defects; and the marijuana use rates were significantly higher for 21 (39%) of the birth defects. The researchers found that prenatal marijuana use increased the risk for gastrointestinal abnormalities in newborns.

Kennare *et al.* (2005) used the South Australian Perinatal Data Collection (1998–2002) to study the outcomes of mothers using a variety of illicit drugs during their pregnancy. Of 89 080 women, 707 (0.8%) indicated use of drugs: marijuana (38.9%), methadone (29.9%), methamphetamines (14.6%), heroin (12.5%), and polydrug use (18.8%). The women tended to be smokers, single, indigenous, of lower socioeconomic status, have psychiatric conditions, and living in metropolitan areas. Risks for various complications of pregnancy were calculated: placenta abruptio, OR 2.53; antepartal hemorrhage, OR 1.41; preterm birth, OR 2.63; small size for age, OR 1.79; congenital abnormalities, OR 1.52; nursery stays longer than seven days, OR 4.07; stillbirth, OR 2.54; and neonatal death, OR 2.92. Only a small amount of the variance in outcomes could be attributed to substance abuse. The author suggested that maternal health and psychosocial lifestyle factors need further study as risks for negative birth outcomes.

Torfs *et al.* (1994) studied the incidence of gastroschisis (abdominal wall defects) in infants in a case–control study using data from the California Birth Defects Monitoring Program; 110 mothers with children with gastroschisis were identified and 220 age-matched controls were used. Univariate analyses found significant associations between gastroschisis and a number of variables, including education, yearly family income, marital status, short interval between menarche and pregnancy, and use of drugs in the trimester before pregnancy. Polysubstance use was found to be more of a risk factor than single drug use. Drugs studied included cocaine, amphetamines, marijuana, LSD, alcohol, and tobacco. The ORs calculated for gastroschisis and drug use were 2.21 (95% CI 1.21–4.03) for the mother, 1.66 (95% CI 1.02–2.69) for the father, and 3.05 (95% CI 1.48–6.28) for use by both mother and father. The authors concluded that young, socially disadvantaged women with a history of substance abuse were at a higher risk of having a child with gastroschisis than non-users.

Forrester & Merz (2006) used a Hawaiian registry (1986–2002) to study the incidence of gastroschisis. They found that the incidence of gastroschisis in children of maternal marijuana users (but not methamphetamine or cocaine) was significantly higher than in the total population. The highest number of cases of gastroschisis was found in the youngest mothers. The authors suggested that, since the gastroschisis incidence increased while the rate of substance abuse did not follow the same trend, substance abuse is not likely to be a major factor in development of this abdominal wall defect.

Scher *et al.* (1988) reported on a longitudinal study of neonatal sleep cycles in children of maternal alcohol and marijuana users. Neonatal EEGs were used to monitor sleep cycles. The authors found disturbed sleep cycles and motility in infants whose mothers used marijuana throughout the pregnancy, while alcohol abuse during the first trimester was associated with sleep cycling disturbances and altered arousal. A small case size was a limitation in this study; however, the study did suggest that there was a substance-specific link to trimester use and outcomes.

The studies on congenital abnormalities are summarized in Table 4.19.

Table 4.19 Congenital abnormalities

Study	Method	Sample	Incidence	Results
Day & Richardson (1991)	Literature review Marijuana use and birth outcomes			Women who smoked marijuana during pregnancy: less well-educated, lower social class, much more likely to use other substances, more likely to be African American Study results: marijuana and birth outcomes equivocal; prospective studies showed no relationship between marijuana use and birthweight; small effect on birth length; small size reported in some studies but no control for other drug use; no consistent correlation with prenatal marijuana use for growth outside neonatal period; morphological studies mostly reported no association
Forrester & Merz (2007)	Population-based study from the Hawaiian Birth Defects Project Registry Drug use and birth defects	Children with 54 birth defects (1986–2002)	Methamphetamine use rate 0.52%, higher than expected for 14 (26%) defects; cocaine use rate 0.18%, significantly higher than expected for 13 (24%) defects; marijuana use rate 0.26%, associated with 12 (39%) of defects	Increased risk of variety of birth defects in drug users, particularly in organ systems; marijuana users had increased risk for gastrointestinal abnormalities
Kennare et al. (2005)	Database description	89 080 women in database, 707 (0.8%) used drugs: marijuana, 38.9%; methadone, 29.9%; methamphetamines, 14.6%; heroin, 12.5%; polydrug, 18.8%	Users more likely smokers, psychiatric conditions, single, indigenous, lower socioeconomic status, metropolitan dwellers; increased risks for placenta abruptio (OR 2.53), antepartal hemorrhage (OR 1.41), preterm birth (OR 2.63), small for age (OR 1.79), congenital abnormalities (OR 1.51), nursery stays > 7 days (OR 4.07), stillbirth (OR 2.54), neonatal death (OR 2.92)	Only small amount of risks associated with substance abuse; need to look at health, psychosocial lifestyle factors

Table 4.19 *Cont.*

Study	Method	Sample	Incidence	Results
Torfs *et al.* (1994)	Case–control study Gastroschisis	110 mothers with children with gastroschisis, 220 age-matched controls	Univariate analysis showed significant association with variety of demographic variables, including use of recreational drug during trimester before pregnancy Risk and drug use by mother, OR 2.21 (95% CI 1.21–4.03); father, OR 1.66 (95% CI 1.02–2.69); both, OR 3.05 (95% CI 1.488–6.28)	Polydrug use more of a risk than one drug; young, socially disadvantaged women with history of substance abuse have highest risk for gastroschisis
Forrester & Merz (2006)	Descriptive study from Hawaiian Registry database, 1986–2002 Gastroschisis and drug use		Maternal marijuana use: significantly more children with gastroschisis than total population; highest number of cases in youngest users	Gastroschisis increase not proportional to drug abuse rate; substance abuse not likely to be a major factor
Scher *et al.* (1988)	Longitudinal study Neonatal sleep cycles Electroencephalography	Children of maternal alcohol and marijuana users	Marijuana user throughout pregnancy: infants have altered sleep cycles, motility Alcohol abuse in first trimester: infant sleep cycle disturbances, altered arousal	Link apparent to substance, trimester use, outcome

CI, confidence interval; OR, odds ratio.

Table 4.20 Neonatal disease

Study	Method	Sample	Incidence	Results
Giese (1994)	Literature review Ocular disease			Physical abuse and illicit drug use can cause ocular dysfunction in children
Fried (1989)	Prospective study Prenatal drug use	Infants of cigarette, marijuana users	Infants of cigarette users: hypertonicity, nervous system excitement at 1 month; decreased mental scores, altered auditory response at 12 months; questionable findings at 24 months Infants of marijuana users: mild narcotic-like withdrawal at 1 month; no association with motor, mental, language outcomes at 1 and 2 years; some cognitive, language change at 3 years	Persistent effects in cigarette smokers; inconclusive in marijuana users

Neonatal diseases

One review and one longitudinal study considered neonatal diseases (Table 4.20).

Giese (1994) reviewed the literature related to ocular findings in infants born to drug-abusing mothers. He discussed some of the long-term effects as well as ocular and systemic sequellae of marijuana and other abused substances.

Fried (1989) reported on a prospective study of the neurobehavioral and teratogenic effects of cigarette and marijuana use by pregnant women. At one month, infants of cigarette-smoking mothers exhibited hypertonicity and increased nervous system excitation; at 12 months, the children had decreased mental scores and altered auditory responses. At one month, the children who had been exposed to marijuana exhibited mild narcotic-like withdrawal symptoms. At 24 months, the continued use of cigarettes by the mothers made it difficult to assess the effect of current use compared with use during pregnancy. The children of marijuana-using mothers showed no association between prior drug use and motor, mental, and language outcomes at age two years; however, at three years of age, the children did exhibit some cognitive and language disorders, as did the children of cigarette smokers.

Comments

A variety of studies are included in this subsection on the possible risk of congenital, hereditary, and neonatal diseases in children of marijuana users. As cited in several review articles, many of the studies present contradictory or inconclusive evidence for risk. In some cases, there are too few studies or too few subjects to make generalizations on the findings. Some studies may also not control for important confounders, including use of other abused substances.

Despite some of the limitations of these studies, some risk evidence is beginning to emerge. It appears that use of marijuana during pregnancy is associated with decreased birthweight and length in newborns. One research group suggested that IUGR may be related to fetal hypoxia. Most studies only interviewed or used existing databases to determine maternal use of abused substances. Many of the marijuana-using mothers with infants with alterations at birth were younger than other mothers, were socially and economically disadvantaged, and often had psychological and delinquent behavioral problems. Many of the mothers were also polydrug users. Longitudinal studies seem to indicate that by six years of age, most children no longer had growth deficits.

Only three studies reported on cardiovascular abnormalities: one on simple ventricular septal defect, one on single ventricle, and one on transposition of the great arteries. In two of these studies, paternal use of marijuana increased the risk for the disorder (single ventricle, transposition of the arteries). Two studies reported on increased cases of gastroschisis in newborns of young marijuana-using mothers. Since this disorder is more common in young women than in older mothers, more research needs to assess potential factors that increase risk of having children with gastroschisis.

Since it is difficult to generalize the findings based on the studies described here, more studies are needed to explore further the risks of abnormal neonatal conditions and the potential for long-term consequences.

Cardiovascular disease

Nine epidemiological studies were found on PubMed published between 1988 and 2008 related to cardiovascular disease and marijuana use: two review articles focused on the cardiovascular consequences of marijuana use; three articles discussed arteritis in marijuana users; a prospective study described drug-induced palpitations; one study looked at the effect of marijuana in increasing cardiovascular risks; and three studies reported on incidents of AMI and marijuana use.

Sidney (2002) described the physiological effects of marijuana use in a review article. Acute effects tend to be dose dependent and include increased heart rate, a mild increase in blood pressure, and decreased vascular resistance, which can precipitate orthostatic hypotension. Exercise tolerance is decreased after smoking marijuana, with users' heart rates increasing to submaximal levels. Marijuana users appear to develop a tolerance to the acute effects of THC after several days or a few weeks.

According to Sidney (2002), there is very little information in the literature on the chronic effects of marijuana use and cardiovascular disease. Some studies indicated that individuals with angina pectoris had an earlier onset of chest pain when using marijuana. Individuals with CAD should be cautioned not to use marijuana because the drug may precipitate clinical cardiac events and increase risk of an AMI. Sidney suggested that more research is needed to study any association of marijuana use and cardiovascular risk factors, the metabolic and physiological effects of chronic use and cardiovascular risk, the cannabinoid cardiovascular system and blood pressure control, and possible neuroprotection associated with strokes.

Aryana & Williams (2007) also reviewed the literature and discuss the physiological effects of marijuana use. They reported on research and case studies that supported marijuana use as a trigger for tachyarrhythmias and acute coronary syndrome. They also reviewed studies involving vascular complications and congenital heart defects.

In a review of cannabis arteritis, Peyrot et al. (2007) reported that over 50 cases of arteritis – similar to thromboangiitis obliterans – had been reported since 1960 by marijuana users who did not smoke cigarettes. They described a 36-year-old male without any cardiovascular risks who experienced necrosis in the toes of his right foot and who later developed popliteal artery occlusion and had his left leg amputated. Peyrot et al. (2007) suggested that cannabis arteritis may be analogous to thromboarteritis obliterans seen in cigarette smokers. They suggested that cannabis arteritis may be a cause of juvenile peripheral obstructive arterial disease, which is often underdiagnosed.

Disdier et al. (2001) described recent cases of cannabis arteritis seen in 10 males, median age 23.7 years. All had distal ischemia in their fingers or toes. Two also had venous thromboses and three had Raynaud's phenomenon. None had classical risk factors for cardiovascular disease, although all were moderate tobacco users and regular marijuana users. Five amputations were necessary in four of the patients. Arteriographic studies found distal abnormalities similar to Buerger's disease (thromboangiitis obliterans), with changes in the architecture of the vasonervorum. Arterial atherosclerotic lesions were also found. Since both Δ^8- and Δ^9-THC cause peripheral vasoconstriction, the authors suggested that use of marijuana adds to the risk for juvenile and young adult arteritis.

An article by Noel et al. (2008) described a case of cannabis arteritis in a young adult that was reversed with complete arterial revascularization after initiation of aspirin therapy. The authors suggested that prompt identification and treatment of cannabis-related arteritis could prevent irreversible damage and tissue death.

Petronis & Anthony (1989) carried out a prospective study in five communities, enrolling 6702 subjects in a multisite study of mental disorders. Using interviews, they found that marijuana and cocaine users were more likely to experience cardiac palpitations than non-users, but that the greater risk was with cocaine users (estimated RR 3.41; 95% CI 1.60–7.29; $p < 0.001$).

Rodondi et al. (2006) reported on data collected in the 15-year longitudinal Coronary Artery Risk Development in Young Adults (CARDIA) study to explore the relationship between marijuana use and diet, BMI, and cardiac risk factors. Other studies have shown that marijuana use can increase appetite and increase the likelihood of eating a high calorie diet. Subsequently, there may be a rise in blood pressure and a decrease in triglycerides and high density lipoproteins. From a database of 3617 subjects, 1365 (38%) had used marijuana. Most of the users were male, tobacco smokers, and used other illicit drugs as well. Extensive marijuana users were more likely than other users and non-users to have a higher caloric intake, drink more alcohol, and have elevated systolic blood pressure and a lower plasma triglyceride level. Multivariate analyses showed that alcohol use was the main confounder that affected systolic blood pressure and triglyceride level and that marijuana use was not independently associated with cardiovascular risks. However, marijuana use was associated with unhealthy behaviors with long-term consequences, including eating a high calorie diet, smoking tobacco, and using other illicit drugs.

In a case-crossover study, Mittleman et al. (2001) studied the effect of smoking marijuana one hour before experiencing an AMI and compared the expected frequency with self-matched control data. Marijuana use has been found to increase heart rate, increase supine hypertension, and cause postural hypotension. They utilized participants in the Determinants of Myocardial Infarction Onset Study (DMIOS) and interviewed patients four days after experiencing an AMI. Of 3883 patients, 124 (3.2%) were marijuana users. Nine had smoked marijuana one hour before symptoms of an AMI, 34 within the previous 24 hours, and 124 (3.2%) within the previous year. The marijuana users tended to be male, current cigarette smokers ($p < 0.001$), obese ($p < 0.008$), and less likely to experience angina signs or symptoms of hypertension. They had a 4.8% (95% CI 2.4–9.5) increased risk of experiencing an AMI one hour after smoking marijuana. After one hour, the risk decreased rapidly. This study suggests that marijuana smoking can trigger an AMI in susceptible populations; however, more studies are needed to determine the physiological mechanisms.

Caldicott *et al.* (2005) provided a review of the literature after describing the case of a 21-year-old male with an AMI after smoking marijuana despite no apparent risk factors for CAD.

Mukamal *et al.* (2008) used an inception cohort study to explore the mortality rate of marijuana users experiencing an AMI. The subjects were 1913 adults hospitalized with an AMI at 45 hospitals in the USA from 1989 to 1994; of these 52 had used marijuana in the year previous to the attack. Compared with non-users, use of marijuana less than weekly had a hazard ratio of 2.5 (95% CI 0.9–7.3), and for weekly use a hazard ratio of 4.2 (1.2–14.3). The age- and sex-adjusted hazard ratio with any drug use was 1.9 (95% CI 0.6–6.3) for cardiovascular mortality and 4.9 (95% CI 1.6–14.7) for non-cardiovascular mortality. The authors suggested that smoking marijuana after an AMI was hazardous and could potentially result in fatal outcomes.

Table 4.21 summarizes these studies.

Comments

Physiological laboratory studies have shown the presence of an endogenous cardiac cannabinoid system involving both CB1 and CB2 receptors. The cardiac EC system is thought to involve cardioprotective mechanisms, including reduction of myocardial infarct size, most likely through CB2 receptors. The EC system has a role in a number of peripheral tissues, including adipose tissue, muscle, the liver, and the gastrointestinal tract. In adipose cells, ECs decrease adiponectin and increase lipogenesis – both conditions that can lead to dyslipidemia. Insulin resistance can develop secondary to a decrease in insulin-stimulated glucose uptake. The CB receptors in the liver, may increase the action of a number of enzymes involved in fatty acid synthesis, leading to dyslipidemia and insulin resistance. In the gastrointestinal tract, the ECs decrease satiety signals, thus stimulating appetite and potentially leading to high calorie diets and obesity.

Based on the research on the EC system and the cardiovascular implications, it would seem that more studies are needed to look at the long-term effects of the phytocannabinoids on cardiovascular health and risk factors for cardiovascular disease. However, in the past 20 years, only six epidemiological studies have been published addressing incidence of MI and cardiac risk factors (hypertension, hyperlipidemia, obesity, insulin resistance) in marijuana users. Vascular studies would be important to explore the effect of THC and other phytocannabinoids on peripheral resistance. Some of the studies reviewed here, including some on pregnancy complications reviewed in an earlier section, suggest that vasoconstriction and peripheral resistance are increased in marijuana users. However, orthostatic hypotension has also been found, especially in acute marijuana use. Studies are needed to determine whether the fall in blood pressure is related to vasodilatation or a decrease in heart rate, perhaps secondary to vagal stimulation, but also to explore whether these situations occur in acute or long-term use.

Since it is known that ECs can bind to CB2 receptors on inflammatory and immune cells and lead to immune dysfunction, the articles on cannabinoid arteritis may be significant to explore with larger populations of marijuana users.

Overall, more studies are needed to determine the cardiovascular risks associated with marijuana use in acute, occasional, and long-term use, and to determine whether various confounders (alcohol and other illicit drug use, metabolic dysfunction, obesity) have an effect on potentiating the effects of marijuana.

Table 4.21 Cardiovascular diseases

Study	Method	Sample	Incidence	Results
Aryana & Williams (2007)	Literature review Marijuana and cardiovascular event triggers			Research, case reports support marijuana use as a trigger for tachyarrhythmias, acute coronary syndrome, vascular complications, congenital heart defects
Caldicott et al. (2005)	Literature review, case report AMI and marijuana user	21 year old with AMI after smoking marijuana; no cardiovascular risk factors		AMI can occur in young marijuana users
Disdier et al. (2001)	Case report Cannabis arteritis	10 males with arteritis, median age 23.7 years; 2 also had venous thrombosis; 3 also had Raynaud's phenomenon	No classical cardiovascular risk factors; 5 amputations in 4 patients; arterial evaluation showed distal abnormaties similar to Buerger's disease, opacification of vasanervosum, some proximal atherosclerosis, venous thrombosis	Prolonged use of marijuana may be an additive risk for juvenile and young adult arteritis
Mittleman et al. (2001)	Case-crossover study Marijuana use and AMI Interview 4 days after AMI	3882 patients from DMIOS: 124 (3.2%) users smoked marijuana 1 h before symptoms; 9 smoked within previous 24 h	Marijuana users more likely to be male ($p < 0.001$), current cigarette smokers ($p < 0.001$), obese ($p < 0.008$), less likely to have angina, high BP; 4.8 times increased risk (95% CI 2.4–9.5) of AMI in recent (1 h) marijuana use	Marijuana use is a rare trigger for AMI
Mukamal et al. (2008)	Inception cohort study Mortality in marijuana smoking patients with AMI Self-report of marijuana use	1913 adults with AMI at 45 hospitals, 1989–1994, follow-up for median of 3.8 years; 52 patients used marijuana in year prior to AMI	Compared with non-users, risk for AMI and marijuana use less than weekly, HR 2.5 (95% CI 0.9–7.3); weekly use, HR 4.2 (95% CI 1.2–14.3)	The age- and sex-adjusted HR with any drug use was 1.9 (95% CI 0.6–6.3) for cardiovascular mortality, 4.9 (95% CI 1.6–14.7) for non-cardiovascular mortality; smoking marijuana after an AMI is hazardous and could potentially result in fatal outcomes
Noel et al. (2008)	Case report Marijuana-induced arteritis	Single marijuana user	Arteritis reversed with early aspirin treatment	Suggests marijuana-induced arteritis can be reversed with early aspirin treatment; atherosclerotic peripheral vascular disease not reversible.

Table 4.21 Cont.

Study	Method	Sample	Incidence	Results
Petronis & Anthony (1989)	Prospective study Palpitations in marijuana and cocaine users Interview data	6702 subjects from 5 communities	Greater risk with cocaine use: RR 3.41 (95% CI 1.60–7.29; $p < 0.001$)	Marijuana and cocaine users more likely to report palpitations than non-users
Peyrot et al. (2007)	Literature review and case report Cannabis arteritis	36-year-old male with no cardiovascular risks	Had digital necrosis, segmental vascular lesions, popliteal artery occlusion, ultimate amputation of left leg	50 cases of cannabis arteritis reported since 1960, similar to thromboangiitis obliterans in cigarette smokers; disorder likely to be underdiagnosed, particularly juvenile peripheral obstructive arterial disease
Rodondi et al. (2006)	Longitudinal study (15 years), CARDIA database Marijuana use with BMI and cardiovascular risk	3617 subjects, 1365 (38%) ever used marijuana	Marijuana users also frequently used tobacco, other drugs; extensive marijuana users were more likely than others to have higher caloric intake, drink more alcohol, have elevated systolic BP, lower triglyceride level; alcohol use major confounder affecting systolic BP and triglycerides	Marijuana use not independently associated with cardiovascular risks; marijuana use associated with eating high calorie diet, smoking tobacco, using other illicit drugs
Sidney (2002)	Literature review Cardiovascular consequences of marijuana use			Acute effects of marijuana dose dependent: increased heart rate, mild hypertension, decreased vascular resistance, decreased exercise test duration with increased submaximal heart rate; tolerance develops after several days, weeks; THC effects mediated by autonomic nervous system Chronic marijuana effects, few data available: decreased perception of anginal pain, possible trigger for AMI

AMI, acute myocardial infarction; BP, blood pressure; CI, confidence interval; HR, hazard ratio; RR, relative risk.

Dermatological disease

No relevant material was found regarding marijuana use and dermatological disease.

Nutritional and metabolic disease

Only two epidemiological studies on marijuana use and nutritional or metabolic disorders were found in the PubMed literature published between 1988 and 2008 (Table 4.22). Both of the articles were reviews of the literature. The first study, by Mohs *et al.* (1990), reviewed the literature on nutritional effects of illicit drugs. Besides marijuana, cocaine and nicotine were also targets of this study. The authors suggested that the three drugs affect food and liquid intake, taste perception and preferences, and body weight. Articles reviewed indicate that during the use of marijuana, or during withdrawal, there can be major changes in food selection and intake – including either weight gain or loss. The authors suggested that more research is needed to explore the relationship between marijuana use and nutritional status.

The second article (Matias & Di 2007) was also a review of the literature, although it is a review of marijuana and energy balance. They described the role of the CB1 and CB2 receptors and their action on nutritional and energy balance. The CB1 receptors are found in the CNS in areas regulating energy intake. Peripherally, CB1 receptors are also found in hepatocytes, adipocytes, and pancreatic islet cells. The ECs associated with these sites are regulated by metabolic hormones and peptides that affect the action of other modulators associated with metabolism. Matias & Di (2007) found studies suggesting that overactivity of the cannabinoids may lead to abdominal obesity, dyslipidemia, and hyperglycemia. Using CB1 antagonists, clinical trials show a decrease in food intake, decreased adipose cell volume, and a return of more functional metabolic balance.

Comments

Recent laboratory studies support a role for the EC receptors – both CB1 and CB2 – in a variety of nutritional and metabolic conditions. The major EC, anandamide, appears to have a role in modulating energy homeostasis and metabolism, including an effect on lipid metabolism (oxidation, lipolysis in adipose tissue, lipogenesis in both the liver and adipose tissue, triglyceride metabolism, and activation of peroxisome proliferation activator receptors). The ECs and their CB1 receptors also affect carbohydrate metabolism (glycolysis, gluconeogenesis, insulin stimulation of glucose uptake, and activation of peroxisome proliferation activator receptor-gamma). These effects are associated with CNS action, particularly in the hypothalamus, forebrain, and brainstem. A number of enzymes and peptides are also involved in the energy homeostatic activity. Overactivity of the endocannabinoid system has been linked to obesity – either as a cause or an effect. Increased fat storage, as seen in obesity, is associated with increased CB receptor expression and EC levels. The ECs are potent appetite stimulators, as is THC found in the phytocannabinoids.

Several other reviews have recently been published related to the role of the ECs in metabolism. Use of rimonabant, a CB1 antagonist, in management of obesity in type 2 diabetes mellitus was described in a review by Davis & Perkins (2007). Cota (2008) also discussed the role of EC hyperactivity in the development of obesity, dyslipidemia, and diabetes mellitus. Vemuri *et al.* (2008) reviewed the role of CB receptor antagonists on the management of obesity and metabolic syndrome.

Two clinical trials will also provide information about the use of rimonabant in control of atherosclerosis and morbidity and mortality in cardiovascular disease. The first results of

Table 4.22 Nutritional and metabolic disorders

Study	Method	Sample	Incidence	Results
Mohs et al. (1990)	Literature review Nutritional effects of illicit drugs			Cocaine, marijuana, nicotine affect food, liquid intake; taste preference, body weight; use of marijuana, or withdrawal, causes major changes in food selection, intake
Matias & Di (2007)	Literature review Metabolic changes, energy balance, and ECs			CB1 receptors in brain areas controlling energy intake, also in hepatocytes, adipocytes, pancreatic islet cells involved in energy homeostasis; level of ECs regulated by metabolic hormones, peptides; overactivity of ECs in metabolic and eating disorders contribute to abdominal obesity, dyslipidemia, hyperglycemia; clinical trials with CB1 receptor antagonists show decreased food intake, abdominal adiposity, metabolic sequelae

EC, endocannabinoid; CB, cannabinoid.

the STRADIVARIUS trial were published in the spring of 2008 (Nissen *et al.* 2008). In this randomized, double-blinded, placebo-controlled trial, 676 patients received either rimonabant or a placebo for 18 months along with dietary counseling. An intravascular coronary ultrasound was done at the beginning and end of the study. The percentage of atheroma volume did not decrease statistically; however, the normalized total atheroma volume did decrease in the subjects taking rimonabant. These individuals also had statistically significant decreases in their body weight and waist circumference, an increase in high density lipoproteins, and a decrease in median triglyceride levels. Both C-reactive protein and glycated hemoglobin also decreased. One negative outcome of rimonabant treatment was more common psychiatric adverse effects, which were not seen in the subjects not receiving the drug. The CRESCENDO trial is due to be completed in the spring of 2009. This clinical trial is studying the effect of rimonabant on the first occurrence of a myocardial infarct, stroke, or death from cardiovascular disease.

With evidence of a relationship between the ECs and obesity, lipid dysfunction, and hyperglycemia, it seems that epidemiological studies of marijuana use and these three conditions would be useful to describe clinical events. Long-term use of marijuana may be linked to or increase the risk of conditions such as metabolic syndrome, hypertension, and cardiovascular disease. There appears to be an opportunity for more clinical research in this area.

Endocrine system disease

Only one case–control study was found in the review of PubMed literature between 1988 and 2008. That study (Holt *et al.* 2005) was discussed above under Female genital disease. The study found an inverse relationship in functional ovarian cysts and BMI in current marijuana users.

Table 4.23 Endocrine diseases

Study	Method	Sample	Incidence	Results
Holt et al. (2005)	Case–control study Functional ovarian cyst in marijuana users and BMI	586 with ovarian cysts; 757 age-matched controls	Multivariate analyses, controlled for age, education, reference year giving risk for functional ovarian cyst in marijuana users: BMI < 20, OR 2.05 (95% CI 0.89–4.75); BMI 20–25, OR 1.78 (95% CI 1.00–3.17); BMI > 25, OR 0.72 (95% CI 0.36–1.42)	As BMI increases, risk of functional ovarian cyst decreases; lower BMI associated with increased risk of ovarian cyst; similar decline in risk with increased BMI in cigarette smokers
Evans et al. (2002)	Case study Breast enlargement in HIV-positive males with antiviral drug use	13 HIV-infected males with breast enlargement	Causes: 9 with gynecomastia (8 unilateral, 8 exposed to protease inhibitors; 6 had potentially other causes [liver disease, marijuana use]); 1 with lipomastia; 3 with lymphoma (2 non-Hodgkin's lymphoma, 1 Hodgkin's lymphoma)	Many others causes can be identified in males treated with antiretroviral drugs who have breast enlargement; marijuana use may be related to gynecomastia

BMI, body mass index; CI, confidence interval; HIV, human immunodeficiency virus; OR, odds ratio.

A second study was by Evans et al. (2002). Their case series explored breast enlargement in 13 HIV-positive males who had exposure to antiretroviral therapy. Nine had gynecomastia, eight unilaterally. Eight had been exposed to prolonged use of protease inhibitors. Six had other potential causes of their breast enlargement, including liver disease and marijuana use; four other cases of breast enlargement were associated with lipomastia (one) or lymphoma (three). Two of the patients with lymphoma had NHL, and one had Hodgkin's disease. The authors suggested that gynecomastia in males treated with antiretroviral drugs may occur for a number of reasons, including lymphoma and long-term marijuana use.

These two studies are summarized in Table 4.23.

Comments

As indicated in the subsection on Nutritional and metabolic disorders, the ECs and their receptors have been implicated in regulation of lipid and carbohydrate metabolism. The relationship between obesity, metabolic syndrome, and insulin resistance point to increased development of diabetes mellitus, particularly type 2. Exploration of the incidence of type 2 diabetes in long-term marijuana users might provide some insight into risk for diabetes in these users.

The study by Evans et al. (2002) suggested that long-term marijuana use was a cause of gynecomastia in two patients. Neither of these two males had lymphoma. Given the research data emerging in the literature, more epidemiological studies involving larger numbers of marijuana users are needed to explore the risks for hematopoietic and immune dysfunction. No other studies were found relating marijuana use to gynecomastia.

Immune system disease

No relevant material was found regarding marijuana use and diseases of the immune system; however, one study was found in the PubMed literature related to the lymphatic system and marijuana use.

Table 4.24 Immune system

Study	Method	Sample	Incidence	Results
Holly *et al.* (1999)	Case–control study Non-Hodgkin's lymphoma Blood tests for viruses and lymphocytes	1281 women + heterosexual men, 2095 controls	Multivariate analysis found decreased risk in long-term marijuana users	Marijuana not identified as a positive risk factor for development of non-Hodgkin's lymphoma

The study by Holly *et al.* (1999) used data from two studies (1988 and 1995) to consider risk factors for NHL in women and heterosexual men. Interviews were conducted and blood samples were tested for viral infection and lymphocyte counts. There were 1281 patients and 2095 controls. Using multivariate analyses, the researchers found that there was a decreased risk for NHL in lifetime marijuana users. Besides marijuana use, other confounders were analyzed. For five confounders, there was a decreased risk of developing NHL, while a number of other confounders increased the risk of developing lymphoma. Marijuana was the only illicit drug considered in the analysis (Table 4.24).

Comments

Very few epidemiological studies have occurred in the last 20 years related to marijuana use and disorders of the immune, hematopoetic and lymphatic systems, despite strong research evidence that CB2 receptors are found predominantly on cells involved in immunity and inflammation. Galiegue *et al.* (1995) described the expression of cannabinoid receptors (CB2) in human immune tissues and leukocytes subtypes. At that time, it was thought that the cannabinoids mediated action of the immune system through these receptors. A recent publication by Ziring *et al.* (2006) suggested that the CB2 receptors are required for the development of both T and B lymphocytes. Though CB2 receptors may not be normally found on normal T cells, Rayman *et al.* (2007) found high CB2 expression on T cells in T-NHL.

Environmental disease

Trauma

Twenty epidemiological articles relating to marijuana and trauma were found in a PubMed search from 1988 and 2008. Four groups of articles were found: five related to injury risk and marijuana use, 12 related to substance abuse in trauma victims, one on crash culpability, and two miscellaneous articles, one on head injuries in substance abusers and a second on the effect of disasters on changes in substance abuse.

Injury risk and marijuana

One review by Macdonald *et al.* (2003) analyses articles describing the relationship between use of cannabis and cocaine and injury risk. They reviewed laboratory studies, epidemiological literature – both descriptive and analytical – and clinical and non-clinical cases of injured drug users. When drug tests, rather than self-report, were used to assess drug use, there were no significant differences in marijuana users involved in fatal and non-fatal situations, nor those involved in collisions, violent situations, or injuries in general. Cocaine users, by comparison, were involved in a greater number of intentional injuries and homicides (28.7%) and injuries while driving (4.5%). Marijuana and cocaine use were both related to more intentional injuries and injuries in general. Although the authors suggested that more studies are needed to consider alternative explanations for injuries, they also suggested that users in treatment are more at risk than other users of being injured.

Vinson (2006) carried out a case–control study with age- and sex-matched controls to determine the risk of injury in users of marijuana and other illicit drugs. He found that use of marijuana in the seven days prior to the injury decreased the risk of injury, while use of other illicit drugs increased the risk of injury.

In a case–control study by Blows et al. (2005), acute use of marijuana increased the risk of injury significantly (OR 3.9; 95% CI 1.2–12.9). This analysis controlled for a number of demographic variables (e.g., age and gender) and also for driving exposure and time of day. When additional confounders were considered (blood alcohol level, seatbelt use, speed, and sleepiness), the risk was insignificant (OR 0.8; 95% CI 0.2–3.3). However, the greatest risk for injury was in the habitual users, even when acute use before driving and all the other confounders were considered (OR 9.5; 95% CI 2.8–32.3). The authors suggested that further research is needed to assess risk-taking characteristics of users, especially habitual drug abusers.

An earlier study by Woolard et al. (2003) did address risk-taking behavior in marijuana-using problem drinkers. In a post-hoc analysis of prospective data, 433 sets of data were reviewed from a larger sample of 3776 injured patients visiting the emergency room. They found 48.3% of injured individuals had smoked marijuana at least three months prior to the injury. Many marijuana users were also problem drinkers with higher Alcohol Use Disorders Identification Test (AUDIT) scores than others (14.0 vs. 11.4; $p < 0.001$) and also used other drugs as well (69.7% vs. 30.3%; $p < 0.001$). With regression analyses comparing with non-use, marijuana use was an independent predictor of prior injury (OR 2.16; 95% CI 1.25–3.75). Marijuana use was also a predictor of alcohol-related injury (OR 2.26; 95% CI 1.45–3.53) and motor-vehicle-related injury (OR 1.69; 95% CI 1.03–2.79). A non-significant finding was the readiness to change score between users (4.14) and non-users (4.22). Their study suggested that injured problem drinkers are also likely to be marijuana users.

In a case–control study, Borges et al. (2005) interviewed 653 injured patients aged 18–65 years using the Whole Mental Health Version of the Composite International Diagnostic Interview. Controls were 1131 urban residents. A 12-month substance abuse dependence on alcohol was found in 12.3% of the patients compared with 1.8% in the control group. There was also a 2.5% dependence on marijuana and other illicit drugs, compared with 0.3% in the controls. The AOR for alcohol use and injury was 4.95 (95% CI 2.87–8.52), and an AOR for illicit drugs use and injury was insignificant, 2.58 (95% CI 0.73–9.17).

Substance abuse in trauma victims

Table 4.25 compares the drug findings in 12 articles found in a PubMed search for publications related to marijuana and traumatic injury. Most of the articles involved patients admitted to an emergency room or trauma unit. Although most of the articles support known evidence related to alcohol and injury, the focus of many of the studies was to determine the risk associated with marijuana use and traumatic injury. These articles are not included in Table 4.27, below, since the information is similar.

Soderstrom et al. (1988) reported on 1023 patients involved in vehicular (67.6%) and non-vehicular (32.4%) accidents. In this prospective study, most of the patients were male (72.8%), under 30 years of age, and had elevated THC levels (34.7%). One-third had

Table 4.25 Comparison of alcohol and illicit drug use in hospitalized trauma victims

Author, Study type	Country	Subjects	Focus	Raised blood alcohol (%)	Marijuana or THC (%)	Cocaine (%)	Drugs + alcohol (%)	Drugs ± alcohol (%)	1 drug (%)	2+ drugs (%)
Soderstrom et al. (1988), prospective	USA	1023	Trauma	33.5 (n = 1006)	34.7					
Rivara et al. (1989), descriptive	USA	452 ER, 160 autopsy	Trauma	33	Most common	8.0, 5.0			40.3, 18.7	
Soderstrom et al. (1995), descriptive	USA	225 Car, 106 MC	MV accident	35.2, 47.1	2.7, 32					
Levy et al. (1996), prospective	USA	628	Orth trauma	25	21	22		56		24
McDonald et al. (1999), descriptive	Jamaica	111	Trauma	32	46	6		62		20
Peden et al. (2000), prospective/ descriptive	SA (Cape Town)	254	Trauma	60	Most common				40	
Bowley et al. (2004), descriptive	SA (Johannesburg)	105	Trauma	59	43.7					

Study	Country	Sample size	Group						
Walsh *et al.* (2004b) descriptive	USA	322	MV	15.8	Most common	9.9	59.3	33.5	
Giovanardi *et al.* (2005), descriptive	Italy	115	MV drivers	10	19	6	40	66	25
Michael *et al.* (2005), descriptive	USA	168 MV (108 drivers)	MV accident	30.6	25	33	65.7	50.9	
Parry *et al.* (2005), descriptive	SA (3 sites)	1565	Trauma	Most common	Most common			33–62	
Reis *et al.* (2006), prospective	Brazil	353	Trauma	11	13.6 (of 242)	3.3 (of 242)			

ER, emergency room; MC, motorcycle; MV, motor vehicle; orth, orthopedic; SA, South Africa; THC, Δ^9-tetrahydrocannabinol.

Table 4.26 Drug use in automobile and motorcycle accidents

Vehicle	THC positive (%)*	Alcohol (%)*	Cocaine (%)	Phencyclidine (%)
Automobile	2.7 (6 of 225)	35.2	8.0	3.1
Motorcycle	32 (34 of 106)	47.1	5.0	1.5

THC, Δ^9-tetrahydrocannabinol.
* $p < 0.001$.
Source: Soderstrom *et al.* (1995).

elevated blood alcohol. There was no significant difference in marijuana use in the number of vehicular compared with non-vehicular accidents, but most vehicular crashes involved use of alcohol.

Rivara *et al.* (1989) used information from 452 trauma patients visiting the emergency room and 160 autopsies of fatally injured individuals to determine the level of alcohol and illicit substance use. Blood alcohol levels and urine samples measured marijuana, cocaine, opioid, and benzodiazepines. Marijuana was the most commonly found abused drug and mostly found in young males; alcohol was found in one-third of both emergency room patients and autopsies. Alcohol and illicit drug use was found more often in injuries caused by assaults or traffic accidents.

Soderstrom *et al.* (1995) compared marijuana use in two types of vehicular accidents. Blood samples were obtained from 225 automobile drivers and 106 motorcycle drivers. The study found that marijuana and alcohol were more likely to be found in accidents involving motorcycles than in other vehicular accidents. Table 4.26 summarizes their findings. The authors concluded that motorcyclists were more likely to be using marijuana and alcohol prior to their injury.

Levy *et al.* (1996) carried out a prospective study looking at the relationship between orthopedic trauma and alcohol and illicit drug use. The study was carried out in a two-year period. From a population of 766 patients, 628 (82%) had complete drugs screens used in the study: 56% tested positive for drug or alcohol use, 24% for two or more drugs, and 9% for three or more drugs. Alcohol (25%), cocaine (22%), and marijuana (21%) were the most commonly found illicit drugs. Most of the abused substances were found in males and patients aged 31–40 years. The abusers' hospitalizations were 1.3 days longer, they had more severe fractures (particularly open fractures or fractures of the tibia), and injuries were more likely to be related to gunshot incidents or altercations. Individuals involved in pedestrian/automobile accidents were also more likely to have detectable levels of alcohol and drugs.

In a 1999 study, McDonald *et al.* examined the urine and serum results of 111 trauma patients: 69 (62%) tested positive for at least one drug, and marijuana was the most commonly detected drug (46%). Marijuana was also the most common drug found in individuals involved in road accidents (50%) and violent injury (55%). The users were typically younger (30–40 years) than non-users. There was no significant difference in length of hospital stay or severity of injury in users and non-users.

Peden *et al.* (2000) studied 254 trauma patients using the CAGE questionnaire to assess alcohol chronicity, an alcolmeter to measure alcohol level, and urinalysis to assess marijuana, morphine, opiate, and methaqualone use. A Drugwipe was also used to test sweat for marijuana. Most of the subjects were male, black, with an average age of 31.3 years. While self-report of alcohol use correlated with laboratory-confirmed alcohol levels, drug self-report did not match with laboratory values. Forty percent of the patients tested positive for at least one drug, most commonly marijuana and methaqualone. However, alcohol was the most abused substance found in this study, with 152 (60%) of the patients testing positive with a breathalyzer test.

Bowley *et al.* (2004) looked at the prevalence of alcohol and drug use in a study of 105 trauma patients; 62 (59%) tested positive for alcohol and 46 (43.8%) tested positive for marijuana. Unlike findings in many of the other studies, more females than males were marijuana users ($p = 0.039$). Only three patients tested positive for methaqualone or amphetamines.

In another study, Walsh *et al.* (2004b) reported on 322 trauma patients involved in motor vehicle accidents. Blood and urine tests showed that 191 (59.3%) tested positive for alcohol or drugs. Marijuana and benzodiazepines were the two drugs most commonly found in these patients. The results of a point-of-collection test piloted in this study correlated with the results of laboratory tests.

Giovanardi *et al.* (2005) reported on the results of urine samples assessed for alcohol and drugs from 115 drivers involved in motor vehicle accidents. The majority of patients were male (85%) and aged 21–40 years. Marijuana was the drug most commonly found in the urine (19%), followed by alcohol (10%). Benzodiazepines (10%) were more commonly found in older patients (41–70 years).

Walsh and coworkers (Michael *et al.* 2005) carried out a study of drug use in trauma victims. Blood and urine samples were available for 168 victims of motor vehicle accidents. Of the 108 drivers involved in trauma, 71 (65.7%) tested positive for either drug or alcohol use. One in four used marijuana, and one in three users of drugs were also using alcohol. Compared with other motor vehicle accident victims, pedestrians involved in accidents had a higher incidence of alcohol use.

Parry *et al.* (2005) reported on three cross-sectional surveys of trauma victims carried out in three cities during 1999 to 2001. Over 50% were involved in violent injury. In the three surveys, 33–62% tested positive for at least one drug, with the majority testing positive for marijuana and/or methaqualone. More males than females were drug users. Of the three years of the study, 2001 was the year reporting the largest drug use.

Reis *et al.* (2006) carried out a prospective cross-sectional study of non-fatal injuries and substance abuse in 353 patients admitted to an emergency room within six hours of injury. The researchers used a standardized WHO questionnaire, a drug consumption questionnaire, a drug abuse screening test, and urine and blood alcohol tests. The blood alcohol level was positive in 11% of the patients. Marijuana use was found in 13.6%. Other drugs found were cocaine (3.3%) and benzodiazepines (4.2%). Rates of drug abuse were similar in the victims.

Problem drinkers and marijuana

Woolard *et al.* (2003) carried out a post-hoc analysis on data obtained prospectively from injured problem drinkers. Complete data were available on 433 injured problem drinkers, including blood alcohol levels and either a self-report of drinking or AUDIT score. Marijuana use during the three months prior to the injury was reported by 209 (48.3%) of the drinkers. The study found that, compared with other drinkers, marijuana-using problem drinkers were often hazardous drinkers and had higher AUDIT scores (14.0 vs. 11.4; $p < 0.001$), higher risk-taking scores (12.4% vs. 10.1%; $p < 0.001$), and used other drugs as well (69.7% vs. 30.3%; $p < 0.001$). Using regression analyses, marijuana use was an independent predictor of each of the following: prior injury (OR 2.16; 95% CI 1.25–3.75), alcohol-related injury (OR 2.26; 95% CI 1.45–3.53), and motor-vehicle-related injury (OR 1.69; 95% CI 1.03–2.79). A Readiness to Change test was also administered, and both users and non-users had similar scores that were non-significant.

Other studies

Walker *et al.* (2003) studied 661 drug-abusing inmates with self-reported histories of traumatic brain injuries. They found that inmates with head injuries had significantly more health problems, higher alcohol and marijuana use, and more mental health problems than those inmates not reporting head injury. The authors suggested that treatment of substance abuse may need to be modified to take the effects of head injury into consideration.

Vlahov *et al.* (2004) used two random digit-dial surveys one and six months after the September 11, 2001 disaster in the USA to explore how disasters affect substance abuse. An increase in use of cigarettes, alcohol, and marijuana were reported one month after September 11, 2001 (30.8%) and six months later (27.3%). The authors suggested that disasters can have long-term health effects on individuals.

The summary of these trauma studies is found in Table 4.25 and Table 4.27.

Comments

The 20 studies reviewed for this trauma subsection included a variety of articles on the relationship or consequences of marijuana use and injury, and also an article on the impact of a disaster on increasing substance abuse. These studies add to the available literature on marijuana use and risk for injury. However, because of the variety of studies, it may be difficult to generalize many of the findings.

The 12 studies on substance abuse in hospitalized trauma patients offer different conclusions based on their subjects and results. Some of the trauma studies used patients involved in motor vehicle accidents, and some of these were automobile, motorcycle, or pedestrian–automobile accidents. Some of the injured patients were involved in violent crimes, intentional injuries, motor vehicle accidents, or some combination of all types of injury. Some studies assessed substance abuse at the point of entry into the healthcare system; others considered risk of injury with long-term use or acute intoxication. Some studies used self-report as a means of judging substance use; others relied on various breath or fluid samples (blood, sweat, and urine) to validate use. These 12 studies were carried out in five different countries (Brazil, Italy, Jamaica, South Africa, and the USA). The number of subjects in the 12 studies varied from 105 to 1565. Alcohol was the most common abused substance in six studies, while marijuana was the most commonly abused drug in seven studies. Polydrug use was fairly common, with three studies reporting use of two or more drugs, and several studies indicating a common finding of both drug and alcohol use. Demographic information suggested that individuals involved in injury are likely to be young males, typically 40 years old or younger and predominantly under 30. Only one study found a greater proportion of female marijuana users than male users. Geographical and cultural differences may have a role in the results of some of the studies.

In those studies reporting risk of injury, at least one study suggested that confounders such as alcohol use, lack of seatbelt use, vehicle speed, and level of sleepiness affected the risk of injury more than marijuana use alone. Some studies suggested that problem alcohol drinkers using marijuana and habitual marijuana users increased their risk of injury significantly. Only one study found that marijuana use in the week prior to injury was actually associated with a decrease in injury risk compared with controls.

Table 4.27 Trauma

Study	Method	Sample	Incidence	Results
Macdonald et al. (2003)	Literature review Risk of injury Laboratory studies, descriptive and analytical epidemiological studies	Intentional injuries, injuries in general		Marijuana users: similar proportions found in fatal, non-fatal injuries, collisions, violent injury, injury in general Cocaine users had large difference in injuries: 28.7% intentional/homicides; 4.5% injured drivers Marijuana and cocaine users associated with intentional injury and injury in general Higher risk for all types of injury in users in treatment More rigorous studies needed; focus on alternative explanations for injury
Blows et al. (2005)	Population-based case–control study Risk injury Self-report about marijuana use 3 h before crash	571 car crash victims, 588 controls from random sample of cars on the road	Acute marijuana use risk for crash, OR 3.9 (95% CI 1.2–12.9), controlled for age, gender, ethnicity, education, passengers, driving exposure, time of day; acute marijuana use risk for crash with additional confounders (blood alcohol content, speed, seat-belt use, sleepiness), OR 0.8 (95% CI 0.2–3.3; n.s.); habitual use of marijuana, adjusted with all confounders and acute use, OR 9.5 (95% CI 2.8–32.3)	Habitual use of marijuana strongly associated with crashes; more studies needed to look at association with risk taking
Borges et al. (2005)	Case–control study Substance abuse with injury World Mental Health interview	653 injured patients aged 18–65 years, 1131 controls	Alcohol use and injury, AOR 4.95 (95% CI 2.87–8.52); drug use and injury, AOR 2.58 (95% CI 0.73–9.17); comorbid alcohol and drugs also found	Substance abuse, dependence for 12 months: alcohol 12.3%, control 1.8%; marijuana and other drugs 2.5%, control 0.3%
Vinson (2006)	Case–control study Risk injury with illicit drug use Phone interview	ER trauma patients, age-, sex-matched controls		Marijuana use 7 days prior to injury associated with decreased injury risk; use of other drugs increased risk

Table 4.27 Cont.

Study	Method	Sample	Incidence	Results
Vlahov et al. (2004)	2 random digit-dial surveys 1 and 6 months after September 11 2001(9/11)		1 month after 9/11, 30.8% increased use of alcohol, marijuana, cigarettes; 6 months after 9/11, 27.3% increased use of alcohol, marijuana, cigarettes	Suggested there may be increased long-term health problems associated with disasters
Walker et al. (2003)	Case–control study Self-report	661 drug-abusing inmates with self-reported head injury: 1 head injury, ≥ 2 head injuries, no history of head injuries	Those with head injuries: increased mental health and general health problems; more alcohol and drug use	Inmates with head injuries experienced more health problems than those without head injuries; head injury could affect treatment plan
Woolard et al. (2003)	Regression analysis of post-hoc analysis of data Problem drinking Blood tests, interview scores	433 injured patients with data for blood alcohol level: report of drinking or AUDIT score, report of use of marijuana 3 months prior to injury	Marijuana-using problem drinkers compared with non-using problem drinkers: more hazardous drinkers; higher AUDIT scores; higher risk-taking scores (12.4 vs. 10.1; $p < 0.001$); more use of other drugs (69.7% vs. 30.3%; $p < 0.001$) Marijuana predictor of prior injury (OR 2.16; 95% CI 1.25–3.75); prior alcohol-related injury (OR 2.26; 95% CI 1.45–3.53); motor vehicle-related injury (OR 1.69; 95% CI 1.03–2.79) Similar readiness to change scores in users, non-users	Marijuana-using problem drinkers, more hazardous drinkers; marijuana use in injured problem drinkers is prevalent

AOR, adjusted odds ratio; AUDIT, Alcohol Use Disorders Identification Test; CI, confidence interval; ER, emergency room; n.s., not significant; OR, odds ratio.

Two studies reported on the consequences of injury: one, a study of head-injured inmates, the second a phone survey of individuals after September 11, 2001. In both studies, long-term health consequences were found, including increased substance abuse in the subjects studied.

Several studies pointed out the need for further study on risky behavior in the substance-abusing population and the consequences of substance abuse on personal and public health resources. Others noted that, in some cases, trauma victims are not screened for abused drugs and that health providers have an opportunity to counsel and educate substance abusers on the consequences of their risky behavior.

Other pathological conditions

No relevant material was found regarding marijuana use and pathological conditions not discussed earlier in the chapter

Marijuana: summary and overview

Much of the research cited in this chapter provides insight into marijuana use and the risk for various health problems from publications cited in PubMed from 1988 to 2008. Prior to 1988, the epidemiological research on marijuana and disease conditions described acute toxic effects and cognitive and psychomotor impairment. Studies also suggested that marijuana had a role in suppressing immune function and was a risk factor for respiratory disease and lung cancer. For this review, the earlier studies were not critiqued and the basis (laboratory and clinical research) of marijuana's relationship to medical disease was not explored. As use of the drug escalated during the past two decades, more studies describe these conditions and others where marijuana use may influence development of acute and chronic disease. As ongoing laboratory studies help to clarify the cell and molecular role of ECs and phytocannabinoids, epidemiological studies are beginning to identify the risk to marijuana users in developing various pathological conditions.

In some cases, the research findings described in this chapter are equivocal and do not clearly indicate that marijuana use is a disease risk factor. In other cases, the research suggests that marijuana use may be associated with certain conditions, but the cause and effect relationship is unclear. A great deal of research, particularly epidemiological research, still needs to be done. As laboratory research begins to clarify the effect of marijuana at the cellular level, epidemiological research is needed to determine clinical findings and to provide a research basis for evidence-based medicine.

The text that follows is a brief summary of the evidence supporting an association between marijuana and a specific topic. A more detailed critique of the research is found in the individual summaries in the preceding subsections. Table 4.28 at the end of this summary illustrates the topics covered in this chapter and the level of evidence based on the studies found in the epidemiological research published and cited in PubMed from 1988 to 2008.

Infections

Bacterial infections

Overall association: supported by some evidence

Only one large cross-sectional study on STDs and marijuana use was reviewed, along with four case studies and two literature reviews. Although there was an increased association between marijuana and gonorrheal and chlamydial infections, risky behavior of the marijuana user appears to be the major factor influencing acquiring an STD. Likewise, TB and meningitis were related more to close contact and risky behavior than use of marijuana. However, the two reviews address the effect marijuana has on inflammation and the immune system, including dysfunction of the T helper cells and B lymphocytes, as well as the natural killer cells and macrophages. The effect of marijuana on these cells may make marijuana users more susceptible to various infections.

Mycoses

Overall association: not supported by evidence

Only one case–control study was reviewed. The study found no difference in the incidence of oral *Candida* in a group of polydrug users and non-users.

Viral (non-HIV) infections: liver damage and hepatitis C virus

Overall association: supported by strong evidence

One case–control and one prospective study were found in the literature. Both fairly large studies involved subjects with chronic HCV infections. In both studies, marijuana use was a predictor of steatosis or fibrosis. Daily use of the drug was more likely to cause liver disease than occasional use. Since the liver has CB1 receptors, marijuana can interact with these receptors and stimulate cellular changes. Because alcohol also can affect the hepatocytes, individuals using marijuana should refrain from use of alcohol to prevent cumulative effects from both abused substances.

Neoplastic disease

Respiratory cancer

Overall association: supported by some evidence

A number of studies addressed marijuana use and oral and lung cancer; however, the evidence is equivocal. Some studies found an increased risk with frequency and length of marijuana use; other studies found no statistically significant association between marijuana and oral–respiratory cancer. The findings of some studies that identified a link between the drug and respiratory cancer were limited because many of the marijuana users were also cigarette smokers. Since it is known that tobacco use can lead to lung cancer, evidence of cancer in these dual smokers could be attributed to cigarette use. A recent (Hashibe et al. 2006) case–control study of 1212 marijuana users found a positive correlation between long-term (over 30 years) marijuana use and respiratory cancer, but the results were not significant for the subjects who were also tobacco smokers. That study found no increase in oral, laryngeal, lung, pharyngeal, or esophageal cancer in marijuana users compared with non-users.

Urinary bladder cancer

Overall association: supported by some evidence

Many of the marijuana users and controls in the single case–control study reviewed had bladder cancer. In this convenience sample of individuals with bladder cancer, it was unclear whether the subjects were also tobacco users. Since tobacco use is associated with the development of TCBC, the marijuana users who used tobacco could have developed the disease through their tobacco use. Self-report was also used to determine marijuana use, so there is the question whether the subjects were truthful in acknowledging or denying the use of the drug.

Musculoskeletal system disease

Propriospinal myoclonus

Overall association: not supported by evidence

In a propriospinal myoclonus study, a case report described one marijuana user who developed myoclonus. No other case reports or epidemiological studies were found in the literature reviewed linking marijuana and propriospinal myoclonus.

Spasticity

Overall association: supported by some evidence

Two studies were found linking marijuana to spinal cord dysfunction. One group of patients with spinal cord injuries self-reported that marijuana helped to decrease their spasticity. These subjects also indicated use of marijuana prior to their injury. The second study compared marijuana and alcohol users with spinal cord injuries. The researchers found marijuana users tended to be younger at the time of their injury, more depressed, and more stressed than the alcohol users.

Stomatognathic disease

Overall association: supported by some evidence

Two reviews and three case–control and prospective cohort studies were reviewed. In two case–control studies, an increase in *Candida*, ulcers, leukoedema, and xerostomia were found in marijuana users; however, these subjects were also tobacco and methaqualone users. A similar number of infections were found in the marijuana users, tobacco users, and non-users.

Although a prospective cohort longitudinal study with 903 subjects found a higher level of dental incident attachment loss and did control for tobacco use, additional studies are needed to show an increased risk of periodontal disease in marijuana users.

Respiratory system disease

Change in pulmonary function tests

Overall association: supported by some evidence

A number of studies were reported that researched changes in pulmonary function tests in marijuana users. Two studies were reviews; two were cohort studies. Some of the findings in the reviews include the following: one would need to smoke four to five joints a day for 30 years before seeing changes typical of chronic obstructive disease, and although bronchodilation (and an increase in FEV_1) occurred in short-term users, there were no significant changes in long-term use of marijuana. The two cohort studies found no significant negative effect when age, weight, and tobacco use were controlled for in the analyses, and changes seen in marijuana users were similar to those seen in tobacco smokers.

Pulmonary inflammation, chronic respiratory signs and symptoms

Overall association: supported by some evidence

Although lung function did not appear to decline over time in marijuana users, a number of studies did find that more airway inflammation appeared in both marijuana users and tobacco users compared with non-smokers. Marijuana users had increased signs and symptoms of chronic bronchitis and an increase in cough and sputum production, but these changes were similar to tobacco users. Many of the studies did not control for tobacco use, which limits the findings in these studies. The studies also used different criteria for "long-term" and "short-term" use of marijuana, and also used different criteria for smoking habits (joints/day or cigarettes/day; one to five a day; 900/year). This makes comparison of findings difficult. More studies, including large prospective studies, are needed to determine the risk associated with marijuana use and chronic respiratory signs and symptoms. Exposure to occupational and environmental substances that might affect respiratory function also needs to be considered.

Marijuana allergen

Overall association: supported by some evidence

One study used a cannabis skin test to determine whether marijuana allergy could be a possible cause of asthma or allergic rhinitis. Although about half of the 127 subjects tested positive on the cannabis skin test, the researchers suggested that the risk of marijuana allergen might be limited to a specific group of susceptible individuals.

Nervous system disease

Neurodevelopment

Overall association: supported by some evidence

One review and four small case–control studies examined the effect of marijuana on neurodevelopment. The review presented animal research findings that motor control, neuroendocrine function, and nociception may be affected by marijuana. However, the author suggested that human studies also need to consider the influence of genetics and environment on these findings. The four case–control studies looked at brain volume changes in marijuana users. Some of the users were also alcohol abusers; others were "frequent" or "heavy" marijuana users. Collectively, they found either no significant change in brain volume or evidence of atrophy, some increase and decrease of gray and white matter in some areas of the brain, and more changes in long-term, heavy users.

Because these studies were small and had conflicting findings, plus there was a lack of standardization of the subjects or confounders, more studies are needed to determine the risk of marijuana damage to the brain.

Neuropsychological changes

Overall association: supported by some evidence

Two reviews, one meta-analysis, and two case–control studies found that marijuana use did not cause significant, long-term effects on cognitive or psychomotor function. Where subtle changes did occur, the researchers suggested that the changes were likely reversible. One meta-analytical study reviewed 1014 studies but could only use 11 in their analysis. The findings suggested that there was an association between marijuana use and learning and forgetting. Functional MRI was used in the case–control studies; both were small studies with equivocal findings. More studies are needed to determine the effect of marijuana on cerebral function.

Central nervous system dysfunction

Overall association: supported by some evidence

The studies reviewed did not show statistically significant evidence that marijuana use is a risk for CNS dysfunction. Several small case reports provided some incidences of ischemic stroke, cerebellar infarcts, and temporary loss of CNS function. One vascular study suggested that there was more resistance in the anterior and middle cerebral arteries of abstaining marijuana users. No studies showing changes in blood flow in individuals currently using marijuana were found. It is possible that the abstaining marijuana users had pre-existing changes in cerebral vessel flow and that the changes were not related to marijuana use.

The authors of the review exploring the safety of the use of marijuana and alcohol by patients prescribed antiepileptic drugs suggested that alcohol withdrawal might lower the seizure threshold, but that marijuana may have an antiepileptic effect. However, there are few studies on the effect of marijuana on seizure activity. They suggested poor short-term memory can interfere with antiseizure drug compliance in seizure-prone marijuana users.

One study did find a strong correlation between marijuana use and the development of tardive dyskinesia in schizophrenic patients receiving neuroleptic drugs. Two other studies described a case of transient amnesia and one of ataxia and seizures developing in marijuana users. Too few studies are available to make judgements about the risk for these conditions.

Chronobiology and sleep disorders

Overall association: supported by some evidence

One study found a difference between hashish users and controls when studying cognitive styles and cerebral hemisphere communication. Another case–control study suggested that sleep disturbances are more common in heavy marijuana users. However, the results were based on polysomnography results with just two days of drug abstinence. Too few studies are available to suggest that marijuana use has an effect on sleep or biological rhythms.

Ocular disease

Overall association: supported by some evidence

Only two case reports suggested marijuana users may have recurring visual distortions, including shimmering, streaking, altered movements; visual spots; or altered depth perception. Too few studies were found to suggest any direct effect or risk of marijuana use on visual changes.

Male urological disease

Male infertility

Overall association: not supported by evidence

Although a literature review suggested that marijuana may be a risk factor for male infertility, a study of pyospermia in infertile males found no significant association between marijuana use and increased leukocytes in seminal fluid. Many of the subjects in this study were also alcohol and/or tobacco users. However, a large survey found inhibited orgasm and painful sex in self-reporting males who were both alcohol and marijuana users.

Bladder and renal disease

Overall association: supported by some evidence

A seven-year follow-up of over 600 patients with hypertension found that illicit drug users were at risk for declining renal function. However, the marijuana users were not shown to have a statistically significant individual risk for renal disease based on blood creatinine analyses.

Although a large case–control study of males with TCBC who used marijuana suggested that they appeared to be at greater risk of developing the cancer, the study also found a number of individuals who did not use marijuana who were equally at risk. The role of tobacco use, a known TCBC risk factor, or other environmental carcinogens could also significantly increase risk.

Female genital and neonatal/congenital disease

Female genital infections

Overall association: supported by some evidence

The marijuana user appears to be more at risk for vaginal infections than non-users. Two fairly large studies found an increased risk of vaginal yeast and trichomonal infections in marijuana users. Given that CB2 receptors are found on leukocytes and immune cells, and activation can lead to disruption of cell function, it is reasonable that women exposed to bacteria, fungi, or protozoa may be more likely to develop infections. However, risky sexual activity can also influence the development of infections, including unprotected sex and promiscuity.

Female infertility

Overall association: supported by some evidence

One case–control study provided some support for ovarian dysfunction in marijuana users. The study showed that there was an increased risk of interference with ovulation with marijuana use, congruent with animal studies showing that marijuana can transiently disrupt ovarian function. The second study found that marijuana users with a low or high BMI were less at risk for functional ovarian cysts. This could be related to the appetite-stimulating effect of marijuana or lack of a healthy diet in drug users. Tobacco use was also associated with ovarian cysts and a decreased BMI.

Pregnancy complications

Overall association: supported by some evidence

Since many pregnant women who use marijuana are also alcohol, tobacco, and polydrug users, it is difficult to determine risk of pregnancy complications in marijuana users. Also, many studies of pregnancy complications used self-report of marijuana use. Self-report of marijuana use is often under-reporting, as found by several studies reviewed for this chapter. Urine or blood tests for illicit drug use are not always carried out by healthcare professionals.

Nevertheless, some information about pregnancy complications can be derived from the research reviewed. Some studies found an increased risk of placenta abruptio in marijuana users. Other studies found no relationship between marijuana use and prematurity. Risk for placenta abruptio was also found in those with hypertension, an older age during pregnancy, and low maternal BMI. Non-compliance with prenatal care was a risk in many pregnancy complications, including placenta abruptio and preterm membrane rupture. Spontaneous abortion was more likely to occur in women carrying loads of > 9 kg, drinking coffee, or reaching over their shoulders than with marijuana use. Marijuana use was also associated with domestic violence, which could affect pregnancy outcomes.

Neonatal outcomes

Overall association: supported by some evidence

There is some evidence in some of the studies reviewed that there is a risk of LBW and shorter body length in newborns of women who used marijuana during their pregnancy. It is unclear, though, whether this risk reflects only marijuana use, or whether other factors influence neonatal outcomes, including polydrug, alcohol, and tobacco use by the mothers; non-compliance with or lack of prenatal care; or the young age of the mothers.

Long-term negative outcomes in neonates

Overall association: not supported by evidence

Some longitudinal studies reported on negative outcomes from prenatal exposure to marijuana in children that could be identified at six years of age. One study reported that these children at six years were more likely to be of short stature, while another study found no growth and development changes in other six year olds. A limitation of longitudinal studies is that it is difficult to control for the environment during the child's development. If the household is socially and economically disadvantaged, what effect does lack of adequate nutrition or life in a chaotic, unstable home have on a child's growth and development? If the adults in the household are continuing to use marijuana, what effect does exposure to marijuana smoke from infancy to age six have on growth and development? More studies are needed to clarify some of these concerns.

Chromosomal and congenital disease

Overall association: supported by some evidence

One study reviewed assessed infants' karyotypes. In the large study, the risk of spontaneous abortion and abnormal chromosomes was studied in marijuana users. The study found that

237

there was not a significant link between risk of normal or abnormal chromosomes in spontaneously aborted fetuses and marijuana use.

The prevalence of cardiac malformations was assessed in three research studies. In a case–control study, simple ventricular septal defects were twice as common in children of marijuana-using pregnant women than in controls. Regular marijuana use (three or more/ week) was associated with an increased risk. Another study reviewed eight types of cardiac malformations in a large database. Only transposition of the great arteries with an intact ventricular septum was associated with marijuana use. Use of marijuana by the paternal partner carried an increased risk. Interestingly, paternal use of alcohol and marijuana also was associated with all cases of single ventricle ($n = 55$) in another study. How paternal marijuana use increases risk of two different types of cardiac anomaly is an area for further study.

A study of birth defects found that infants of marijuana-using mothers were more likely to have gastrointestinal defects than infants of other mothers. Gastroschisis was found to be increased in two other studies, but these studies also acknowledged that polydrug use was more of a risk than use of marijuana alone. One group of researchers suggested that young, socially disadvantaged women were more at risk of having a child with gastroschisis than non-users. Another group found while gastroschisis incidence increased, the use of marijuana did not increase, suggesting that other factors are involved in the development of this gastrointestinal disorder.

Cardiovascular disease

Acute cardiovascular effects

Overall association: supported by strong evidence

A review of the literature described the acute effects of marijuana on the cardiovascular system. They include a mild increase in blood pressure and decreased vascular resistance, with the potential for developing orthostatic hypotension. The cannabinoids also appear to decrease exercise tolerance. Another review on acute marijuana effects indicated that cardiac arrhythmia was a sequela of marijuana use. A prospective study involving over 6700 subjects confirmed that palpitations were a likely consequence of marijuana use. These cardiovascular signs and symptoms are often minimized after use of marijuana for a few days or weeks. These studies support findings in earlier studies reporting marijuana's cardiovascular effects.

More studies could be done to determine the vascular effects of marijuana. Some studies in this chapter have suggested that marijuana, and particularly THC, is a vasoconstrictor and can increase peripheral resistance, leading to elevated blood pressure. However, other studies have found that marijuana use can cause decreased peripheral resistance and orthostatic hypotension, especially in acute marijuana use. Studies are needed to determine the relation of hypotension and marijuana use in acute and long-term users.

Cannabis arteritis

Overall association: supported by strong evidence

Several studies addressed the development of arteritis in marijuana users. Over 60 cases of cannabis arteritis have been described since the 1960s. A review of the literature described most of these cases and suggested that cannabis arteritis is similar to the thromboangiitis obliterans seen in cigarette smokers. They suggested that cannabis arteritis may be underdiagnosed in juveniles with peripheral obstructive disease.

The signs of cannabis arteritis may vary, but can include distal ischemia in the fingers and toes. According to one study, the median age of 10 arteritis victims was 23.7 years. In this study, amputation was necessary in four patients. Since both Δ^8- and Δ^9-THC can cause vasoconstriction, the authors suggested that young marijuana users may be at risk for cannabis arteritis. Another study found that aspirin therapy was able to reverse the tissue damage and lead to revascularization. Some, but not all, studies found atherosclerotic lesions in vessels of those with cannabis arteritis. Further case–control or prospective studies may be able to provide more evidence for the development of this condition in marijuana users.

Cardiovascular risk

Overall association: supported by some evidence

A variety of studies have been conducted to determine the risk for cardiovascular disease in marijuana users. The CARDIA study is a 15-year longitudinal study designed to explore cardiac risk factors and the use of marijuana. Approximately one-third of the over 3600 patients had used marijuana, but they also used tobacco, alcohol, and other illicit drugs. The marijuana users were more likely to have a higher systolic blood pressure and a lower triglyceride level than non-marijuana users. They also had a higher caloric intake and drank more alcohol. Multivariate analysis found that marijuana was not independently associated with several of these findings, but it was associated with eating a high calorie diet, smoking tobacco, and using other illicit drugs.

Since marijuana does increase appetite, some smokers may have diets that are high in calories and high in lipids. More studies are needed to explore the risks for marijuana users in developing obesity, hypertension, hyperlipidemia, and insulin resistance – all conditions that increase the likelihood of developing cardiovascular disease.

The epidemiological literature was very limited for AMI as only two studies were reviewed that addressed AMI in marijuana users. The paucity of AMI–marijuana studies suggests that AMI in these smokers is a rare event. Recent laboratory studies indicate that an endogenous cannabinoid cardiac system includes CB1 and CB2 receptors in cardiac tissue. Ongoing animal studies are exploring the potential cardioprotective effect of CB2 receptors in decreasing infarct size after ischemia.

One case study described a 21 year old who developed an AMI after smoking marijuana. With no evidence of risk factors for CAD, marijuana use was suspected as the cause. In a case-crossover study, participants in DMIOS were interviewed within four days of experiencing an AMI. Fewer than 4% of the participants had used marijuana in the year previous to their infarct. The study found that the risk for an AMI decreased rapidly one hour after smoking the drug. Most of the marijuana users were obese and cigarette smokers at the time of the infarct. Only 7% of the marijuana users smoked a joint within one hour of experiencing an infarct.

Although an inception cohort study found that smoking marijuana is hazardous and can result in a fatal outcome, other studies and literature reviews showed that the risk of an AMI is low but may occur in susceptible populations. More studies, especially long-term studies, are needed to determine the risk of AMI in marijuana users who have or do not have cardiovascular risk factors.

Nutritional and metabolic disease

Overall association: supported by some evidence

Only two reviews of the literature were found related to the appetite stimulant effect of marijuana. One review suggested that weight gain and weight loss are possibilities during active marijuana use and periods of drug withdrawal, respectively. The other review focused on the CB1 and CB2 receptors and their role in nutritional and energy balance. In the CNS, these receptors have a role in appetite and regulation of energy intake. Peripheral CB receptors in hepatocytes, adipocytes, and pancreatic cells interact and may be regulated by metabolic hormones and peptides. Stimulation of these CB receptors may lead to obesity, dyslipidemia, and hyperglycemia. These outcomes can contribute to the increased risk of cardiovascular disease, including atherogenesis and metabolic syndrome.

Use of a CB1 receptor antagonist in recent clinical trials may provide some information about the role of these receptors in morbidity and mortality associated with cardiovascular disease. There appears to be ample opportunity for clinical research in this area.

Endocrine disease

One study related to the use of marijuana by women with ovarian dysfunction was discussed above under Female infertility. A small case report of males with gynecomastia suggested that breast enlargement may be related to administration of antiviral drugs, lymphoma, and long-term marijuana use. No other epidemiological studies were found related to the endocrine system and marijuana use. Since CB receptors are found on the pancreas, studies of the prevalence of diabetes mellitus in marijuana users may help to determine the risk of developing metabolic syndrome, diabetes mellitus, and both renal and cardiovascular disease.

Immune system disease

Overall association: not supported by evidence

Only one epidemiological study was found in the literature review. A large case–control study found a decreased risk for NHL in lifelong marijuana users. Studies are needed related to marijuana use and hematopoietic and immune dysfunction. Since CB2 receptors are found on natural killer cells, macrophages, and the lymphocytes, studies are needed to determine whether marijuana users are more at risk for disorders related to inflammation and immune responses. There appears to be opportunities to link bench science with clinical studies that may be helpful in practicing evidenced-based medicine.

Environment disease

Trauma risk

Overall association: supported by strong evidence

Many studies have been published since 1988 that describe the increased risk of injury in marijuana users. The increased risk appears to be associated with marijuana use, but also with concurrent use of alcohol and other illicit drugs. Marijuana users were involved in motor vehicle accidents, including automobile, motorcycle, and pedestrian incidents. They were also involved with violent crimes and intentional injuries. Marijuana use was the primary drug of abuse in 7 of 12 studies reviewed, with alcohol the next most abused drug. Individuals involved in trauma of any type typically were young males, predominantly under the age of 30, polydrug users, and alcohol users.

In addition to the cognitive or psychomotor effects of illicit drug use, marijuana users also demonstrated the risky behavior that can result in trauma. Lack of wearing a seatbelt in a vehicle, misjudging vehicle speed, and an altered level of attention may also be consequences of marijuana use at the time of trauma.

Research concerns

There appear to be many research opportunities for those interested in marijuana use and its risk for various illnesses. Some of the research reviewed could be improved by enhancing the methodology. Many of the studies described single cases or small numbers of cases of marijuana use and untoward outcomes. Many studies lacked controls. Self-report of drug use, which can have recall bias and may not be accurate, was often used. Verification of drug use by drug screening tests would help support the individual's report of marijuana use.

Many of the studies involved individuals who used marijuana; however, there were variations among the studies on the length of use (months/years) and amount of use (daily/weekly/monthly). Sometimes the subjects were abstaining, but the length of abstinence varied from 24 hours to several weeks. Polydrug, tobacco, and alcohol use was very common. This substance abuse could have an effect on risk analysis, particularly if other drug use was not identified as a confounder. For example, if subjects were tobacco and marijuana users, the risk of marijuana use and bladder cancer could be blurred if adjustments were not made in the statistical analysis for tobacco use.

A meta-analysis of research findings is difficult, as one group of researchers found, because of the lack of standardization of terms and inclusion criteria. "Recreational use," "short-term user," and "long-term user" were not always defined in the same way in many of the studies. As a result, comparing outcomes becomes problematic.

Many of the studies, particularly those with small sample sizes or methodology flaws, need to be replicated. This would enhance the value of the research and allow for better generalizability and the opportunity to use the research to make clinical decisions.

There are some areas where there is a dearth of research, including studies of the hematopoietic and immune systems, neoplastic disease, and endocrine dysfunction. Many other subsections in this chapter had only a few studies on various topics. With so few studies, it is not possible to make generalizations about the risk of disease and marijuana use.

Table 4.28 summarizes the association of marijuana with research covering various body systems described in this chapter. The "Topic" column indicates the condition described, followed by the rating for the evidence of association in parentheses. The term "strong" suggests there is a significant body of knowledge supporting a direct or indirect association between marijuana and the condition (e.g., a significant number of studies, cohort or case–controlled studies, clinical laboratory studies, or a single seminal

Table 4.28 Marijuana summarye

Body system	Topic and evidence of association
Infections	Bacterial (some), viral (liver damage and hepatitis C virus) (strong)
Neoplastic	Respiratory cancer (some), transitional cell bladder cancer (some)
Musculoskeletal	Spasticity (some)
Digestive	None
Stomatognathic	Oral health (some)
Respiratory	Chronic inflammatory change (some), allergen (some)
Otorhinolaryngological	None
Nervous	Atrophy, decreased brain volume (some); cognitive, psychomotor function (some); cerebral ischemia (some); safety: drug use, and antiepileptic drugs (some); tardive dyskinesia (some); sleep disturbances (some)
Ocular	Visual changes (some)
Urological	Transitional cell bladder cancer (some)
Female reproductive and congenital/neonatal	Female genital infections (some); female infertility and ovarian dysfunction (some); placenta abruptio (some); altered newborn growth and development (some); infant cardiac abnormalities (some); infant gastrointestinal abnormalities (some)
Cardiovascular	Acute cardiovascular effects (strong); cannabis arteritis (strong); cardiovascular risk (some)
Dermatological	None
Nutritional and metabolic	Effect on food intake, metabolic syndrome (some)
Endocrine	None
Immune system	None
Environment	Trauma (strong)
Other pathologies	None

study). "Strong" suggests the clinician may find this condition in a marijuana user. "Some" suggests that there are some studies supporting a direct or indirect association between marijuana and the condition (e. g., a smaller number of studies, case–control or case reports, or a study reporting a rare or under-reported condition). In many cases, "some" suggests more evidence is needed to support a strong association with a condition.

Results: opioids

Introduction

Opioids have a long history of medicinal use. References to opium among the writings of the Ancient Greek and Arab civilizations have shown that it was used in various preparations and for many conditions. Opium and its preparations currently are used primarily for the management of pain. In the modern era, the addictive effects of opioids have been studied and are well known to many clinicians, and the acute signs and symptoms of opioid intoxication also are well described in many sources, textbooks, and review articles. Prolific biomedical research over the past 20 years has elucidated the invisible – the structural and functional physiology of opioids and their signaling mechanisms. However, there is not nearly as much known about how opioids affect various body systems. Opioids are prescribed and administered daily in both inpatient and outpatient settings and patients who have had opioid dependence and abuse disorders frequently are found in these settings, so it is important for clinicians to understand these effects. The focus of this chapter is to explore the epidemiological research on opioid use and diseases of the body systems.

Abstracts concerning epidemiological research on opioid use and human disease were selected from the PubMed database. Over 50 abstracts published from 1988 to 2008 were reviewed. These were divided into subchapters based upon MeSH categories. The "best fit" was chosen for discussion when an abstract might have been categorized into several subchapters. A summary of the opioid research is presented at the end of the discussion. All research articles are listed in the References.

Background

The term opioid refers to substances related to opium and includes two major groups: natural substances and fully synthetic substances. This is in contrast to the term opiates, which refers only to the former, that is, drugs naturally or semi-synthetically derived from opium. Opium itself is the powdered juice of the unripe seed capsules of the opium poppy plant, *Papaver somniferum,* and is a collection of more than 20 peptide alkaloids, divided into two classes: phenathrenes, examples of which are morphine, codeine and thebain; and benzylisoquinolines, such as papaverine (a smooth muscle relaxant). These are the medically important naturally derived opioids and they act mainly upon the opioid mu receptor. It is important to note, for clarity, that the term "narcotic" is both medically (substances which induce sleep) and legally (substances which have addictive potential) defined and the term does not refer specifically to opioids.

The semi-synthetic opioids are produced through modification of the naturally derived opioids. Examples include oxycodone and naloxone, modified from thebain, and heroin, formed from the addition of acetyl groups to morphine. The semi-synthetic opioids, like the naturally derived opioids, act through the mu receptor, but they have different pharmacological properties. The fully synthetic opioids, structurally or functionally analogous to opiates, were developed, mostly unsuccessfully, to be effective analgesics with limited addictive potential and few other side effects. Examples of synthetic opioids are tramadol (Ultram) and dextromethorphan. These may interact with a variety of opioid receptors.

Since the 1970s, researchers have uncovered a variety of endogenous opioids. These are sometimes referred to as endorphins, although this term can be non-specific because it also refers to a specific endogenous opioid, beta-endorphin, and also to a subgroup of the endogenous opioids. There are three groups of endogenous opioids: endorphins, enkephalins, and dynorphins. Endogenous opioids are important neuropeptide messengers, with three primary mechanisms; they are neurotransmitters, modulators of neurotransmission, and also neurohormones.

There are three classical opioid receptors, mu, kappa and delta, and a more recently discovered receptor, the nociceptin (N/OFQ) receptor. Most opioid drugs and medications are specific for the mu receptor, but endogenous opioids act upon all three classical receptors. Subtypes of each receptor exist but their actions have not yet been fully clarified. The receptors are coupled to G-proteins and are associated with intracellular adenylyl cyclase, potassium channel activation, and suppression of voltage-gated calcium channels. It is thought that they may also be coupled to other second messenger systems. The receptors range from being moderately selective (kappa) for a specific ligand to being only mildly selective (mu and delta). Acute desensitization of the mu and delta receptors occurs through endocytic internalization, and this is thought to account for acute tolerance to opioids. It is hypothesized that chronic tolerance occurs through increased activation of adenylyl cylcase.

The anatomic distribution of opioid receptors in the CNS matches the effect of opioids on the CNS. Opioid medications and drugs act primarily through activation of the mu receptor, which is distributed within pain pathways. This causes the desired effect of analgesia through inhibition of ascending nociceptive pathways and activation of descending pain control pathways. The analgesic effect is reported as making pain feel less intense, causing a blunting of the visceral pain reaction as well as drowsiness and possibly euphoria. Opioids also modify affect and the inherent reward system through the presence of endogenous opioids and opioid receptors in the nucleus accumbens (which is involved in the reward system) and the ventral striatum (which affects limbic/affective function). Euphoria, and blunting of anxiety, is thought to occur via opioid receptors in the primarily adrenergic locus ceruleus, which has sympathetic nervous system output. Further, depression of the respiratory drive and stimulation of coughing and of nausea/vomiting occur through opioid receptors in the CNS (in brainstem respiratory centers, cough center in the medulla, and the chemoreceptive trigger zone in the area postrema, respectively).

Through the presence of opioid receptors in many other systems, opioids have a variety of effects: receptors present in the hypothalamus regulate temperature set point and endocrine function; receptors present in the stomach and small intestine decrease gastric and enteric secretions and peristaltic waves; those present in the large intestine decrease propulsive motion. Morphine, specifically, causes the release of histamine, which is thought to account for its cardiovascular vasodilatory effects (reducing preload reduces the workload of the heart during an MI) and its integumentary vasodilatory and urticarial effects (causing flushing and itching).

By taking advantage of the widely distributed opioid receptors, medicinal opioids have numerous uses besides analgesia, including as antitussives (dextromethorphan), antidiarrheals (loperamide), and anesthesia adjuncts (fentanyl). This is a double-edged or even triple-edged sword. Because of the distribution of the receptors in vital reward, euphoric, and anxiolytic functional areas of the CNS, opioids have a great abuse potential. Similarly, opioid receptors are so widely distributed among the organ systems (and opioid receptors are quite non-specific for a ligand) that abused opioids may have far-reaching effects, some elucidated and many probably still unknown, throughout the body.

Infections

Intravenous use

The following three articles provide a general overview of infections occurring in intravenous opioid users.

Cherubin and Sapira (1993) updated a prior literature review they had completed 25 years before this 1993 study. They performed a literature search of both internal medicine and subspecialties over a 30-year period and identified studies that conformed to three classifications: studies describing the baseline medical complications for the year 1968, studies from after 1968 showing changes from this baseline, and studies from after 1968 showing this change in addition to the conceptulization of this change. Cherubin and Sapira (1993) specifically focused upon the epidemiology of diseases, including the changes in diseases, appearance of new diseases, and disappearance of diseases. Through this literature review, they found a number of patterns. First, there was an increased prevalence of disease among drug abusers. Second, some diseases, tetanus and malaria, were becoming rare. Third, a major new occurrence was the rise of HIV. Finally, drug use patterns changed, with an increase in the use of cocaine. They conclude that the disease landscape among intravenous drug users has become more complex.

Makower et al. (1992) became interested in studying intravenous drug-abusers because of the increasing number presenting to their emergency department. They focused upon the workload generated by intravenous drug-using patients, their presenting conditions, and the resultant management of these patients. In a prospective study over three months, all patients were requested to fill out a survey including demographic information and drug use history. Makower et al. (1992) identified 177 drug users, who presented a total of 215 times to the emergency department. Of these 215 visits, 112 (52.1 %) resulted in admission, 41 (36.6%) to surgical services. The patients used multiple drugs, with the top three being buprenorphine (142), heroin (120), and benzodiazepine (105). The top drug-related diagnoses included abscess (22), cellulitis (20) and opiate overdose (17). The top non-drug-related diagnoses were head injury (11), other medical conditions (11), and lacerations (10). Of the 112 admissions, 59 were to the emergency ward, 25 to the medical ward, and 18 to the surgical ward. In total, 72.3% of patients were admitted for reasons directly attributed to intravenous drug use. An unexpected finding was the wide distribution of drugs abused and the high percentage of patients admitted for reasons related to drug use, especially the number of injection site infections.

O'Donnell and Pappas (1988) described the pulmonary complications of intravenous drug use, including airway and interstitial disease, respiratory failure, pulmonary edema, and HIV and the acquired immunodeficiency syndrome (AIDS). To determine the frequency of these conditions, the authors performed a retrospective study over 22 months, from 1985 to 1987, of the Georgetown Pulmonary Service. They completed 423 inpatient consultations in an inner-city hospital and identified 53 charts showing history of intravenous drug use; 51 of these were available for review. They collected demographic data, HIV status, and pulmonary diagnosis.

The sample included mostly black men in their mid 30s who used heroin; some additionally injected cocaine and amphetamines. Twenty-five of the forty subjects tested positive for HIV (62.5%). Fifteen patients required mechanical ventilation and 13 (84%) survived. Pulmonary diagnoses included septic pulmonary embolism (23.5%), most commonly caused by *Staphylococcus aureus*; community acquired pneumonia (19.6%); TB (9.8%), mostly cavitary; AIDS (9.8%); acute respiratory distress syndrome (7.8%); pleural disease (5.8%); and pulmonary edema (1.9%). A diagnosis of AIDS was based on *Pneumocytis carinii* (now *P. jiroveci*) pneumonia in three cases and *Mycobacterium intracellulare* in one patient. Respiratory failure occurred in only three patients. Interstitial and bullous lung disease occurred in four.

O'Donnell and Pappas (1988) concluded that intravenous drug users continued to develop lung infections in large numbers and that this is likely related to seeding of lung tissue through contaminated needles. The risk of TB in their drug-abusing sample appeared to be higher than among the general population. They found a higher rate of infectious versus non-infectious complications and that infectious non-AIDS pulmonary complications were the most common pulmonary complication of intravenous drug use.

Horsburgh *et al.* (1989) performed a retrospective case–control study to describe the incidence of infection among intravenous drug users. They identified 270 intravenous drug users and 562 matching controls with no drug use over a period from 1978 to 1985. They found that drug users had a significantly higher incidence of infections, most notably hepatitis ($p < 0.001$). Endocarditis and disseminated gonococcal infection were more frequent among drug users ($p < 0.05$). There was no increased incident of abscess, cellulitis, AIDS, TB, *P. jiroveci* pneumonia, viral infections, or fungal infections. Heroin users, uniquely when compared with other intravenous drug users, had higher incidence of infection unrelated to needle use. The authors hypothesized that this may indicate impaired immunity among heroin users.

These studies are summarized in Table 5.1.

Comments

The review by Cherubin and Sapira (1993) provides background information about disease among intravenous drug users and illustrated how the disease landscape changes over time and that disease was becoming more prevalent. The prospective descriptional study of Makower *et al.* (1992) showed that numerous drugs were abused by the intravenous route and that cellulitis and abscesses were common infections among those using this route. O'Donnell and Pappas (1988) found that intravenous drug users have a high rate of pulmonary infection, especially *S. aureus*-associated pulmonary embolism, community acquired pneumonia, and TB. They suggested that the use of contaminated needles allows bacteria to enter the bloodstream and seed the lung. The case–control study by Horsburgh *et al.* (1989) found that intravenous drug users have higher infection rates than non-users, especially for hepatitis, endocarditis, and disseminated gonococcal infection. It appears that there is an association between intravenous route of drug use and increased infection rates; it is not possible to determine a specific association of intravenous opioids and infection rates from these studies.

Table 5.1 Infections and intravenous drug use

Study	Method	Sample	Incidence	Results
Cherubin & Sapira (1993)	Internal medicine and subspecialty literature review 1968–1993 Disease prevalence in drug abusers	Literature selected by authors	Increased prevalence of disease in drug abusers; decreased prevalence of previously common diseases (tetanus, malaria), increase in HIV	Over the 25 year analysis, treatment of diseases associated with IV use became increasingly complicated; the introduction of HIV, as well as shifts in usage, has caused a change in disease and patient management
Makower et al. (1992)	Prospective study Attendance at emergency department	All new attendances at Glasgow Royal Infirmary: 177 IV drug users seen 215 times over 3 months (1.14% of all patients)	72.3% admitted for reasons directly attributed to IV drug use: abscesses (22), cellulitis (20), opiate overdose (17)	Increased risk to staff and significantly increased department workload with increased admissions for drug abuse
O'Donnell & Pappas (1988)	Retrospective study 1985–1987, Georgetown Pulmonary Service Pulmonary complications of IV drug use	53 charts showing history of IV drug use; 40 tested for HIV, 25 (62.5%) positive; 15 required mechanical ventilation; 84% survived Pulmonary diagnoses: septic pulmonary embolism (23.5%), most commonly caused by S. aureus; community acquired pneumonia (19.6%); tuberculosis (9.8%); AIDS (9.8%); acute respiratory distress syndrome (7.8%); pleural disease (5.8%); pulmonary edema (1.9%)		IV drug users continued to develop lung infections in large numbers and this was likely related to seeding of lung tissue through contaminated needles and drug supplies; higher rate of infectious versus non-infectious complications
Horsburgh et al. (1989)	Retrospective case–control Study Incidence of infection in IV drug users	270 IV drug users; 562 matching controls with no drug use over a period from 1978 to 1985	IV drug users, compared with controls, had higher incidence of infections, most notably hepatitis ($p < 0.001$); endocarditis and disseminated gonococcal infection more frequent ($p < 0.05$)	Compared with other IV drug users, heroin users had higher incidence of infection unrelated to needle use, possibly related to impaired immunity; increased incidence of infection among IV drug users, particularly opportunistic infections

AIDS, acquired immune deficiency syndrome; HIV, human immunodeficiency virus; IV, intravenous.

247

Table 5.2 Bacterial infection

Study	Method	Sample	Incidence	Results
Dressler & Roberts (1989a)	Case study Heart infection in opiate addicts Necropsy	Necropsy of 80 hearts of opiate addicts	Cardiac valves were anatomically normal in 65 patients (81%) and abnormal in 15 patients (19%) before the onset of IE; 59 with evidence of active IE Valve infections in 80 with healed or active IE: tricuspid 35 (44%); mitral 34 (43%); aortic 32 (40%); pulmonary 2 (3%);	IE found by pathological evidence in patients with history of opioid use

IE, infective endocarditis.

Bacterial infections

One relevant citation was found on a PubMed search for bacterial infections and opioids: this was a necropsy study of the hearts of 80 opioid-addicted patients. In their study, Dressler and Roberts (1989a) found that 59 of the patients had anatomical evidence of active infective endocarditis, 11 patients had healed infective endocarditis, and 10 had both. The valves affected were tricuspid ($n = 35$, 44%), mitral ($n = 34$, 43%), aortic ($n = 32$, 40%), and pulmonary ($n = 2$, 3%). Overall, damage was sufficient to cause cardiac dysfunction in 70 (68%) of the infected valves. The authors determined by gross examination that, prior to infection, the infected valves most likely had been anatomically normal in 65 patients (81%) and abnormal in 15 patients (19%) (Table 5.2).

An additional study on the modes of death from cardiac disease is covered below under Cardiovascular disease and includes additional information about the prevalence of infectious endocarditis in opioid drug abusers.

Comments

The one study reviewed is merely descriptive but suggests that opioid use is associated with infective endocarditis, with equal effect on tricuspid, mitral, and aortic valves, and that the infection can be associated with significant cardiac dysfunction. It is impossible to ignore that the intravenous use of the drug is very likely to have provided access for bacteria to the blood, with subsequent seeding of the heart. Future research would need to control for this confounder and perhaps may include use of opioids abused by an alternative route or routes.

Mycoses

Only one study was found that addressed the association between mycosis and prescription opioid use. Yewell *et al.* (2002) reported a case series of five patients with history of intranasal abuse of prescription opioid medication. The authors reported the symptoms and physical findings of these patients: nasal and/or facial pain; nasal obstruction; chronic foul-smelling drainage; nasal septal perforation; erosion of the lateral nasal walls, naso-pharynx, and soft palate; and mucopurulent exudate. Two of five patients were diagnosed with invasive fungal rhinosinusitis (Table 5.3).

Table 5.3 Mycoses

Study	Method	Sample	Incidence	Results
Yewell et al. (2002)	Case series	5 patients with history of intranasal prescription narcotic use	Evidence of invasive fungal rhinosinusitis in 2; symptoms included nasal and/or facial pain, nasal obstruction, chronic foul-smelling drainage; common physical findings were nasal septal perforation; erosion of the lateral nasal walls, nasopharynx, and soft palate; mucopurulent exudate on affected nasal surfaces	Invasive fungal rhinosinusitis as well as other symptoms and signs indicative of rhinosinus irritation are found in patients with history of inhaled narcotic use

Comments

An association between opioid drug use and mycosis is not supported by the literature. The case study reviewed does not address the impact of the intranasal route of drug use on invasive rhinosinusitis and the signs and symptoms reported. For example, sniffing cocaine has been found to be related to midline lesions while other methods of cocaine administration do not show the same effect. The lack of other studies describing fungal infections and opioid use further strengthens the need for more studies, particularly to assess the relationship between invasive fungal rhinosinusitis and intranasal prescription opioid abuse.

Viral infections: HIV

One abstract was reviewed that discussed the relationship between methadone use and upregulation of HIV activity in a laboratory setting. Li et al. (2002) performed an in vitro study looking at effect of methadone when added to human fetal microglia from fresh human fetuses at 14–17 weeks of gestation and blood monocyte-derived macrophage cultures from six HIV-infected patients, aged 22–28 years. They found that methadone enhanced the upregulation of CCR5 expression, a coreceptor for HIV entry into monocyte-derived macrophages. They also looked at addition of methadone in microglial monocyte-derived macrophages and latently infected monocyte-derived macrophages and found that methadone enhanced viral activation and replication in all three cell types (Table 5.4).

Comments

Although not clinically relevant, this study shows that in vitro methadone enhanced HIV activation and replication and also posits a possible mechanism for increased HIV transmission in the presence of methadone. However, this study does not demonstrate an in vivo effect of methadone or other opioids on HIV transmission, activation, or replication. The study also does not indicate whether the concentration of methadone used would be similar to a bioavailable concentration in vivo. With no other studies found reviewing the affect of opioids on HIV, further study clearly is needed. Since methadone is often used to treat opioid addiction in patients who may be infected with HIV, the potential for increased transmission and enhanced activation and replication of HIV with methadone use is compelling.

Table 5.4 HIV infection

Study	Method	Sample	Incidence	Results
Li et al. (2002)	In vitro laboratory study Methadone added to human fetal microglia and blood monocyte-derived macrophage cultures	Fresh human fetal brain tissue (14–17 weeks of gestation) from Anatomic Gift Foundation; peripheral blood mononuclear cells from 6 HIV-infected patients, aged 22 –28 years	Not described	Methadone upregulates CCR5 in monocyte-derived macrophages and enhances viral activation and replication in microglia and monocyte-derived macrophages

HIV, human immunodeficiency virus.

Neoplastic disease

No results concerning opioid use and neoplastic disease were identified.

Musculoskeletal system disease

Three case studies were reviewed discussing musculoskeletal effects of opioids.

Klockgether et al. (1997) described a 30-year-old male who developed gluteal compartment syndrome with complete sciatic nerve palsy after intravenous administration of heroin. The patient also had an elevated serum CK and rhabdomyolysis, which was likely the cause of the compartment syndrome.

Melandri et al. (1996) performed a cardiac biopsy on a patient with prolonged hypoxic coma who developed rhabdomyolysis secondary to opiate use. They found myocardial damage similar to damage seen with drug overdoses complicated by muscular effort or hypoxic coma, including focal lesions of inflammatory cells, apoptotic myocardial cells, and vascular congestion. They hypothesized that an opiate overdose led to rhabdomyolysis and hypoxic coma, with resulting myocardial damage.

Yang et al. (1995) discussed a 29-year-old male who was initially found comatose after a heroin overdose. Awake upon admission, he initially was diagnosed with transverse myelitis or vasculitis of the spinal cord, based upon bilateral lower extremity paralysis, absent deep tendon reflexes and positional sense in lower extremities, and tenderness and swelling of all four limbs. With an elevated serum CK and transient ARF, rhabdomyolysis was suspected as the cause of the neurological findings, which subsequently resolved with minimal residual effects.

These studies are summarized in Table 5.5.

Comments

There is a plausible association between opioid use and rhabodmyolysis. The three case studies reviewed each described rhabdomyolysis occurring after opioid use, especially in high concentrations. Studies with larger sample sizes, perhaps starting with case–control studies, should be performed to further evaluate this possible association.

Digestive system disease

No results concerning opioid use and digestive disease were identified.

Table 5.5 Musculoskeletal disease

Study	Method	Sample	Incidence	Results
Klockgether et al. (1997)	Case report Gluteal compartment syndrome	30-year-old male IV heroin user	Symptoms: painful swelling of right leg, complete sciatic nerve palsy following IV injection of heroin Elevated serum CK, rhabdomyolysis	Neurological recovery after 4 weeks; rhabdomyolysis suspected as cause
Melandri et al. (1996)	Case report	Opioid user with hypoxic coma	Myocardial biopsy showed damage: focal lesions formed by small mononuclear inflammatory cells with a few neutrophils, associated with degenerated and necrotic myocardial fibers, interstitial edema and congestion of intrinsic blood vessels	Suggested that hypoxic coma following opioid overdose led to rhabdomyolysis and myocardial damage
Yang et al. (1995)	Case report	29-year-old male 1 day after heroin overdose	Symptoms: paralysis of lower extremities, swelling and tenderness of the four extremities, absent lower extremity deep tendon reflexes and positional sense Elevated plasma CK; transient acute renal failure	Resolution of most neurological signs and symptoms in 4 weeks

Stomatognathic disease

No results concerning opioid use and diseases of the mouth and jaw were identified.

Respiratory system disease

Multiple studies were reviewed describing respiratory dysfunction with opioid use, including five studies associated with asthma and heroin use, two that described non-cardiogenic pulmonary edema associated with heroin and buprenorphine use, and one that described respiratory depression in a patient receiving buprenorphine.

Krantz et al. (2003) described two studies, in one article, examining the association between asthma exacerbations requiring intensive care and heroin use. The first was a case series of 23 patients admitted to the intensive care unit with asthma. Of these, 13 self-reported asthma exacerbation after heroin use, and this was correlated with a positive urine drug screen. The second study was a retrospective case–control study comparing patients in intensive care with asthma and with DKA. In this study, they found asthmatics to have a significantly higher incidence of heroin use (41.3% vs. 12.5%; $p = 0.006$) and higher positive urine drug screen for opiates (60% vs. 7%; $p = 0.001$). Both studies indicated an increased incidence of severe asthma attacks after heroin use.

Boto de los et al. (2002) performed a prospective case–control study of bronchial diseases and the use of rebujo (inhalation of a vaporized heroin–cocaine mixture) in

91 subjects (62 from a drug rehabilitation center and 29 admitted to the hospital for other reasons); 122 individuals chosen from the general population who had not inhaled the drugs served as the control group. All subjects completed a questionnaire, had lung function tests performed, and had IgE levels measured. Of the 62 subjects in the drug rehabilitation group, there was a 41.9% one-year wheezing prevalence, 44.4% one-year bronchial hyper-reactivity prevalence, and 22.02% asthma prevalence. In the control group, these values were 32.7% ($p = 0.22$), 15.57% ($p < 0.0001$) and 8.19% ($p < 0.01$), respectively. No wheezing was experienced before rebujo drug use, but the subjects began to experience wheezing after drug use. Of these patients, there was a mean latency of 4.09 months before wheezing began. Wheezing stopped after discontinuation of the heroin–cocaine mixture in only 7.6% of these subjects. The researchers concluded that the rebujo mixture was related to the onset of bronchial hyperreactivity.

Cygan *et al.* (2000) provided a small case series of five patients who developed status asthmaticus following inhaled heroin use. Four of the five required mechanical ventilation.

Hughes & Calverley (1988), described three patients with asthma exacerbations requiring mechanical ventilation soon after inhalation of heroin. Two of the three died.

Two abstracts were reviewed that discussed opioid use and non-cardiogenic pulmonary edema. Sporer & Dorn (2001) conducted a retrospective chart review of 27 patients who had developed significant hypoxia – not attributed to other causes – within 24 hours of apparent heroin overdose; 26 (96%) had developed symptoms prior to emergency department arrival or within the first hour. Twenty (74%) of the patients had classical radiographic pulmonary alveolar edema. Nine (33%) patients required mechanical ventilation and 18 (66%) were treated only with supplemental oxygen. Twenty patients (74%) had no hypoxia 24 hours after admission and the remaining cases resolved within 48 hours.

Thammakumpee & Sumpatanukule (1994) reported a case of a 21-year-old woman who developed non-cardiogenic pulmonary edema following sublingual administration of 0.2 mg buprenorphine.

Jain & Shah (1993) reported a case of a 48–year-old male who developed severe post-operation respiratory depression after receiving 30 mg ketorolac intramuscular two hours after 150 μg epidural buprenorphine. The patient had a thoracotomy for esophageal cancer. The authors noted that the risk of respiratory depression is likely associated with a cumulative effect of these two drugs.

These studies are summarized in Table 5.6.

Comments

There appears to be a relatively well-supported assocation between heroin and asthma exacerbation. Based upon the four small studies reported here, inhaled heroin may facilitate severe asthma exacerbations. It would be interesting to place this association into context by performing studies of larger sample size that assess the incidence of heroin-associated asthma exacerbations compared with heroin-unassociated asthma exacerbations; the severity of heroin-associated asthma exacerbations compared with heroin-unassociated exacerbations; and prospectively whether there is an increased risk of asthma exacerbations among heroin users. The studies described here did not control for confounders, especially cigarette use or other inhaled drug use, which future studies that look into respiratory complaints should address.

There is limited support for an association between non-cardiogenic pulmonary edema and opioids. The study by Sporer & Dorn (2001) is particularly useful to clinicians because

Table 5.6 Respiratory disease

Study	Method	Sample	Incidence	Results
Krantz et al. (2003)	Case series and retrospective case–control study. Heroin use and asthma. Self-report of heroin use and asthma exacerbation	Case series: 26 admissions to ICU for asthma in 23 patients aged 16 to 50 years. Case–control subjects aged 15–50 years: 84 cases with asthma (104 ICU admissions), 42 controls with diabetic ketoacidosis	Case series: 13/23 (56%) described asthma exacerbations associated with heroin insufflation. Case–control: compared with subjects with diabetic ketoacidosis, asthmatics were significantly more likely to report heroin use (41.3% vs. 12.5%; $p = 0.006$), had a significantly higher prevalence of –positive urine drug screen results for opiates (60% vs. 7%; $p = 0.001$)	Increased incidence of heroin use and acute asthma requiring ICU admission
Boto de los et al. (2002)	Case–control. Inhalation of rebujo (heroin– cocaine mixture vaporized on aluminum foil)	91 rebujo users (69 from drug rehabilitation, 29 admitted for other reasons), 122 non-user controls from general population	Drug rehabilitation patients compared with controls: prevalence of wheezing over the past 12 months, 41.9% vs. 32.78% ($p = 0.22$); prevalence of bronchial reactivity, 44.4% vs. 15.57% ($p < 0.001$); prevalence of asthma, 22.02% vs. 8.19% ($p < 0.01$)	Increase in bronchial reactivity and asthma exacerbation in subjects who inhaled rebujo
Cygan et al. (2000)	Case series and review of literature	5 patients with status asthmaticus triggered by inhaled heroin	Not defined	4 required mechanical ventilation
Sporer & Dorn (2001)	Retrospective chart review August 1994 through December 1998. Heroin and NCPE	27 patients presenting to an urban academic hospital with NCPE within 24 h of heroin overdose	20 (74%) were hypoxic on emergency department arrival; 6 (22%) had symptoms develop within the first hour; 20 (74%)with classic pulmonary alveolar edema on radiography; 9 (33%) requiring mechanical ventilated; 18 (66%) requiring: supplemental O_2; hypoxia resolved in 20 (74%) in first 24 h, in all within 48 h	NCPE was clinically apparent either immediately or within 4 h of the overdose; mechanical ventilation is necessary in a minority of patients; signs and symptoms resolve within 48 h

253

Table 5.6 Cont.

Study	Method	Sample	Incidence	Results
Thammakumpee & Sumpatanukule (1994)	Case study	21-year-old woman without existing cardiovascular disease	Developed NCPE 70 min after sublingual administration of 0.2 mg buprenorphine	Pulmonary edema resolved spontaneously with conservative treatment; allergic response to buprenorphine suspected
Jain & Shah (1993)	Case study	Respiratory depression in 48-year-old male after thoracotomy for esophageal cancer	Developed severe postoperative respiratory depression after 150 µg epidural buprenorphine and 30 mg intramuscular ketorolac	Cummulative effective of both drugs probably led to respiratory depression
Hughes & Calverley (1988)	Case series	3 patients (19-year-old female, 23-year-old male, 17-year-old female) with asthma	All required mechanical ventilation after heroin use	2 died of acute severe asthma

ICU, intensive care unit; NCPE, noncardiogenic pulmonary edema.

of the potential for the use of the results in a clinical setting: most patients developed symptoms before arrival at the emergency department or within one hour; most could be managed by supplemental oxygen alone; all episodes resolved within 48 hours; and most cases could be confirmed by a chest radiography. However, further study is needed to support an association between non-cardiogenic pulmonary edema and opioids because the association is based upon this single chart review of small sample size, possibly affected by selection bias, and upon a case study. The case study examined non-cardiogenic pulmonary edema occurring after buprenorphine use, and with the increasing clinical use of buprenorphine, clinicians may want to further pursue research into this possible side effect of the medication.

The last study reviewed indicated that respiratory depression can occur as a result of the combined use of epidural bupranorphrine and non-steroidal anti-inflammatory drugs, but, as a case study, the meaning of this finding is not clear.

Otorhinolaryngological disease

The review yielded no results associating opioid use with diseases of the ear, nose, and/or throat. (The section above on Mycoses discussed nasal disease and mycotic infection.)

Nervous system disease

Central nervous system: seizures

Three abstracts were identified that describe opioid use and seizures. Alldredge *et al.* (1989) performed a retrospective chart review of 49 patients who experienced recreational drug-induced seizures over a 12-year period. They found that most patients had a generalized tonic–clonic seizure; however, multiple seizures and status epilepticus were also seen. While in most cases cocaine was the drug used ($n = 32$), seven of the cases were associated with heroin use. Ten of the patients had a history of prior seizures associated with drug use. All but one had no neurological deficits after the seizures.

Jovanovic Cupic *et al.* (2006), in a prospective study of 57 patients with a mean age of 22.3 years who had a history of tramadol abuse or intoxication for over three years, found that 31 (54.4%) patients developed tonic–clonic seizures after a tramadol dose ranging from 250 to 2500 mg. Of these, 26 (84%) developed a seizure within 24 hours of drug use; 14 (45%) had single seizures and 17 (55%) had multiple seizures. Abusers with seizures were statistically significantly ($p < 0.05$) younger than those who did not have seizures, who used the drug over a longer time span, and who also tended to abuse alcohol and tramadol together.

Tobias (1997) reported a case of an adverse drug event when 4 mg/kg tramadol was administered to a child and led to seizure activity.

Table 5.7 summarizes these studies.

Comments

The association between seizures and opioids is only minimally supported. Alldredge *et al.* (1989) found that only some of the seizures were associated with heroin use and that heroin was not one of the more common drugs associated with seizures. This study may be influenced by confounding factors, such as polydrug use and pre-existing seizure disorder, and also by selection bias. The study would have been strengthened with a larger sample size and perhaps if reviews of charts occurred at multiple sites.

Table 5.7 Central nervous system: seizures

Study	Method	Sample	Incidence	Results
Alldredge et al. (1989)	Retrospective chart review 1975–1987, San Francisco General Hospital Drug-induced seizures	47 patients with 49 recreational drug-induced seizures	7 with multiple seizures; 2 developed status epilepticus; all others had a single seizure; drugs implicated: cocaine (32), amphetamine (11), heroin (7), phencyclidine (4)	All but one patient recovered without neurological sequelae; patient with status epilepticus had some neurological deficit
Jovanovic-Cupic et al. (2006)	Prospective cohort study over 3 years Tramadol and neurotoxicity	57 patients with history of tramadol abuse and intoxication	31 (54.4%) had tonic–clonic seizures, single in 14 (45%), multiple in 17 (55%); seizures occurred within 24 h after tramadol intoxication in 26 (84%) patients; compared to addicts without seizures, those with seizures abused tramadol over a longer period of time, were more likely to take tramadol with alcohol, and were younger	The neurotoxicity of tramadol commonly manifests as generalized tonic–clonic seizures occurring most frequently within 24 h
Tobias (1997)	Case study Tramadol and seizures	Child with seizure activity after administration of 4 mg/kg tramadol	Not defined	Seizure likely an overdose or adverse drug event

Published in 1989, the study's population may not be representative of the current drug-abusing population.

Specifically for tramadol, there appears to be more potential for an association with seizures than for heroin. The recent prospective study by Jovanovic-Cupic et al. (2006) may be very timely and useful to the clinician because tramadol is increasingly being used by drug users and clinicians may see seizures related to this. Importantly, for seizures occurring beyond a 24-hour period after tramadol use, tramadol is unlikely to be the cause. This study would have been greatly strengthened by the use of a control group. Also interesting in its analysis would have been a more detailed comparison between tramadol users who had seizures and those who did not have seizures. The case report (Tobias 1997) further supports an association between tramadol and seizures. Additional studies are needed.

Brain pathology

One study was reviewed that focused on an opioid effect on cerebellar brain function. Ropper & Blair (2003) reported a case of a middle-aged male with acute onset cerebellar signs that included ataxia. Symmetric deep cavitational cerebellar damage was identified by MRI. The patient admitted that he had inhaled heroin just prior to symptom onset. The authors suggested that the cavitation was a toxic reaction to heroin use.

Two additional studies were found that suggest that microvascular ischemic changes and spongiform leukoencephalopathy can occur in users inhaling heroin vapors. Borne

Table 5.8 Brain pathology

Study	Method	Sample	Incidence	Results
Ropper & Blair (2003)	Case report Heroin and cerebellar lesions MRI	Middle-aged male developing cerebellar signs and ataxia after heroin use	Pronounced cerebellar signs appeared acutely 1 day after heroin use; MRI showed symmetrically deep cavitational cerebellar lesions	Temporal relationship between heroin use and symptoms of ataxia, cerebellar lesions suggestive of toxic reaction
Borne et al. (2005)	Literature review CNS pathology in heroin users Diagnostic imaging	Heroin users	CNS pathology associated with heroin abuse: neurovascular ischemia, ischemic stroke, leukoencephalopathy, CNS atrophy, infections	Opiate abusers can have a variety of CNS pathologies associated with their drug use
Hagel et al. (2005)	Pictorial review of the literature Spongiform leukoencephalopathy in heroin inhalers MRI	Heroin inhalers	MRI findings: white matter change in posterior cerebrum, cerebellum, cerebral peduncles, corpus callosum, internal capsule, corticospinal tract, medial lemniscus, tractus solitarius	Long-term use of heroin can lead to CNS changes associated with a lethal outcome

CNS, central nervous system; MRI, magnetic resonance imaging.

et al. (2005) described the diagnostic imaging of individuals abusing opioids and solvents reported in the medical literature. They found a number of CNS pathologies associated with heroin abuse, including neurovascular ischemic changes and ischemic stroke. Inhalers of heroin vapors have been found to have a rare form of leukoencephalopathy and CNS atrophy and infections have also been found in opiate abusers.

Hagel et al. (2005) used a pictorial essay format to describe the types of cerebral changes seen in spongiform leukoencephalopathy. This rare condition has been found in individuals who inhale the heroin vapors that form when free-based heroin is heated. The MRI findings include pathological changes in the white matter of the posterior cerebrum and cerebellum, cerebellar peduncles, and the corpus callosum. The internal capsules were also affected. Pathological changes also were found in the corticospinal tract, medial lemniscus, and tractus solitarius. These changes appear to develop over a long period of heroin use, with symptoms developing in three distinct stages and ending with death.

These studies are summarized in Table 5.8.

Comments

The study by Ropper & Blair (2003) suggests the possibility that inhaled heroin is associated with cavitational cerebellar damage and ataxia. The two other studies also support the association between heroin use and brain pathology. These three publications, a case report and two reviews, suggest that heroin use is associated with cerebral and cerebellar pathology, particularly when heroin is inhaled. However, more studies are needed to provide additional evidence that there is a significant risk of cerebral–cerebellar pathology when inhaling heroin or using other opioids.

Ocular disease

Three papers were found in a PubMed search from 1988 to 2008 that describe ocular pathology associated with opioid use. Two of these studies look at strabismus and opioid use. One is a retrospective study in adults, while the other is a retrospective cross-sectional review looking at infants born to opiate-dependent mothers. The third paper is a collection of case reports of ocular candidiasis among intravenous buprenorphine users.

Strabismus

The first paper (Sutter & Landau 2003) was a retrospective study of seven patients found to have acute strabismus related to heroin and/or methadone abuse. Acute esotropia (convergent squint) was the most common oculomotor abnormality and was associated with heroin withdrawal. The two cases of exotropia (divergent squint) were associated with heroin or methadone intake rather than withdrawal. Treatment with prism lenses was used in some cases; the remaining problems cleared spontaneously or corrected with resumption of heroin use. The researchers suggested that poor binocular function may be a predisposing factor to the development of either esotropia or exotropia as a sequela of sudden changes in drug levels.

The second study (Gill et al. (2003) was a retrospective cross-sectional study of infants of opiate-dependent mothers who were recalled for an ophthalmic examination: 71 infants (mean age 21 months) were identified; 29 had a full ophthalmological examination and 20 were surveyed by a questionnaire. Seven (14%) of the infants had strabismus on examination, and four (8%) required glasses or patching. Seven additional infants (14%) had a history of intermittent strabismus but were not formally examined. Multiple maternal variables were analyzed, but none was found to predict which infants would be susceptible to strabismus other than opiate use. The prevalence of strabismus found in this study was approximately 10 times the expected rates of strabismus in the general population and presumed to be caused by antenatal opiate exposure.

Ocular candidiasis

Cassoux et al. (2002)) provided a collection of four case reports of ocular candidiasis developing in four individuals who used high-dose sublingual buprenorphine in an intravenous injection. Three dissolved the buprenorphine in lemon juice prior to injection, while the fourth used saliva as the solvent. The authors compared their findings with those from a prior outbreak of candidiasis in France related to heroin use. At that time, the lemon juice used to dissolve the heroin was found to be contaminated with Candida albicans. This study seems to support the previous observation that the lemon juice was the source of the candidal contaminant rather than the buprenorphine.

These studies are summarized in Table 5.9.

Comments

The first two studies suggest that there is a relationship between opiates and strabismus in both adults and infants. The absolute risk of developing strabismus secondary to opioid use is difficult to gauge given the small size of the studies and the retrospective design. That said, the finding of a 10-fold increase in the incidence of strabismus in infants of opiate-dependent mothers suggests that this risk is real. Binocular vision deficits prior to drug use

Table 5.9 Ocular manifestations

Study	Method	Sample	Incidence	Results
Sutter & Landau (2003)	Retrospective study Strabismus and opioid use	7 patients with acute strabismus after opioid withdrawal	5 with esotropia (convergent squint) after heroin withdrawal; 2 with exotropia (divergent squint) after heroin or methadone intake	Strabismus cleared spontaneously or after resumption of drug use in 3 patients; 4 patients required corrective lenses; poor binocular function may be predisposing factor
Gill *et al.* (2003)	Retrospective cross-sectional study Strabismus in infants of opiate-dependent mothers	71 infants born within an 18-month period; 49 recalled for ocular examination	29 received ophthalmic examination; 20 surveyed by questionnaire; 7/49 (14%) had strabismus on examination; another 7 (14%) had a history of strabismus but declined examination	No confounders other than opiate use; rate of strabismus in infants of opiate-dependent mothers was 10 times that seen in the general population
Cassoux *et al.* (2002)	Case reports Candida endophthalmitis and buprenorphine	4 with candida endophthalmitis and a history of buprenorphine injection	Sublingual buprenorphine was dissolved in lemon juice or saliva prior to injection	Ocular infection most likely related to contaminated lemon juice/saliva rather than buprenorphine itself

may also be a predisposing factor. The mechanisms of the observed association of opiate use and strabismus are unknown; however, since opiate use and withdrawal impacts CNS function, the effect of varying blood levels of abused opioids could influence parasympathetic and cranial nerve function. Further studies are needed to assess whether screening at-risk infants is cost-effective and improves outcomes. Healthcare providers also need to be aware that heroin use and withdrawal may be related to strabismus.

The increasing misuse of sublingual buprenorphine as an intravenously administered drug is highlighted in the third paper. The four case reports suggest that use of contaminated solvents can lead to various infections. In this study, *C. albicans* led to ocular infections; however disseminated fungal and bacterial infections could also occur. More studies describing the prevalence of infections in intravenous drug users who dissolve their drugs in contaminated solvents are needed. However, the causative agent of the ocular fungal infections is not likely to be the buprenorphine itself.

Male urological disease

In a review of studies published between 1988 and 2008, a PubMed search revealed four papers linking opioid use and urological pathology. A variety of renal dysfunction is shown. Rhabdomyolysis is presumed to be the source of kidney failure in some cases, while in others there is not a clear cause.

Renal disease

A review article (Dettmeyer *et al.* 2005) summarized numerous articles published since the 1960s that showed a relationship between renal diseases and chronic parenteral abuse of heroin, cocaine, morphine, amphetamine, and other abused drugs or adulterants.

"Drug-addict nephropathy" is an important cause of ESRD today. It is unknown whether it is the injected substance itself or associated infections such as HBV, HCV, or HIV that leads to the pathological kidney findings in heroin users with renal disease.

Rice *et al.* (2000) carried out a retrospective case–control study that analyzed predisposing factors predicting the need for dialysis in patients with heroin-related rhabdomyolysis and renal failure. Twenty-seven patients were identified who had developed renal failure after intravenous heroin use. Renal failure was likely caused by rhabdomyolysis in all cases, and 8 out of 27 patients required dialysis for an average of 14 days (range, 3–26). Those who required dialysis had a higher admission CK and a higher admission serum creatinine, higher peak CK, lower urine output in the initial 24 hours, and a longer length of hospitalization (all significant at $p \leq 0.05$). Most patients had significant comorbidities that predisposed them to serious complications and long-term disability. Twenty patients had positive serology tests for viral infection: HIV (5%), HBV (10%), and HCV (74%). Some patients had pneumonia and respiratory failure, compartment syndrome, and residual muscle weakness. The authors concluded that significant renal recovery should be expected in this population despite these complications since none of these patients required treatment for chronic renal failure. However, some serious complications can occur.

Lynn *et al.* (1998) reported a case series in which five intravenous opiate drug users were found to have renal disease following illicit drug use. Three patients presented with nephrotic syndrome, one had ARF, and one had hypertension with urinary sediment with red and white blood cells, casts, and proteinuria. All but one of the patients was positive for HCV, and all were negative for HBV and HIV. Pathological findings in the renal biopsied tissue found large vacuolated areas, suggesting lipid-like deposits in the glomerular cells, and infiltrating macrophages. Acute tubular necrosis or focal glomerular sclerosis was evident in three patients. The authors suggested that the renal pathology was related to the available drugs used and the solvents used (lemon juice or acetic anhydride and sodium bicarbonate).

Uzan *et al.* (1988) discussed 13 heroin users. All had used heroin with or without other drugs for 3 to 12 years. Two sniffed heroin intranasally while the remaining 11 were intravenous drug users. Six patients were found to have acute tubular necrosis, with this resulting from rhabdomyolysis in five and after gentamicin antibiotic therapy for bacterial endocarditis in the sixth. Renal biopsy showed various forms of glomerulonephritis in the five patients with nephrotic syndrome. Two patients had hypertension with intrarenal vascular lesions. Both patients were positive for HBV antigen. Out of these 13 patients, two with glomerulonephritis required treatment with chronic dialysis and/or renal transplantation. The other 11 patients recovered normal serum creatinine and renal function.

These studies on renal disorders are summarized in Table 5.10.

Comments

These four articles show an association between chronic opiate use and kidney disease. The renal damage is likely from rhabdomyolysis secondary to opiate use, concurrent comorbidities, or the opiate use itself. The review article mentioned that it was unclear whether it was the injected substance itself, adulterants, or associated diseases such as HBV, HCV, or HIV that caused the kidney damage.

Rhabdomyolysis is often found in opiate users with ARF. As detailed above, renal failure in this setting is usually reversible, with no residual renal deficit, but dialysis may

Table 5.10 Urological pathology

Study	Method	Sample	Incidence	Results
Dettmeyer et al. (2005)	Literature review, 1960s to 2000 Renal disease and parenteral opiate use		End-stage renal disease associated with drug addict nephropathy and associated with a variety of abused drugs	Some correlation between parenteral opiate use and renal disease; abused drug, solvents, disease comorbidity (HBV, HCV, HIV) may all be implicated in renal pathology
Rice et al. (2000)	Retrospective analysis Risk factors associated with renal failure from heroin-induced rhabdomyolysis and predictors of needing dialysis	27 with ARF after recent IV heroin use	Rhabdomyolysis was the likely cause in all patients; 8 required dialysis (average of 14 days); 20 had comorbidities, including HIV (5%), HBV (10%), HCV (74%); pneumonia, respiratory failure, compartment syndrome	Dialysis-predicting factors: high admission CK, high serum creatinine, high peak CK, low initial 24-h urine output ($p = 0.05$); patients experiencing IV heroin-induced renal failure should be expected to regain full function but may require dialysis if their kidney function is poor; long-term disability related to complications can occur
Lynn et al. (1998)	Case study Renal disease in IV opiate use	5 IV drug users with pathological renal biopsy findings	3 with nephrotic syndrome; 1 with ARF; 1 with high blood pressure, urine containing red and white blood cells, cells/casts; proteinuria; all positive for HCV Biopsy findings: vacuolated areas suggestive of lipid deposits, infiltrating macrophages; 2 with acute tubular necrosis; 1 with focal glomerular sclerosis	IV opiate use, or solvents used for injection, may contribute to the deposition of lipids and macrophage infiltration, and resulting renal disease
Uzan et al. (1988)	Case study ARF and heroin use	11 IV heroin users, 2 intranasal heroin users	5/11 patients showed glomerulonephritis, 2 needing dialysis/transplant; all patients with ARF from rhabdomyolsis and gentamicin therapy regained normal renal function	Heroin use, IV or nasal routes, is associated with ARF; those developing glomerulonephritis may be at increased risk of needing dialysis/transplant

ARF, acute renal failure; CK, creatine kinase; HAV, hepatitis A virus; HBV, hepatitis B virus; HCV, hepatitis C virus; HIV, human immunodeficiency virus; IV, intravenous.

be required in some patients. Poor renal function tests, high CK, low urine output, and significant comorbidities are often predictors of those drug users who might require dialysis.

Since multiple pathological features are noted in two of the studies (Lynn *et al.* 1998, Uzan *et al.* 1988), there does not seem to be a clear consensus on the most common pathology seen. Additionally, clinical presentations are variable, ranging from hypertension to nephrotic syndrome. Further studies are needed to investigate whether opiates are nephrotoxic, or if this damage is secondary to rhabdomyolysis and other associated conditions. The statistical risk of developing kidney failure secondary to opioid use alone remains unknown.

Female genital and neonatal/congenital disease

Seven articles showing the relationship between opioids and pregnancy were found in the literature search. The topics include complications with pregnancy, adverse fetal outcomes, and neonatal abstinence syndrome (NAS). One additional paper was found that investigated congenital diseases and maternal opioid use.

Pregnancy complications

In (2008), Binder & Vavrinkova published a prospective randomized controlled trial to evaluate the effect of substitution therapy in heroin-addicted pregnant women involving 117 women, who were randomized to three groups: 47 received no substitution therapy (maintained ongoing heroin use), 32 received methadone substitution therapy, and 38 received buprenorphine substitution therapy. Thirty other women initially qualified for the study failed to participate because of non-compliance with the study guidelines. Substitution therapy was initiated in the first trimester, and all groups were followed throughout their pregnancy and postnatally at a perinatal care unit. Birthweights were compared with national birthweight tables, and severity of NAS was evaluated by Finnegan's score scale. The lowest infant birthweight, the highest number of newborns with IUGR, and the most numerous placental changes were found in the heroin-using group ($p < 0.05$, compared with the two substitution groups). However, the severity and course of NAS were most severe in newborns of women from the methadone-substitution group ($p < 0.001$). The authors noted that while comparison of groups is difficult because of the confounding impact of lifestyle choices, substitution therapy provided social stability, increased access to prenatal care, and decreased street heroin consumption. As methadone protracted the NAS, they recommend focusing more attention on buprenorphine substitution therapy.

Kuczkowski (2007) reviewed all drugs of abuse and the management of patients during the perinatal period. Medical complications similar to those observed in non-pregnant women who abuse opioids are also seen in pregnant women (cellulitis, skin abscesses, septic thrombophlebitis, hepatitis, AIDS, endocarditis, and malnutrition). Under specific effects on pregnancy, IUGR and various forms of fetal distress are mentioned as known consequences of intrauterine drug exposure. Methadone is mentioned as the current recommendation for the treatment of pregnant patients addicted to opioids. For peripartum care, opioid replacement is recommended throughout labor to avoid acute withdrawal. Administration of antagonists or agonist–antagonists should be avoided to prevent precipitation of withdrawal symptoms. Should these develop, they may be effectively managed with the sympatholytic clonidine hydrochloride. Epidural and spinal anesthesia may be safely used, but these patients have shown an increased tendency for hypotension. Peripheral intravenous access may be difficult and necessitate a central line. Finally, these patients may require larger doses of pain medication postpartum because of cross-tolerance resulting from chronic receptor stimulation.

Jansson *et al.* (2007) published an observational study of 50 methadone-maintained pregnant women aimed at predicting the severity of NAS. Prior studies have shown that NAS occurs in a subset of methadone-exposed infants, who require medication to treat the syndrome. The women were attending a comprehensive substance abuse treatment facility. Monitoring by ECG occurred at 36 weeks of gestation at the times of trough and peak maternal methadone levels. Vagal tone was used as an estimate of the individual's respiratory sinus arrhythmia and an indicator of autonomic control. The occurrence of NAS was found to be unrelated to maternal substance abuse history, methadone maintenance history, or psychotropic medication exposure. Male infants were more likely than female infants to develop NAS and to require drugs postnatally ($p < 0.05$). Maternal vagal responders were more likely than vagal non-responders to have infants with NAS ($F_{2,44} = 4.15$; $p < 0.05$). The infants of maternal vagal responders were also more likely to require medication for treatment ($F_{2,44} = 3.39$; $p < 0.05$). Jansson et al. (2007) suggested that those women on methadone therapy who show vagal tone changes are more likely to have infants with NAS than are non-responders.

Fajemirokun-Odudeyi et al. (2006) published a retrospective study of 110 babies born to 108 women on either methadone maintenance therapy or using heroin in late pregnancy. Compared with offspring of women substituting methadone for heroin, offspring of women who used heroin were more likely to require morphine (40% vs. 19%), had higher mean maximum NAS scores (5.8 vs. 4.7), and stayed in the neonatal unit significantly longer (17.2 vs. 11.8 days).

Lam et al. (1992) published a retrospective case–controlled study involving 51 pregnant Chinese women who abused narcotics (primarily heroin). Very few substituted methadone for heroin. Some of their infants displayed prematurity (41%) and were small for gestational age (27.5%); infants of drug-abusing mothers were 629 g lighter at birth, had a 5 cm smaller head circumference, and were 7 cm shorter in length. The drug-abusing mothers had a higher prevalence of antepartum hemorrhage (13.7%) and venereal disease (23.5%). Compared with the control group, the perinatal mortality rate was 2.5 times higher in the drug-exposed infants (19.5/1000) and there was one maternal death. The NAS occurred in 83% of the drug-exposed infants

Little et al. (1990) published a retrospective case–control study evaluating the effects of "T's and blues" (pentazocine and tripelennamine) abuse during pregnancy. Pentazocine is a synthetically prepared narcotic, and tripelennamine is an antihistamine. Infants of 23 abusers were compared with infants of 100 unexposed women. Compared with non-users, T's and blues abusers were found to have infants with significantly reduced birthweight, length, and head circumference, and increased congenital anomalies. Of the three infants with major congenital anomalies, one anomaly was associated with moderate to heavy maternal alcohol use during pregnancy and one infant experienced in utero anoxia; therefore neither of these two anomalies were thought to be related to the T's and blues abuse.

Levy and Koren (1990) published a review of drugs of abuse and their effects on obstetric and neonatal health. They identified two trends as barriers to understanding the adverse effects of drugs, including cocaine, cannabinoids, alcohol, cigarettes, and opioids. They suggested that clustering of many other risk factors in the context of drug abuse can confound results. Moreover, there is a tendency to publish studies showing adverse fetal effects while reports of no effects by drugs and chemicals are discouraged. This would lead to a skewing of the available pool of data. The authors concluded that more studies need to be done to determine the long-term effects of in utero exposure to drugs of abuse.

These studies are summarized in Table 5.11.

Table 5.11 Pregnancy complications

Study	Method	Sample	Incidence	Results
Binder & Vavrinkova (2008)	Prospective randomized comparative study Opioid replacement therapy in pregnancy and infant outcomes	117 women, randomized to 3 groups: 47 no replacement (on heroin), 32 methadone substitution, 38 buprenorphine substitution Infants: no premature delivery prior to 34 weeks	Heroin-exposed infants: highest incidence of LBW, IUGR, placental changes ($p < 0.05$); NAS most severe in methadone-exposed infants ($p < 0.001$)	Confounding variables may account for some findings; buprenorphine substitution therapy recommended rather than methadone
Kuczkowski (2007)	Literature review Risks associated with drugs of abuse and pregnancy	All drugs of abuse and management of patients in perinatal period	Maternal medical complications opioid use: cellulitis, skin abscesses, thrombophlebitis, hepatitis, AIDS, endocarditis, malnutrition Infant outcomes: IUGR, fetal distress	Methadone recommended for replacement therapy; anesthesia can precipitate hypotension, and larger doses of pain medication are needed because of cross-tolerance
Jansson et al. (2007)	Descriptive study Severity of NAS in infants ECG	50 methadone-maintained pregnant women	Vagal tone response to methadone during times of trough or peak (effect on respiratory sinus rhythm, autonomic control): maternal vagal responders more likely to have infants with NAS ($p < 0.05$); NAS: unrelated to substance abuse history, methadone maintenance, exposure to psychotropic drugs; male infants more likely to develop NAS, require medication ($p < 0.05$)	Maternal vagal tone's response to methadone may be a predictor of NAS severity
Fajemirokun-Odudeyi et al. (2006)	Retrospective study NAS symptoms in infants born to women who used heroin or methadone during late pregnancy	110 newborns from 108 mothers using heroin or on methadone maintenance during late pregnancy	Comparing infants of heroin-using group with methadone group, morphine therapy needed by 40% vs. 19%; length of stay 17.2 vs. 11.8 days	Heroin use in late pregnancy is associated with increased need for morphine therapy for the newborn, higher NAS scores, and longer hospital stays when compared with infants born to mothers on methadone maintenance

Lam et al. (1992)	Retrospective case–control study. Gravidas pregnancy outcomes in narcotic abusers	51 gravidas who had abused narcotics, heroin being the most common; non-abusing controls	Perinatal mortality was 2.5 times higher in abusing group than in the control group	Narcotic use in pregnancy increases the risk of prematurity, small for gestational age babies antepartum hemorrhage, and is associated with high prevalence of venereal disease and late antenatal care
Little et al. (1990)	Retrospective case–control study. Materal use of "T's and blues" (pentazocine and tripelennamine)	23 "T's and blues" abusers; 100 unexposed women	3 infants had congenital anomalies, although 2 were attributable to other sources	Lower birthweights, shorter length, smaller head circumference, and possible increase in congenital abnormalities in infants of mothers who used T's and blues
Levy & Koren (1990)	Literature review Obstetric/neonatal effects of drug abuse	Trends and barriers to understanding obstetric/neonatal effects of drug abuse	Lack of studies showing adverse effects of drugs may influence implications of published literature	Barriers include clustering of risk factors in the drug-abusing population, and a tendency to only publish studies showing adverse effects

IUGR, intrauterine growth retardation; LBW, low birthweight; NAS, neonatal abstinence syndrome.

Comments

Based on the evidence discussed above, it seems clear that opiates can be associated with decreased fetal growth (measured by birthweight, IUGR, head circumference, and body length). All of the papers that looked at this subject were in agreement that heroin use likely caused more growth restriction than methadone substitution therapy.

The prospective randomized comparative study of Binder & Vavrinkova (2008) also demonstrated an increased prevalence of placental changes in heroin users when compared with women on substitution therapy, but this has not been reported in any other studies reviewed. Also mentioned in the one review paper (Kuczkowski 2007), but not verified in other recent articles, are recommendations on the clinical care of opiate-addicted mothers in the antepartum and postpartum period.

Less clear is the impact of heroin, methadone, and buprenorphine on NAS. Fajemir-okun-Odudeyi et al. (2006) compared infants of mothers using heroin in late pregnancy and infants of mothers on methadone maintenance therapy and showed that infants of mothers who took heroin in late pregnancy required more morphine, had higher NAS scores, and required longer hospital stays. Kuczkowski's (2007) review article supports this observation, recommending methadone pre- and postnatally for all pregnant patients addicted to opioids. This article also specifically warns against the use of agonist–antagonist drugs (such as buprenorphine) in pregnancy because of the risk of precipitating acute withdrawal. This is in conflict with the randomized controlled trial that showed bupre-norphine substitution therapy in pregnancy to be an effective and promising option (Binder & Vavrinkova 2008). Also in this study, methadone maintenance was found to be associated with more severe NAS when compared with ongoing heroin use and buprenorphine therapy. Although other studies disagree with this observation that methadone mainten-ance seems to worsen NAS, the fact that the Binder & Vavrinkova (2008) study is a randomized comparative study does give it some greater significance. These authors sug-gested that buprenorphine might be a better maintenance medication, but further study is needed before this finding could be extended as a standard of care. A larger study with direct comparison between methadone and buprenorphine could help to resolve this debate

Congenital disease

One paper (Fulroth et al. 1989) was found that examined perinatal outcomes with respect to congenital problems in infants exposed to heroin and/or cocaine in utero (Table 5.12). Eighty-six infants who were born to women with a history of cocaine and/or heroin use during pregnancy were observed. Infants were divided into four groups depending on their mother's drug use. These groups included a cocaine-only group, a heroin-only group, a heroin plus cocaine group, and a group whose urine tests were negative but the mother admitted to cocaine use during pregnancy. Microcephaly and growth restriction were frequent in the infants in the cocaine group (17% and 27%, respectively). Microcephaly was also significant in the heroin plus cocaine group. All groups experienced mild withdrawal symptoms, but the highest percentage of infants showing symptoms was in the heroin plus cocaine group. Furthermore, withdrawal requiring treatment also occurred most frequently in this group. The authors concluded that heroin and cocaine have a synergistic effect on the growth and development of the newborn.

Comments

This study showed an increased incidence of mild withdrawal symptoms and an increased incidence of symptoms requiring treatment in the heroin plus cocaine group. Although this

Table 5.12 Congenital malformations

Study	Method	Sample	Incidence	Results
Fulroth et al. (1989)	Comparative study	84 infants born to mothers who used different combinations of heroin and cocaine while pregnant	Infants of cocaine users showed microcephaly in 17% and growth retardation in 27%; 47% of infants born to heroin and cocaine-using mothers showed withdrawal symptoms	Highest incidence of treatment-requiring withdrawal in cocaine and heroin group, suggesting a synergistic effect

Table 5.13 Neonatal disorders

Study	Method	Sample	Incidence	Results
Reynolds et al. (2007)	Case report	2 infants	Both infants exposed in utero to maternal use of codeine-containing cough syrup: developed perinatal arterial strokes	Arterial stroke may be associated with maternal usage of codeine-containing medication

study was small in size, it does suggest that there may be a synergistic effect of cocaine and heroin with respect to the newborn's withdrawal symptoms.

Based on these findings, there seems to be an association between maternal cocaine use and microcephaly in the infant as there was an increased incidence in the cocaine group and the cocaine plus heroin group. The incidence of microcephaly in heroin-exposed infants requires further study, particularly since cocaine use was a confounder in this study (see Ch. 3).

Neonatal disorders

One paper (Reynolds et al. 2007) was reviewed that presented two case studies. Both patients were newborn infants with perinatal arterial stroke, which may have been associated with in utero exposure to codeine-containing cough syrup (Table 5.13). The authors observed that maternal opioid-containing prescription medication or illicit drug use has been identified as a known cause of perinatal arterial stroke. They suggested that codeine-containing prescription drugs used in pregnancy, such as morphine and methadone, predisposes the infant to NAS and arterial stroke.

Comments

It does seem possible that large amounts or long-term use of codeine during pregnancy could mimic the NAS seen in infants born to mothers on methadone maintenance. Although only two case studies are presented, the similar mechanism of codeine, methadone, and heroin make it feasible to warn pregnant mothers of the potential risk when using medications that contain codeine. Further studies would be needed to assess accurately the true risk of perinatal arterial stroke in infants exposed to codeine in utero.

Cardiovascular disease

Two papers were found in a PubMed search from 1988 to 2008 that describe cardiovascular pathology associated with opioid use. One studied how chronic opioid use may influence development of CAD. The other used cardiac biopsy to assess cardiac damage after clinically evident rhabdomyolysis secondary to opiate use. Three additional articles address modes of death and cardiac disease associated with opiate use and cardiac arrhythmias associated with methadone and buprenorphine.

Coronary artery disease

Marmor et al. (2004) evaluated CAD in two autopsy groups. The first group consisted of 98 decedents with methadone or opiates in their blood at autopsy. The authors made the assumption that finding opiates or methadone in the body at autopsy was an indicator of long-term exposure, which may have an effect on the coronary arteries. Hearts of 97 frequency-matched decedents without methadone or opiates in their blood were also autopsied. Severe CAD was found significantly less often in the first group (5/98) than in the second group (16/97). Using multiple logistic regression analysis, the OR when comparing those with moderate and severe CAD with those with mild or no CAD was 0.43 (95% CI 0.20–0.94) for methadone or opiate use, suggesting that long-term exposure to opiates may in some way decrease the risk of CAD.

Myocardial injury

Melandri et al. (1996) published a descriptive study of a single case report. A patient with clinically evident rhabdomyolysis secondary to opiate use underwent a cardiac biopsy to characterize any evidence of myocardial injury. The biopsy showed inflammatory changes, degenerative and necrotic muscle cells, and interstitial edema. The myocardial damage patterns were similar to damage seen with opiate overdoses complicated by muscular effort or hypoxic coma. They hypothesized that the myocardial damage was a result of rhabdomyolysis occurring after an opiate overdose and severe vascular myohypoxia.

Dressler and Roberts (1989b) examined the modes of death and the prevalence of cardiac disease in 168 autopsied hearts of opiate addicts. They found 20 major modes of death: active infective endocarditis ($n = 67$, 40%), drug overdose ($n = 39$, 24%), CAD ($n = 14$, 8%), pulmonary granulomatosis ($n = 7$, 4%), and other diseases (seven cardiac, eight noncardiac) in 41 (24%). Only 7 of the 168 hearts (4%) were considered normal. Major disease findings included active and healed infective endocarditis ($n = 80$, 48%), cardiomegaly ($n = 114$, 68%), CAD ($n = 35$, 21%), acquired valvular disease ($n = 16$, 10%), myocardial disease ($n = 14$, 8%), and congenital heart anomalies ($n = 19$, 11%). In 30 (80%) of the 35 hearts with CAD, there was severe atherosclerotic plaque and vessel narrowing. This study supports previous findings of major causes of death in opiate addicts (infectious endocarditis, drug overdose, pulmonary granulomatosis from talc); however, a major new finding was evidence of significant CAD in this sample of opiate addicts.

In 2003, the synthetic opioid levacetylmethadol used to treat heroin addiction was withdrawn from the US market because the drug lengthened the QT interval and increased the risk of torsades de pointes and lethal ventricular tachycardia. Methadone has also been found to increase the QT interval and cause torsades de pointes in susceptible individuals. With the increased use of buprenorphine for heroin substitution, the safety of this synthetic opioid has been reviewed. A case study reported by Krantz et al. (2005) described an addict who developed a prolonged QT interval and torsades de pointes when taking methadone. While being carefully monitored, the individual was switched to buprenorphine with no clinically significant change in his QT interval and no evidence of torsades de pointes.

After the safety of buprenorphine was established, Krantz *et al.* (2007) subsequently carried out a national survey, which was sent to US physicians to determine their awareness of the cardiac effects of methadone, levacetylmethadol, and buprenorphine on QT prolongation; 692 (66%) of the physicians surveyed by mail responded. Of these, 519 (75%; 95% CI 72–78) were aware that levacetylmethadol prolonged the QT interval; 284 (41%; 95% CI 37–45) were aware that methadone prolonged the QT interval; only 166 (24%) were aware that methadone use could lead to torsades de pointes ventricular arrhythmia; and 360 (52%) knew that buprenorphine was a safe alternative to methadone and did not cause torsades de pointes. Although physicians associated with programs with a large census or academic settings were more aware of methadone's effects on cardiac rhythms, fewer than 54% of these individuals were aware that methadone could cause torsades de pointes. The authors suggested that since scientific publication and prescribing information has not adequately informed physicians about torsades de pointes and opiate substitution therapy, universal education initiatives are needed to educate physicians.

These studies are summarized in Table 5.14.

Comments

Three articles describe different cardiac phenomena related to opiate use. The first makes a claim that long-term opiate use is associated with decreased severity of CAD. However, the findings of significant CAD in autopsied hearts by Dressler and Roberts (1989b) suggest that opiate use is not cardioprotective. Further epidemiological studies, including those focusing on the amount and length of chronic methadone/opiate use and incidence of severe CAD, could shed more light on this topic.

The case study by Melandri *et al.* (1996) supports the findings of articles described under Musculoskeletal diseases and Male urological diseases, above, which describe the pathology associated with rhabdomyolysis in opioid abusers, particularly in those with heroin overdoses.

The two articles by Krantz *et al.* (2005, 2007) suggest that, although the safety of buprenorphine related to prolonged QT syndrome and torsades de pointes has been studied, many physicians who prescribe opioid substitution therapy are unaware of the potential danger of using methadone in individuals susceptible to prolonged QT syndrome and torsades de pointes.

Dermatological disease

The review yielded no results concerning opioid use and dermatological disease.

Nutritional and metabolic disease

One article (Mohs *et al.* 1990) reviewed the literature for nutritional effects of abuse of marijuana, heroin and other opioids, cocaine, and nicotine (Table 5.15). Morphine was found to be associated with calcium inhibition, decreased gastrin release, hypercholesterolemia, hypothermia, and hyperthermia. Additionally, heroin addiction has been observed to cause hyperkalemia. Two nutritional states were also mentioned with reference to their impact on

Table 5.14 Cardiovascular disease

Study	Method	Sample	Incidence	Results
Marmor et al. (2004)	Retrospective study CAD and opiate use Autopsy	98 decedents with methadone/opiates in their blood at autopsy, 97 frequency-matched control decedents	Severe CAD was found in 5/98 in the methadone/opiates group vs. 16/97 in the control group	Opiates/methadone in the bloodstream may be associated with decreased CAD progression
Melandri et al. (1996)	Case report Opiates and heart damage Biopsy	Biopsy-proven myocardial damage after opiate-induced rhabdomyolysis and myohypoxia	Myocardial focal lesions formed by small mononuclear inflammatory cells with a few neutrophils, associated with degenerated and necrotic myocardial fibers, interstitial edema, and congestion of intrinsic blood vessels	Myocardial damage can occur with rhabdomyolysis and hypoxic coma caused by opiate overdose
Dressler & Roberts (1989b)	Retrospective study Cardiac death in opiate addicts	168 autopsied hearts of opiate addicts	Modes of death: 67 (40%) active infective endocarditis; 39 (24%) drug overdose; 14 (8%) CAD; 7 (4%) pulmonary granulomatosis; 41 (24%) other diseases (7 cardiac, 8 non-cardiac) Prevalence of cardiac disease: 80 (48%) active, healed endocarditis; 114 (68%) cardiomegaly; 35 (21%) CAD (85% of hearts had significant vessel narrowing); 16 (10%) acquired valvular disease; 14 (8%) myocardial disease; 19 (11%) congenital heart anomalies; 7/168 hearts considered normal	Study supports prior studies of major causes of death from opiate use: infectious endocarditis, drug overdose, pulmonary granulomatosis; new finding was significant CAD in this study
Krantz et al. (2005)	Case study ECG	Patient developing torsades de pointes on methadone	Buprenorphine substituted for methadone with no adverse effects	Buprenorphine may be safely used to prevent torsades de pointes in individuals susceptible to developing long-QT syndrome
Krantz et al. (2007)	Descriptive study Physician knowledge questionaire	1040 physicians; 692 (66%) responses	Questionaire assessed physician knowledge of effects of heroin substitutes on long-QT syndrome and torsades de pointes: 75% (95% CI 72–78) knew levacetylmethadol caused long-QT syndrome and torsades de pointes; 41% (95% CI 37–45) knew methadone caused long-QT syndrome; 24% (95% CI 21–27) knew methadone can cause torsades de pointes 52% (95% CI 48–56) knew buprenorphine not associated with long-QT syndrome	Many physicians using methadone-substitution therapy were unaware of the drug's effect on causing torsades de pointes

Table 5.15 Nutrition

Study	Method	Sample	Incidence	Results
Mohs et al. (1990)	Literature review	Articles on nutrient effects of marijuana, heroin, cocaine, nicotine	Heroin use associated with hyperkalemia; morphine use associated with calcium inhibition, impaired gastrin function, hypercholesterolemia, and hypo or hyperthermia	Specific physiological changes are observed in opiate users

morphine metabolism. First, diabetes mellitus has been shown to decrease sensitivity to and dependence on morphine. Second, vitamin D deficiency has been found to decelerate morphine dependency. Major changes in food selection and intake occur during opiate use and withdrawal. These changes have been associated with weight loss and weight gain.

Comments

There are many nutritionally related changes that occur with chronic and acute opiate use. Further epidemiological studies are needed to investigate the effects of opiate drug use on the broad spectrum of nutrient levels and to determine the efficacy of targeted nutrition strategies during drug withdrawal and rehabilitation.

Endocrine system disease

One abstract related to pituitary enlargement and opioid use (Teoh et al. 1993) in a case–control study comparing eight males with current opioid or cocaine abuse by DSM-III criteria with eight healthy male controls with no drug abuse or any indication for MRI. All cases and controls were between 26 and 33 years of age. The average length of opioid use was 7.8 ± 2.0 years and cocaine use 6.9 ± 1.4 years. Pituitary gland volumes were measured by MRI and were found to be significantly larger (730 ± 24 mm^3; $p < 0.01$) in drug-abusing individuals compared with non-drug users. The researchers suggested that the pituitary gland may enlarge prior to any evidence of abnormal pituitary function.

Abs et al. (2000) related intrathecal opioid treatment to endocrine disruption in 73 patients who received intrathecal opioids for non-malignant pain and 20 controls matched with comparable pain syndromes but not treated with opioids. In the opioid group, the serum testosterone of the 29 men was found to be significantly lower than that in the 11 control men ($p < 0.001$). The 18 postmenopausal females in the opioid group were found to have significantly lower serum luteinizing hormone ($p < 0.001$) and follicle-stimulating hormone ($p < 0.012$). Amenorrhea and disrupted menstrual cycles were observed in the 21 premenopausal members of the opioid group. Approximately 15% of those treated with opioids developed central hypocorticism and growth hormone deficiency. The authors concluded that most of the men and every woman treated with opioids demonstrated hypogonadotropic hypogonadism.

A similar study (Finch et al. 2000) observed 30 patients who were being treated for non-malignant pain with intrathecal opioids and 10 men and 10 postmenopausal women as controls. Control subjects maintained expected hormone levels. However, 10 of the men treated with opioids were observed to have lower than expected testosterone ($p = 0.0032$) and free androgen index ($p = 0.0126$). The 12 postmenopausal treated females had significantly low levels of follicle-stimulating hormone ($p = 0.0037$) and luteinizing hormone

Table 5.16 Endocrine diseases

Study	Method	Sample	Incidence	Results
Teoh et al. (1993)	Case–control study MRI	16 males (aged 26–33 years): 8 opioid/ cocaine-dependent (over 6 years), 8 healthy, non-drug users	Opioid- and cocaine-dependent men had significantly larger pituitary gland volumes (730.0 ± 24.4 mm^3) than control subjects (540.0 ± 26.6 mm^3) ($p < 0.01$)	Opiate and cocaine users may have enlarged pituitaries prior to developing abnormal pituitary function
Abs et al. (2000)	Case–control study	29 males and 44 females treated with intrathecal opioids, 11 male and 9 female controls	Treated males: 25 low serum testosterone ($p < 0.001$); 20 low serum LH levels ($p < 0.001$) Treated females: 18 postmenopausal females with low serum LH ($p < 0.001$) and FSH ($p < 0.012$); 21 premenopausal females with disrupted menstrual cycles Male and female 15% developed central hypocorticism and GH deficiency	Number of subjects treated with intrathecal opioids that developed hypogonadotropic hypogonadism suggests association
Finch et al. (2000)	Case–control study	30 patients receiving intrathecal opioid treatment; 20 controls matched with similar pain but no opioid treatment	Treated males: 10 with low serum testosterone ($p = 0.0032$) and free androgen index ($p = 0.0126$) Treated postmenopausal females: 12 with low serum FSH ($p = 0.0037$) and LH ($p = 0.0024$)	Hypogonadotropic hypogonadism is a complication of intrathecal opioid treatment

FSH, follicle-stimulating hormone; GH, growth hormone; LH, luteinizing hormone; MRI, magnetic resonance imaging.

($p = 0.0024$). The authors concluded that this, paired with lower levels of pituitary gonadotropins, demonstrated an association between this form of opioid treatment and hypogonadotropic hypogonadism.

These studies are summarized in Table 5.16.

Comments

While Teoh et al. (1993) did find a larger pituitary gland in cocaine- and heroin-abusing subjects, there are a number of questions that must be answered in order to properly interpret this study. Is a larger pituitary gland clinically significant? Is any hormone dysfunction associated with this enlarged pituitary? Is the size of the pituitary a result of the drug use or is it antecedent to drug use? Since both cocaine and heroin were used by those with larger pituitaries, it would be important to determine whether each drug or concurrent use of both drugs leads to pituitary enlargement. Finally, it is also relevant to know whether the pituitary decreases in size with discontinuation of drug use. This study's sample size was small; a larger study should be conducted to ensure an accurate representation of the larger populations represented by these samples.

Both of the studies concerning hypogonadism found similar results. Within the context of intrathecal opioid treatment, there has been an association demonstrated with hormonal disruption. However, these two observational studies had relatively small populations and the effects observed were relatively mild and limited. What significance such hypogonadism might have within the context of illicit opioid abuse over various periods of time is not discernable at this point.

Immune system disease

Eisenstein *et al.* (2006), in a literature review, focused upon the effect of opioids on the immune system and indicated that there is much evidence in the literature that morphine is immunosuppressive when associated with acute injection. However, they noted that there are fewer studies looking at the effect of subacute or chronic morphine administration. The authors also comment on another important aspect of morphine use, tolerance, and noted that the immune system effect of morphine does, in some but not all cases, show evidence of tolerance. However, their focus was primarily on the effect of morphine withdrawal on the immune system. They found 10 studies that looked at this, which can be summarized as follows: immunosuppression was evident with drug withdrawal and recovery time to baseline immune status varied, although immunosuppression lasted up to three years in the one identified human study. Studies have shown that morphine exposure can sensitize the body to bacterial lipopolysaccharide, thus increasing the risk for sepsis. Morphine exposure had been shown to depress the hypothalamic–pituitary–adrenal axis and may be involved in immunosuppression.

A recent review article by Sacerdote (2008) described findings from both human and animal studies on the immunosuppressant effects of opioids. Morphine is associated with a depression of both natural and acquired immunity and has been found to alter pathways regulating immune function. However, animal studies suggest that not all opioids have the same effect on the immune system. For example, fentanyl has been found to depress immune function, but the synthetic buprenorphine has little effect on the immune system. The author suggested that more clinical studies are needed, particularly since adverse effects of opioids prescribed for the elderly and immunocompromised patients can have deleterious effects.

These two publications are summarized in Table 5.17.

Comments

The review by Eisenstein *et al.* (2006) complements the study of Li *et al.* (2002) in providing support for morphine-induced immunosuppression. It also indicates areas for further study: there is a need to study subacute and chronic effects, as opposed to acute effects, of morphine exposure on the immune system and to examine the effect of morphine withdrawal. It is expected that, to some extent, withdrawal is quite common among morphine users and that these users are also at risk for exposure to infectious agents, especially HIV. Looking at the drug-using population as a whole, the effect of morphine withdrawal-induced immunosuppression may be larger than that of which we are currently aware. The review by Sacerdote (2008) highlighted the role of opioids in immunosuppression and encouraged further research on the effects of each of the opioids since immune responses vary with the drugs.

Table 5.17 Opioids and the immune system

Study	Method	Sample	Incidence	Results
Eisenstein et al. (2006)	Literature review	Focus on morphine withdrawal and effect on immune system	10 studies found immunosuppression lasted as long as 3 years after drug cessation; morphine also can predispose to bacterial sepsis and alteration of hypothalamic–pituitary–adrenal axis's role in immunity	Studies of acute drug injection indicate that morphine is immunosuppressive; studies of subacute or chronic injection of morphine on immune function are limited and have variable results; there are even fewer studies of withdrawal effects on immune function
Sacerdote (2008)	Literature review	Articles related to opioid effect on immunosuppression	Morphine depresses both natural and acquired immune function; animal studies suggest that not all opioids have the same effect on immune function (fentanyl depresses; buprenorphine has little effect)	More clinical studies needed to determine effect of opioids on immune function

Environmental disease

The review yielded no relevant results.

Other pathological conditions

The review yielded no relevant results.

Opioids: summary and overview

The following section provides a brief synthesis of the material on opioids and medical illness outlined above. The strongest evidence is included, as well as interesting papers that, although small in size or weak in design, may provide ideas for future research.

Infections

Overall association: supported by some evidence

Infectious complications secondary to opiate use include bacterial endocarditis and nasopharyngeal mycosis, the latter related to intranasal heroin use. Both of these, however, may be the result of the delivery of the drug as opposed to the drug itself. In the case of intravenous heroin use, evidence of infective endocarditis was found in a majority of the decedents studied. Presumably this results from the introduction of bacteria into the bloodstream. Similarly, the use of narcotics intranasally prior to the onset of nasopharyngeal mycosis and invasive rhinosinusitis raises the strong possibility that the route of delivery is related to the development of the infection as well as any toxic effect of the opioids.

One small basic science research project found that methadone increased HIV transmission and worsened viral burden in vitro. Given that HIV is a common problem in intravenous drug users, and methadone is a common form of maintenance treatment, this finding is certainly of concern. Further research into this interaction could shed light on how methadone enhances viral activation and replication. At this time, however, there is no evidence that these results occur in vivo, nor are there any recommendations to modify the treatment program of methadone-maintained patients with HIV.

Musculoskeletal disease

Rhabdomyolysis

Overall association: supported by strong evidence

Opiate overdose is a well-known risk factor for the development of symptomatic rhabdomyolysis. Sequelae of this complication are varied. The most common findings from this literature search show adverse effects on the musculoskeletal and renal systems, although a case of myocardial hypoxia related to rhabdomyolysis was described under Cardiovascular disease. Rhabdomyolysis secondary to intravenous heroin overdose was shown to cause a compartment syndrome, with resultant paralysis, swelling, tenderness, and absent reflexes. There are several references documenting the development of ARF from the rhabdomyolysis as well, which is perhaps expected from the known nephrotoxic effect of myoglobin. Pathological changes in opioid-induced rhabodmyolysis show a pattern of acute tubular necrosis. Other renal changes have been documented secondary to opiate abuse, but the mechanisms of these injuries are unclear. They are often in the setting of polysubstance abuse and comorbidities (HIV, hepatitis) and, therefore, cannot be specifically tied to the opioid itself.

Respiratory system disease

Further epidemiology studies are needed to determine the specific role of the opioids in the respiratory conditions.

Asthma

Overall association: supported by some evidence

Inhaled heroin does seem to have an association with severe asthma exacerbation. The mechanism of this association is unclear, however, and the inhaled heroin may simply trigger an exacerbation in someone who is already predisposed (one who has baseline moderate/ severe asthma), or it may trigger an asthma attack through bronchial hypersensitivity to the heroin. It also seems to worsen chronic wheezing and bronchial reactivity. Higher levels of inhaled heroin use in those asthmatics who require intensive care also suggests that inquiring about drug use is a key historical piece that should be emphasized in this patient population. Co-use of heroin and codeine was associated with bronchial dysfunction; however, the use of both drugs and wheezing needs to be studied further to determine whether co-use is synergistic or whether only one of the drugs is likely to trigger wheezing.

Non-cardiac pulmonary edema and respiratory depression

Overall association: supported by some evidence

Another respiratory condition, non-cardiac pulmonary edema, was reported in two case studies. Because of the lack of other obvious causes, these instances were thought to be caused by heroin overdose or buprenorphine administration. No further research has substantiated this risk or suggested a mechanistic cause. Respiratory depression has also been reported in a perioperative patient receiving an opioid (buprenorphine) epidurally and a non-steroidal anti-inflammatory drug (intramuscular ketorolac).

Nervous system disease

Seizures

Overall association: supported by some evidence

Opioids in general may increase the risk of seizure when used recreationally. This is documented most convincingly with studies involving tramadol, which when abused seems to approximately double the incidence of seizure when compared with patients who do not abuse tramadol. Heroin is normally not considered to be one of the more common drugs associated with seizures. In spite of this, the presence of seizure in a patient prescribed tramadol (or perhaps other opioids) should certainly raise the clinician's suspicion that the drug has been taken in excess. More epidemiological studies are needed to determine the prevalence of seizures in opioid users who are not abusing other drugs.

Cerebral/cerebellar dysfunction

Overall association: supported by some evidence

Several studies were reported that described the negative effect of inhaled heroin on cerebral and cerebellar function. Cavitational cerebellar damage, spongiform encephalopathy, and ischemic stroke have been described in the recent literature reviewed. More epidemiological studies are needed to determine the risk of cerebral and cerebellar disease associated with opioid use.

Ocular disease

Strabismus

Overall association: supported by some evidence

Opiate use does seem to have an association with adult and infant strabismus, although the mechanism of this association is unknown. The finding of a 10-fold increase in the incidence of strabismus in infants born to opiate-dependent mothers is a significant statistic. It is not known at this time if screening this population is cost-effective or even if interventions are effective. Case studies have also documented acute-onset strabismus in adults following heroin intake, methadone intake, and opiate withdrawal. However, more studies are needed to determine whether strabismus is more likely to occur in individuals with poor binocular function prior to drug use.

Ocular candidiasis

Overall association: supported by some evidence

In addition to strabismus, intravenous administration of high-dose buprenorphine intended for sublingual use put some patients at risk for fungal infections, which were manifested with ocular complaints (blurry vision, floaters). It appears that the solvents used to dissolved drugs can be as dangerous as the drugs themselves. Contaminated lemon juice, for example, has been associated with ocular fungal infections as well as systemic fungal disease. To what extent solvent contamination is the cause of some infections seen in drug users is an area for further research.

Male urological disease

Rhabdomyolysis

Overall association: supported by strong evidence

Rhabdomyolysis was the major cause of renal disease in opioid drugs users described in this review, but other abused drugs are also known to be related to rhabdomyolysis and the onset of renal failure.

Renal pathology: male and female

Overall association: supported by some evidence

Some drug abusers also experienced renal pathology, which may have been related to the toxic effects of the drug or the solvents used for injection: nephrotic syndrome; acute tubular necrosis; and hypertension with renal dysfunction. Further research would be helpful to determine the risk of nephrotic disease in the opioid drug user.

Female genital and neonatal/congenital disorders

Fetal growth

Overall association: supported by some evidence

Opiate effects on pregnancy are well documented. Heroin has been found to negatively impact fetal growth including decreasing birthweight, limiting intrauterine growth, and decreasing head circumference and body length. These outcomes may be exacerbated by concurrent maternal opioid and cocaine use. Opioid replacement therapy has been the mainstay of therapy for addicted mothers, and there is good evidence that methadone has less-deleterious effects on fetal growth than does ongoing heroin use.

Neonatal abstinence syndrome

Overall association: supported by strong evidence

Infants born to mothers who use opioids, methadone or heroin, are subject to classic withdrawal symptoms, which are collectively termed "neonatal abstinence syndrome" (NAS). Treatment typically involves weaning the newborn with morphine. The severity of NAS is determined by Finnegan scores and the amount of morphine needed to control the newborn's hyperarousal. From the literature reviewed, there is some debate regarding the ideal maternal therapy to reduce the severity of NAS in the newborn. Historically, methadone has been the mainstay of treatment. A newer agent for treating opioid addiction, buprenorphine, has started to be used as a maintenance therapy for pregnant women. Only one paper compared the severity of NAS in methadone and buprenorphine groups. It showed that buprenorphine does appear to be a viable alternative to methadone, as it effectively reduced symptoms of NAS. Larger studies with direct comparison between methadone and buprenorphine could serve to resolve this debate regarding the most effective maintenance therapy in opiate-addicted pregnant women.

Congenital disease and perinatal stroke

Overall association: supported by some evidence

The effect of opioid use on neonatal outcomes suggests that opioid-exposed infants are small for gestational age and experience more prematurity. However, many of the studies reviewed failed to consider other factors that can affect infant outcomes, including adequate prenatal care, nutritional status of the pregnant opioid user, polydrug abuse, and use of alcohol and cigarettes. These factors, particularly alcohol and cigarette use, have been shown to increase risk of prematurity and delivery of infants who are small for gestational age. The difficulty in controlling the prenatal environment will continue to challenge the findings of many pregnancy and postnatal studies

Cardiovascular disease

Coronary artery disease

Overall association: supported by some evidence

Although one study suggested that opioids had a protective effect on coronary vessels, another larger study of autopsied hearts showed significant cardiovascular disease in opioid users. The study describing the modes of death and prevalence of cardiac disease highlighted the possible damage to the cardiovascular system when opioids are used. Further epidemiological studies are needed to determine the risk of CAD in the opioid abuser.

Torsades de pointes

Overall association: supported by some evidence

Torsades de pointes is a known lethal consequence of methadone's effect on lengthening the QT interval in susceptible individuals. Of concern is a reported study based on a survey of US physicians indicating less than 50% of the responders knew that methadone prolonged the QT interval and could lead to torsades de pointes. Slightly more than half knew that buprenorphine was a safe alternative to methadone and that buprenorphine did not prolong the QT interval or cause torsades de pointes.

Nutritional and metabolic disease

Overall association: supported by some evidence

A paucity of epidemiological studies on nutritional status and nutrient excess or deficits was found in the PubMed literature reviewed. Although morphine use altered calcium and serum lipid levels, no studies were found that addressed parathyroid or thyroid function, gastrin dysfunction, or triglycerides and hyperlipidemia. Additionally, heroin may be related to elevated serum potassium levels. Further epidemiological studies are needed to address nutritional status of the opioid abuser and risks of adverse nutrient effects related to drug use.

Endocrine disease

Pituitary dysfunction

Overall association: supported by some evidence

Three studies were found that addressed endocrine function in opioid drug users, although, as indicated above, some opioids have been found to affect gastrin release.

One study identified an enlarged pituitary gland in eight opioid and cocaine abusers. Why these individuals were studied and whether there were any altered pituitary hormone levels preceding the MRI studies is unclear. Two studies were found that relate opioid use to hypogonadotropic hypogonadism, but only within the context of intrathecal treatment for chronic pain. However, larger studies with individuals abusing a variety of opioids and comparing the findings to those in non-drug users may be helpful in determining the risk of pituitary dysfunction in the opioid-using population.

Immune system disease

Overall association: supported by some evidence

Few epidemiological studies of the immune system have been reported in the PubMed literature during the past 20 years. Only two review articles were found, and both addressed the immunosuppressant effects of morphine. One review also indicated that morphine may depress the hypothalamic–pituitary–adrenal axis; however, this was not addressed in the opioid-endocrine related findings. Sacerdote (2008) suggested that the opioids vary in their ability to affect immune function. Buprenorphine, for example, appears to have little effect on the immune system, while morphine and fentanyl both depress immune function. Since many of the opioids may be used in the elderly, individuals with chronic pain, and immunocompromised individuals, more epidemiological studies demonstrating risk for infections or increased evidence of malignancy would be helpful in understanding opioid effects on the immune system.

Research concerns

There are many opportunities for further research on the effects of opiates on physical health. Most of the studies were relatively small case reports and series, case–control studies, and retrospective chart reviews. Very few studies indicated the OR or RR values for assertions that certain disorders are associated with opioid use. Prospective studies, cohort and cross-sectional studies, and randomized controlled trials are necessary in order to show whether it is the drug in question that is associated with a dysfunction, and not confounders such as polydrug use, alcohol and cigarette use, nutritional status, socioeconomic status, or other comorbidities.

Many of the studies reviewed could be strengthened by replication studies involving larger sample sizes and in various clinical settings. In this way, the results could be generalized and decisions could start to be made on how new information should affect patient management. It will be valuable for the clinician to be aware of those disorders mentioned in this chapter in order to recognize them when they develop. Further, some of the stronger associations might be investigated in asymptomatic patients who are known opioid users. For these common associations, and also for potentially serious complications that arise

Table 5.18 Opioid summary

Body system	Topic and evidence of association
Infections	Abscesses and cellulitis (some), pulmonary infection (some), bacterial endocarditis (some), invasive rhinosinusitis (some)
Neoplastic	None
Musculoskeletal	Rhabdomyolysis (strong)
Digestive	None
Stomatognathic	None
Respiratory	Asthma (some), non-cardiogenic pulmonary edema (some), respiratory depression (some)
Otorhinolaryngological	None
Nervous	Seizures (some), cerebral/cerebellar dysfunction (some)
Ocular	Strabismus (some), ocular candidiasis (some)
Urological	Renal disease with rhabdomyolysis (strong), other renal pathology (some)
Female reproductive and congenital/neonatal	Fetal growth restriction (some), placental changes (some), neonatal abstinence syndrome (strong), congenital disease (some), perinatal stroke (some)
Cardiovascular	Coronary artery disease (some), infective endocarditis (some), torsades de pointes and ventricular tachycardia (methadone) (strong)
Dermatological	None
Nutritional and metabolic	Calcium inhibition, decreased release gastrin, hypercholesterolemia, hypo- and hyperthermia, hyperkalemia (all some)
Endocrine	Pituitary enlargement, hormone alteration (some)
Immune	Immunosuppression (some)
Environment	None
Other pathologies	None

from opiate abuse, it may be economically sound to initiate screening or early intervention programs. Much more needs to be done before this claim can be made. Nevertheless, the ultimate goal would be the prevention of these medical illnesses in order to achieve a true reduction in the burden of disease.

Table 5.18 summarizes the association of opioids with research covering various body systems described in this chapter. The "Topic" column indicates the condition described, followed by the rating for the evidence of association in parentheses. The term "strong" suggests that there is a significant body of knowledge supporting a direct or indirect association between opioids and the condition (e.g., a significant number of studies, cohort or case–controlled studies, clinical laboratory studies, or a single seminal study). "Strong" suggests the clinician may find this condition in an opioid user. "Some" suggests that there are some studies supporting a direct or indirect association between opioids and the condition (e.g., a smaller number of studies, case–control or case reports, or a study reporting a rare or under-reported condition). In many cases, "some" suggests more evidence is needed to support a strong association with a condition.

Results: hallucinogens, stimulants, and barbiturates

Introduction

Amphetamines

Alpha-Methylphenethylamine (amphetamine, Adderall, Dexedrine), the prototypical phenylethylamine, exerts profound stimulatory effects on the CNS as well as exerting effects on peripheral alpha- and beta-adrenergic receptors. N-Methyl-O-phenylisopropylamine (methamphetamine, Desoxyn) is produced from the amphetamine molecule by the addition of a second methyl group, which serves to increase both lipophilicity and CNS activity of the drug. These drugs exist as both dextro- and levo- stereoisomers, with the former conferring far greater CNS stimulation. Given that the vast majority of studies included for review here explore the relationship between methamphetamine use and the risk for various health problems, the following introduction will focus on providing background solely on this drug.

Methamphetamine was first synthesized in the early 1900s and was widely disseminated to military personnel during World War II for the prevention and reversal of fatigue. By the 1950s, the drug was being used legitimately as treatment for a number of medical conditions including obesity and narcolepsy. Given the drug's desirable euphoric, stimulant, and anorectic effects, within the next decade methamphetamine was being produced in clandestine laboratories for recreational purposes. Since the 1980s, crystal methamphetamine (methamphetamine hydrochloride) use has become increasingly prevalent, initially on the west coast of the USA and now across North America. Users prefer this smokable form of methamphetamine for its increased potency and immediate effects. Methamphetamine has been classified as a Schedule II controlled substance since 1971.

In the CNS, acute administration of methamphetamine stimulates release of monoamine neurotransmitters (dopamine, serotonin, norepinephrine) from storage sites in nerve terminals, thereby increasing levels of these neurotransmitters. This results in feelings of increased alertness, diminished need for sleep, locomotor stimulation, euphoria (at high doses), and anorexia. Long-term administration preferentially affects dopaminergic neurotransmission, primarily in the striatum, resulting in diminished levels of dopamine, reduced dopamine transporter density, and decreased activity of the enzyme tyrosine hydroxylase, which is integral to dopamine synthesis. This results in impairments in both cognitive and motor function.

Methamphetamine also stimulates the cardiovascular system via the release of norepinephrine and dopamine from peripheral adrenergic receptors. This results in tachycardia and vasoconstriction, with an end result of reduction of cardiovascular oxygen supply. Methamphetamine has also been shown to exert cardiotoxic effects that are independent of catecholamine excess. Further, concurrent use of alcohol, cocaine, and opioids exacerbates cardiotoxic effects of methamphetamine.

Peak methamphetamine plasma concentration is observed two to three hours after oral administration and within 30 minutes of intravenous administration. The duration of action may be up to 20 hours. Methamphetamine is metabolized primarily by hepatic oxidative metabolism, primarily through the cytochrome P450 2D6 isoenzyme. The elimination half-life is approximately 10 hours and is pH dependent.

Given the effect of methamphetamine on dopamine neurotransmission and dopamine's role in reinforcement and reward, chronic methamphetamine use is highly addicting. Withdrawal symptoms include fatigue, irritability, anxiety, depression, and intense hunger. Methamphetamine toxicity primarily manifests in the CNS as agitation, anxiety, and hallucinations. Acute episodes of psychosis have been observed in both healthy methamphetamine users and those with pre-existing mental illness. Toxicity also manifests in the cardiovascular system as tachycardia, palpitations, and chest pain.

3,4-Methylenedioxymethamphetamine

MDMA is a ring-substituted amphetamine derivative that is structurally similar to methamphetamine. First synthesized in the early 1900s, MDMA was briefly used as an adjunct to psychotherapy in the 1970s and by the end of the decade MDMA or "ecstasy" was being used recreationally. It exerts a combination of effects including psychostimulation, euphoria, and hallucinogenesis; however, it is unique among stimulants and hallucinogens for its ability to produce feelings of empathy and closeness with others. MDMA is a white, tasteless powder typically ingested orally in tablets containing 50 to 150 mg of drug. MDMA is a racemic mixture: the levo-isomer is primarily responsible for the stimulant and empathic effects and the dextro-isomer is associated with the hallucinogenic effects. Since 1985, MDMA has been classified as a Schedule I controlled substance. It continues to be widely used internationally and in the USA among young drug users, particularly those participating in rave parties and techno-club dance circuits. According to the National Survey on Drug Use and Health (US Substance Abuse and Mental Health Services 2007), lifetime use continues to increase, with 5% of the US population reporting MDMA use in 2006.

MDMA use significantly affects many facets of CNS serotonergic neurotransmission both acutely and chronically. Acutely, there are three major effects: stimulation of serotonin release, inhibition of serotonin reuptake, and inhibition of serotonin metabolism by monoamine oxidase. Together, these result in increased serotonergic neurotransmission, which manifests as elevated mood and euphoria. Long-term effects of MDMA include the inhibition of tryptophan hydroxylase, the rate-limiting enzyme of serotonin synthesis, and the overall increased consumption of serotonin. Together, these effects result in decreased serotonergic neurotransmission. Serotonergic neurotoxicity is most prominent in the striatum, hippocampus, and prefrontal cortex and is thought to manifest as cognitive impairments, including memory deficits and psychiatric diseases such as depression and anxiety.

In addition to its profound effects on serotonin, MDMA also facilitates the release and inhibits the reuptake of dopamine and norepinephrine through its interactions with membrane transporters and storage systems. It has been shown to increase secretion of a number of hormones including cortisol, prolactin, oxytocin, dehydroepiandrosterone, and antidiuretic hormone. It is believed that the MDMA-induced secretion of oxytocin plays an integral role in the prosocial effects of MDMA use.

Peak MDMA plasma concentration and peak effect are observed one to two hours after administration and return to baseline four to six hours after administration. MDMA is metabolized by hepatic oxidative metabolism. The elimination half-life is eight to nine hours for a typical 100 mg dose and up to 20% of a dose is excreted unchanged in the urine.

Chronic MDMA use can be addictive, with some users meeting the diagnostic criteria for dependence. Withdrawal symptoms include fatigue, depression, anorexia, and difficulty concentrating. MDMA toxicity exists along a continuum. Mild intoxication may commonly manifest with palpitations, hyper-reflexia, nausea, and restlessness, while severe intoxication includes symptoms such as cardiac arrhythmias, muscle rigidity, hepatotoxicity, hyperthermia, and seizures.

Benzodiazepines

Substances classified as benzodiazepines are among the most prescribed medications in the USA today. They are a group of depressants that are therapeutic for a wide range of maladies including anxiety, insomnia, seizures, and withdrawal syndromes. The effectiveness and relative safety of benzodiazepines have led to their common clinical usage and public availability. Undoubtedly, such widespread presence contributes to their illicit use and abuse. However, medications such as diazepam or alprazolam are rarely the sole substance of choice for recreational users. Rather, it is common for benzodiazepines to be taken in combination with other drugs or alcohol to enhance sedation or to counteract stimulants.

The benzodiazepines derive their name from a shared chemical structure, which includes both a benzene and a diazepine ring. The group consists of multiple drugs that are typically organized by half-lives. Those considered short acting have a half-life of six hours or less and include clorazepate, halazepam, flurazepam, triazolam, and midazolam. Those with half-lives longer than six hours, but no longer than 24 hours, include chlordiazepoxide, temazepam, oxazepam, lorazepam, alprazolam, estazolam, and flunitrazepam. Finally, those with longer elimination periods include diazepam and quazepam. However, the duration of each drug's effect does not necessarily correspond with half-life. This is determined by the unique enzymatic processing of each into its active internal metabolite (von Mondach 2005).

The general effect of a benzodiazepine is depression of the CNS, though not to the same extent as the barbiturates. After oral or intravenous administration, benzodiazepines undergo modification by enzymes of the cytochrome P450 family. The active metabolites are rapidly absorbed by the brain and perfused organs and redistributed to other organs, muscle, and fat. Once the benzodiazepine metabolites circulate through the CNS, they modulate inhibitory signaling by acting upon neurotransmitter receptors that are sensitive to gamma-aminobutyric acid (GABA). They specifically target $GABA_A$ receptors, which form an integral membrane chloride channel when activated and contribute to the inhibitory signaling. While barbiturates act directly on $GABA_A$ receptors, benzodiazepines affect them indirectly by interacting with GABA itself. Therefore, the presence of GABA moderates the ionotropic effect of benzodiazepines. These interactions and eventual binding to $GABA_A$ receptors by benzodiazepines can be interrupted by chemical antagonists, such as flumazenil. Clinically, these antagonists can be used to negate unwanted benzodiazepine influence in some circumstances.

The physiological effects of $GABA_A$-receptor activation are dose dependent and can range from anxiolytic effects to total sedation. Depression of the CNS eventually leads the user through degrees of sleepiness and a lack of motor skill coordination. Benzodiazepines are often used medically for their anesthetic ability; however, they are not strong enough to replace general anesthesia. They are also capable of crossing the placental barrier and can be passed to the neonate through breast milk. If taken over time, it is possible for the user to develop a tolerance to the calming effects of the drug, which will lead toward dependence if not managed correctly. This dependence, in turn, will cause discomfort and withdrawal when use of the drug is prevented. Therefore, benzodiazepines are listed under Schedule IV of the Controlled Substances Act.

Barbiturates

The barbiturates are a collection of drugs that have been utilized for their sedative effects since the beginning of the twentieth century. Their prescription and use has fallen off markedly since the late 1970s because of the introduction of benzodiazepines. The barbiturates have slowly been replaced in the medical world, and in the illicit market by extension, because benzodiazepines perform similar functions with less risk of overdose, dependence, and abuse.

The barbiturates consist of a wide variety of drugs, all derived from barbituric acid (2,4,6-trioxohexahydropyrimidine). Barbituric acid is inert, but the addition and combination of functional groups allows for a variety of active substances. Like the benzodiazepines, they are often classified by half-lives. Short-acting barbiturates include methohexital and thiopental and affect the user for a matter of minutes. Intermediate barbiturates include amobarbital, butabarbital, and many others. Phenobarbital and mephobarbital are examples of long-lasting barbiturates and take a day or longer to metabolize. These substances in various doses depress the CNS in degrees from analgesia to general anesthesia. Unlike benzodiazepines, barbiturates may also create euphoric effects in some circumstances, which enhance the risk for abuse (von Mondach 2005).

The CNS depressive effect results from barbiturate interactions with $GABA_A$ receptors. GABA is a primary inhibitory neurotransmitter in humans and barbiturates encourage the activity of GABA as well as enhance its effects on cells of the CNS. This potentiation of inhibitory signals is similar to, but distinct from, benzodiazepine mechanisms. It is also believed that barbiturates block excitatory signals by preventing the stimulation of α-amino-3-hydroxyl-5-methyl-4-isoxazole-propionate (AMPA) receptors. Therefore, stimulation is prevented and inhibition is strengthened, resulting in a depressed state (von Mondach 2005).

With the exception of a few barbiturates that have antiepileptic capabilities, the pharmaceutical use of barbiturates is limited. Before any beneficial analgesic or anxiolytic effect is reached, the drug's hypnotic effects prevail. Given this, barbiturates are medically impractical relative to benzodiazepines. Additionally, barbiturates are subject to both psychological and metabolic tolerance. Psychological tolerance occurs more rapidly and increases the risk of barbiturate poisoning. Tolerance to barbiturates may also increase the user's tolerance to other CNS depressants such as alcohol. It is because of these risks that barbiturates have been fading from medical use and their availability for illicit use has decreased.

Lysergic acid diethylamide

In 1938 LSD was first synthesized by Dr. Albert Hofmann while he was working as a chemist for the Sandoz Corporation in Basel, Switzerland. He was experimenting with lysergic acid compounds derived from ergot, a type of fungus that grows on grasses and oats, when he accidentally absorbed a dose of LSD and after further tests experienced its full hallucinogenic effect.

The use of LSD as a recreational drug increased with the counter-culture movement of the 1960s and 1970s, where its "mind-expanding" effects were emphasized. Over time, LSD has taken multiple street names including "acid," "blotter acid," "window pane," "cid," "dots," and "mellow yellow." It is usually ingested orally and is sold in tablet or capsule form. Commonly, a single dose (varying from 50 to 300 μg) of LSD is absorbed on to stamp-sized blotter paper, which may contain elaborate decoration to advertize its effects. At less than five or ten dollars per dose, LSD is relatively inexpensive when compared with other illicit drugs. It is colorless, odorless, and many times more potent than other hallucinogens such as mescaline. Unlike psychedelic mushrooms, samples of LSD sold on the street are reliably potent (von Mondach 2005).

Like MDMA, LSD exerts its effect because of its high affinity for serotonin ($5\text{-}HT_2$) receptors in the nervous system. Different hallucinogens have affinities for different sub-units of the $5\text{-}HT_2$ receptor and the potency of each is correlated to this affinity. LSD is also known to interact with different receptor subtypes in minimal concentrations. It is not known how this combination of interactions accounts for the unique characteristics of LSD (von Mondach 2005).

The effects of LSD, like most hallucinogens, are extremely unpredictable. LSD is rapidly absorbed, with effects beginning 40 to 60 minutes after ingestion and, depending on dose, lasting as long as 12 hours. Experiences vary between users, and individual experiences of a single user depend upon mood, personality, and environment. Physical effects include dilation of pupils, sweating, salivation, lacrimation, sleeplessness, and increases in pulse and blood pressure. Perceptions become distorted and are sometimes accompanied by feelings of elation, depression, arousal, paranoia, or panic. Visual distortion is the most pronounced, with vivid colors and altered shapes. In dark environments or with eyes closed, visions persist. Users also tend to focus attention on unusual details and patterns while intoxicated. In many cases, users will experience crossing of senses, where colors are heard and sounds are seen (von Mondach 2005).

There is no supporting evidence for any possible therapeutic uses of LSD. There are both short- and long-term adverse consequences. In the short term, users may experience a "bad trip" in which hallucinations may accompany severe anxiety or intense depression. Visual disturbances may be accompanied by suicidal thoughts. Although there are no documented accounts of fatalities simply from intoxication, deaths resulting from suicide or trauma as a result of a bad trip can occur shortly after LSD intoxication. Such reactions may require medical intervention in order to calm the user down or manage the user's reaction with reassurance through "talking down" techniques. A possible long-term effect of LSD use is hallucinogen-persisting perception disorder (HPPD), also known as "flashbacks." This disorder occurs in a small proportion of former users up to decades after LSD ingestion has ceased and largely consists of visual disturbances, which include flashes of color, after-images, and peripheral disturbance. These HPPD attacks may be precipitated by mood, environment, and marijuana or alcohol intoxication. The disorder may represent permanent damage or changes to the user's visual system.

Unlike other illicit substances, LSD has little addictive potential. Persistent and repeated use of LSD is uncommon and no withdrawal syndrome has been documented, but tolerance to behavioral effects of LSD does occur after multiple uses. Trends in LSD use have fluctuated over time and it currently appears to be on the wane in today's recreational drug use culture. However, LSD use still occurs in "rave culture" and in combination with other drugs on a limited basis. LSD is listed as a Schedule I substance and monitored in compliance with the Controlled Substances Act.

Infections

No evidence was found in a PubMed search indicating a correlation between hallucinogen, barbiturate, or benzodiazepine use and bacterial or viral infection. However, the search revealed publications examining the relationship between microorganisms and stimulant use, including two case–control studies and a large data analysis. These focused on users of methamphetamine, with the case studies focusing on bacterial infections among methamphetamine users. To date there are no studies examining the relationship between other infectious agents and stimulant use.

Amphetamines

Cohen *et al.* (2007) conducted a case–control investigation to evaluate the relationship between self-reported methamphetamine use and methicillin-resistant *S. aureus* (MRSA) skin and soft tissue infections. The study took place in a community with a large rural population in Georgia, USA. Other risk factors for MRSA skin and soft tissue infection were also assessed. Overall, MRSA was cultured from over two-thirds of all skin and soft tissue infection. Methamphetamine use was reported in nearly 10% of these MRSA positive infections. More patients with MRSA skin and soft tissue infections reported recent methamphetamine use than controls (AOR 5.10; 95% CI 1.55–16.79). No difference in MRSA strain or susceptibility was observed between users and non-users. These MRSA-positive skin and soft tissue infections did not appear to be related to intravenous methamphetamine use as most users reportedly smoked or inhaled the drug.

In the second case–control study, Schafer *et al.* (2006) examined a community-wide pertussis outbreak in Jackson County, Oregon, USA in 2003. The authors sought to identify risk factors for pertussis infection in adults. Confirmed cases were strictly defined and reported to public health authorities. Five overlapping clusters (135 reported cases of pertussis) were recognized. One of these clusters comprised a group of methamphetamine users. However, methamphetamine use was not shown to be a significant independent risk factor for pertussis infection in adults.

Cooper *et al.* (2007) performed an analysis of hospital discharge data contained within the Centers for Disease Control and Prevention National Hospital Discharge Survey Database. The authors used two algorithms – one designed for sensitivity and the other for specificity – to identify cases of IDU-related infective endocarditis. An analysis of the temporal patterns of these cases showed a substantial increase in IDU-related infective endocarditis discharges during 2002–2003; the IDU-related infective endocarditis discharges among the HIV/AIDS population decreased during the study period. Citing an increase in the number of methamphetamine treatment admissions, the stability in treatment admissions for cocaine use and the similar effect of both drugs on the myocardium, the authors hypothesized that the observed increase in IDU-related infective endocarditis may be partly caused by increasing methamphetamine use.

These studies are summarized in Table 6.1.

Comments

The relationship between stimulants and bacterial infections has yet to be well described. Existing work focuses on methamphetamine use. Only one study was designed with the

Table 6.1 Methamphetamine use and bacterial infection

Study	Method	Sample	Incidence	Results
Cohen *et al.* (2007)	Case–control study MRSA skin and soft tissue infections and methamphetamine use	119 with culture-confirmed SSTI, 283 controls	MRSA isolated from 81/119 with SSTI; methamphetamine use in last 3 months reported by 8/81 (10%) and 5/283 (2%) controls; recent methamphetamine use more likely in patients with MRSA SSTI than controls (AOR 5.10; 95% CI 1.55–16.79)	There is an association between MRSA SSTIs and recent methamphetamine use
Schafer *et al.* (2006)	Case–control study Risk factors (including illicit drug use) for reported pertussis infection	135 confirmed cases of pertussis in 1-year period: of eligible adults, 20 cases and 40 matched controls	Three overlapping clusters of cases identified: one cluster involved a jail population linked to methamphetamine users Methamphetamine/illicit drug use was not identified as a risk factor for illness	Cases of pertussis infection cluster in diverse populations; these populations may include methamphetamine users; methamphetamine use is not an independent risk factor for pertussis infection
Cooper *et al.* (2007)	Data analysis of CDC National Hospital Discharge Database Prevalence of IDU-related IE	IDU-related IE identified using two algorithms (one sensitive, one specific); cases were aggregated into 2-year periods from 1996 to 2003	Both algorithms indicate that the number of IDU-related hospital discharges for IE rose by 38–66 during 2001–2002 and 2002–2003; During this same period, IDU-related IE hospital discharges decreased among the HIV/AIDS population and the number of IDU remained stable	Treatment admissions for cocaine use remained stable during 2002–2003 and admissions for methamphetamine use increased; therefore, increase in IDU-related IE may be caused in part by increased methamphetamine use

AOR, adjusted odds ratio; CDC, US Centers for Disease Control and Prevention; CI, confidence interval; IDU, injection drug users; IE, infective endocarditis; MRSA, methicillin-resistant *Staphylococcus aureus*; SSTI, skin and soft tissue infection.

explicit objective of describing the relationship between methamphetamine and a specific bacterial infection (MRSA). Methamphetamine use was self-reported in both case–control studies. In the analysis of hospital data, medical records were screened for diagnosis or procedure that indicated the use of a commonly injected drug (cocaine, heroin, or methamphetamine), but no specific screening was performed for methamphetamine. None of the studies used urine toxicology to confirm methamphetamine use.

Neoplastic disease

No associations were found regarding stimulant, hallucinogen, barbiturate, or benzo-diazepine use and neoplastic disease.

Musculoskeletal system disease

Diseases of the musculoskeletal system were limited in their association with stimulants, hallucinogens, barbiturates, and benzodiazepines. However, tangential connections exist with regard to stimulant and barbiturate use.

Amphetamines and MDMA

Stimulants exert effects on the musculoskeletal system either by direct toxic effect on myocytes or by predisposing myocytes to injury. Rhabdomyolysis is the most common musculoskeletal injury occurring in stimulant users. Numerous single case reports have described rhabdomyolysis in users of both methamphetamine and MDMA; however, only one large case study has attempted to examine the relationship between methamphetamine use and rhabdomyolysis.

Richards *et al.* (1999a) performed a five-year retrospective review of all patients presenting to the emergency department who were given a final diagnosis of rhabdomyolysis. Of 367 patients identified, 166 (45%) tested positive in a urine screen for methamphetamine. When compared with patients testing negative for methamphetamine, these patients had a higher initial CK. No difference in development of ARF was observed between patients testing positive for methamphetamine and those testing negative. The authors concluded that there may be an association between rhabdomyolysis and methamphetamine use, and CK quantification should be performed to assess muscle injury (Table 6.2). Patients presenting with rhabdomyolysis of questionable etiology should be screened for illicit drug use.

Comments

The literature contains a single study examining the relationship between methamphetamine use and rhabdomyolysis. This is fairly large study, conducted at a single university center located in California's Central Valley – an area well known for a high prevalence of methamphetamine use. Limitations of the study include lack of information as to quantity of methamphetamine used and time lapse between use and presentation to the emergency department. Concomitant drug or alcohol use may be a confounding factor.

Barbiturates

Barbiturates may be associated with certain connective tissue disorders. Barbiturate anticonvulsants, including phenobarbital and primidone, were included in a prospective controlled study undertaken by Mattson *et al.* (1989) involving the Veterans Administration Epilepsy Cooperative Study from 1978 to 1983. They sought to determine the validity of a suspected relationship between anticonvulsant drugs and Dupuytren's contractures, frozen shoulder, Ledderhose's syndrome, Peyronie's disease, fibromas, and general joint pain. A total of 622 patients were observed, some of whom were being treated with carbamazepine, phenobarbital, phenytoin sodium, or primidone. None of the patients being treated with carbamazepine or phenytoin developed connective tissue problems. However, 10 (6%) of the 178 patients treated with either barbiturate as their only antiepileptic therapy developed a disorder ($p < 0.001$). Subsequent to this study, one investigator also identified five more cases of phenobarbital-induced connective tissue disorders at a different site.

While reviewing the literature available through PubMed, two case studies were identified that describe barbiturate anticonvulsants being associated with or inducing

Table 6.2 Methamphetamine use and rhabdomyolysis

Study	Method	Sample	Incidence	Results
Richards et al. (1999a)	5 year retrospective review of attenders at emergency department Incidence and risk of rhabdomyolysis in methamphetamine users	367 patients with final discharge diagnosis of rhabdomyolysis	166 (43%) positive for methamphetamine; these patients also with two-fold greater initial creatine kinase; no difference in development of renal failure	Association between methamphetamine toxicity and rhabdomyolysis may exist; measuring creatine kinase can assess potential muscle injury; patients with unclear etiology should be screened for illicit drug use

Table 6.3 Barbiturates and connective tissue disease

Study	Method	Sample	Incidence	Results
Mattson et al. (1989)	Prospective survey Connective tissue disorders with antiepileptic drugs	622 patients being treated with carbamazepine, phenobarbital, phenytoin sodium, or primidone	10 (2.5%) of the 406 patients who were treated for 6 months or more developed a connective tissue disorder; all were being treated with barbiturates	A statistically significant ($p < 0.001$) relationship exists between treatment of epilepsy with barbiturates and onset of connective tissue disorders
Saviola et al. (1996)	Case study Rheumatism and barbiturate use	2 cases of rheumatism induced by phenobarbital	Rheumatism developed 12 months after initiating barbiturate use in one and after 20 years of treatment in the second	
Saviola et al. (2003)	Case study Rheumatism and barbiturate use	1 case of rheumatism induced by phenobarbital	85-year-old male with new-onset rheumatism	
Strzelczyk et al. (2008)	Case study Plantar fibromatosis and barbiturate use	3 cases of barbiturate-induced plantar fibromatosis	Ages 31 to 42 years with long-term use of barbiturates	

rheumatism. Saviola et al. (1996) presented two such cases where phenobarbital induced rheumatism after 12 months and 20 years of therapy. A similar case involved an 85-year-old man (Saviola et al. 2003).

More recently, Strzelczyk et al. (2008) described three case studies in which continuous use of anticonvulsant barbiturates led to plantar fibromatosis. The subjects range from 31 to 42 years in age and had all been treated with barbiturates for extended periods of time. None of the patients had a history of the known risk factors.

These studies on barbituates are summarized in Table 6.3.

Comments

The relationship between barbiturate use and connective tissue disorders has been limited to cases involving barbiturates as anticonvulsant treatment. After our review of the available literature, it is unclear if this relationship would be relevant in the context of illicit use or abuse. However, the studies described do present evidence to make a correlative argument regarding barbiturate-induced connective tissue disorders.

Digestive system disease

The hepatotoxic effect of MDMA is well reported in the literature by numerous single case studies. Among users of MDMA presenting with hepatic disease, the clinical pattern is highly variable, ranging from painless jaundice, malaise, and mildly elevated liver function tests to acute hepatic failure. At present, there are no studies examining the relationship between methamphetamine, barbiturates, hallucinogens, or benzodiazepines and digestive disorders.

MDMA

Two case studies describe relatively small numbers of patients presenting with MDMA-induced liver damage. Ellis *et al.* (1996) reported on eight patients presenting to a single center with liver disease temporally related to MDMA ingestion. These included presentations consisting of a mild hepatitis (two), hyperthermia and liver disease (two) and acute liver failure (four). Bilirubin ranged from 40 to 480 µmol/L and AST from 749 to 2659 µmol/L. With the exception of patients presenting with acute liver failure, all patients recovered. Of patients presenting with acute liver failure, one of four patients survived after a liver transplant. Some patients reported one-time MDMA use while others were regular MDMA users. Use history did not correlate with severity of hepatotoxicity.

Dykhuizen *et al.* (1995) reported on three patients with subacute hepatitis after MDMA use. Patients presented with symptoms of mild hepatitis and lacked history of heavy alcohol use or intravenous drug use. Peak bilirubin ranged from 75 to 371 µmol/L and peak AST ranged from 639 to 1410 µmol/L. All clinical symptoms resolved within five weeks to three months. The authors concluded that MDMA can be hepatotoxic. Young people with painless jaundice should be screened for MDMA use.

Table 6.4 outlines these two publications and one review article.

Comments

The literature contains many single case reports of MDMA-induced hepatic pathology. Two larger case studies included here were performed in the UK, where MDMA use became widespread in the early 1990s. The strength of these studies lies in the thoroughness of the clinical documentation. One difficulty in linking MDMA to hepatotoxicity or any other pathology is the difficulty in quantifying dose or confirming use, given MDMA's short half-life. Drug use in these case reports was self-reported.

Stomatognathic disease

The review found that chronic use of stimulants adversely affects oral health. With MDMA use, this is through clenching of teeth and bruxism secondary to stimulant-induced psychomotor agitation. Chronic and prolonged methamphetamine use is most commonly associated with numerous dental caries. Xerostomia is a common side effect of both drugs. Three studies describe the effect of stimulants on oral health.

Amphetamines and MDMA

Two studies examine the effect of MDMA on tooth wear. In the UK, Redfearn *et al.* (1998) surveyed young people frequenting a peer information network center. Tooth wear of 30

Table 6.4 Clinically varied presentations of hepatotoxicity with MDMA use

Study	Method	Sample	Incidence	Results
Jones & Simpson (1999)	Review of research MDMA-induced hepatotoxicity and management			MDMA-induced hepatotoxicity may be caused by (1) lack of CYP2D6, (2) immune-mediated mechanisms, (3) failure of thermotolerance leading to lipid peroxidation
Ellis et al. (1996)	Case report MDMA and acute liver damage	8 patients with liver disease temporally related to MDMA ingestion	Hyperthermia/liver disease (2), patients survived; mild hepatitis (2), patients survived; acute liver failure (4), one survival after transplant	Severity of liver disease does not correlate with amount or duration of MDMA use; some patients were one-time users, others regular users
Dykhuizen et al. (1995)	Case report MDMA-related hepatitis	3 patients with subacute idiosyncratic toxic hepatitis after MDMA ingestion	Clinical hepatitis, elevated liver function tests in all 3; no association with alcohol or intravenous drug use; complete resolution in 5 weeks to 3 months	There is a relationship between MDMA use and hepatotoxicity; young people with painless jaundice should be screened for MDMA use

MDMA, 3,4-methylenedioxymethamphetamine.

MDMA users and 28 non-users was quantified using a previously established tooth wear index. With respect to back tooth wear, the mean tooth wear scores for the two groups differed significantly ($p < 0.001$). The scores for front tooth wear were not significantly different. The authors concluded that MDMA use increased the likelihood of back tooth wear. They further posited that tooth wear was exacerbated by the consumption of acidic soft drinks.

In the USA, Richards & Brofeldt (2000) also studied the effect of methamphetamine on tooth wear. They identified 43 methamphetamine users presenting to the large hospital emergency department in California's Sacramento Valley. Tooth wear was measured using a standard index and the route of drug delivery was ascertained. Users who inhaled or snorted methamphetamine (33%) showed significantly greater anterior maxillary tooth wear than users who smoked or injected the drug ($p = 0.005$). The authors suggested that inhalation of methamphetamine preferentially vasoconstricts the arterial supply common to both the nasal mucosa and the anterior maxillary teeth, creating an environment of chronic ischemia and resulting in greater anterior maxillary tooth wear.

McGrath & Chan (2005) studied oral sensations experienced during drug use among a group of young people at a drug rehabilitation program in Hong Kong. They employed a questionnaire to investigate various oral sensations as well as to elucidate differences in sensations experienced by users of MDMA and other drugs. The study population comprised 117 men and 7 women, with a mean age of 20 years. All participants were polydrug users, with 95 (77%) reporting methamphetamine use, 69 (56%) reporting MDMA use and

Table 6.5 Stimulant use and oral health

Study	Method	Sample	Incidence	Results
Redfearn et al. (1998)	Case–control Tooth wear Tooth wear index	30 ecstasy users, 28 non-users	Users compared with non-users: mean tooth wear score for back teeth 0.96 (SD 0.16) vs. 0.12 (SD 0.08) ($p < 0.001$); score for front tooth wear not significant	Use of MDMA increases likelihood of tooth wear on back teeth; this is exacerbated by acidic soft drinks
Richards & Brofeldt (2000)	Interview Methamphetamine users and tooth wear	43 methamphetamine users (snorters, inhalers) in emergency department	14 (33%) showed significantly higher tooth wear than users who employed different routes of drug delivery ($p = 0.005$)	There is unique pattern of tooth wear based upon route of drug administration; inhalation may be related to mucosal vasoconstriction
McGrath & Chan (2005)	Self-completed questionnaire Previous pattern of drug use and oral sensations	124 young adult polydrug abusers at a drug rehabilitation program, mean age 20 years	MDMA users reported significantly more chewing ($p < 0.001$), grinding ($p < 0.001$) and tenderness of the temporomandibular joint ($p < 0.001$)	Type of illicit drug used is associated with distinct oral health sensations

SD, standard deviation; MDMA, 3,4-methylenedioxymethamphetamine.

ketamine use, and 57 (46%) reporting heroin use. With a strict focus on MDMA users, 60 users (63%) reported feelings of "chewing something" after drug use, compared with 29 (58%) of drug users reporting no use of MDMA; 48 users (70%) reported feeling "pain or tenderness in jaw muscle or joint after drug use" as well as "grinding their teeth." All of these subjective measures were significantly different when compared with non-users of MDMA ($p < 0.001$). Feeling of "mouth dryness" was reported almost equally among MDMA users and non-users. The authors concluded that this subjective analysis of the types of oral sensations among MDMA users supports the recent concern regarding tooth wear and bruxism among MDMA users.

These studies are summarized in Table 6.5.

Comments

Most of the oral effects of MDMA have been documented as single case reports. Few studies have sought to describe these effects more fully. The small studies described above offer a qualitative perspective on oral sensations experienced by stimulant users as well as two quantitative analyses of the effect of MDMA and methamphetamine on tooth wear. In all of the studies described, drug use was determined by self-report. Both studies assessing tooth wear used the same tooth wear index, which assigned a numeric score for specific enamel characteristics. Tooth wear assessed by this index showed that inhaled methamphetamine preferentially affects front tooth wear while MDMA use affects back tooth wear. Confounders for the studies are described by the authors and include increased tobacco use, increased consumption of carbonated soft drinks, and the reduced attention to oral hygiene that is common among drug users.

Respiratory system disease

No relevant information was found that demonstrated an association between barbiturate, hallucinogen, and benzodiazepine use and respiratory disease. However, some results were obtained for the use of amphetamines and respiratory disease.

Amphetamines

A number of case reports describe an association between stimulant use and the development of pulmonary arterial hypertension (PAH). Chin *et al.* (2006) conducted a retrospective review of 340 patients with PAH to determine whether idiopathic PAH was associated with greater rates of stimulant use when compared with other forms of PAH. Stimulant use was defined as any reported use of amphetamine, methamphetamine, or cocaine. In subgroup analysis, the data showed that methamphetamine use alone was 7.73 times more common in patients with idiopathic PAH than in PAH with known risk factors (95% CI 2.55–23.5; $p < 0.0002$). Methamphetamine use was 11.61 times more common in patients with idiopathic PAH than patients with chronic thrombotic pulmonary hypertension (95% CI 3.34–23.5; $p < 0.0001$). The authors concluded that methamphetamine use is more common in patients with idiopathic PAH than in patients with other types of PAH (Table 6.6).

Comments

This is a single-center retrospective chart review study conducted over 2.5 years that shows an association between methamphetamine use and idiopathic PAH. Drug use was self-reported and took place days to years before patients presented with disease. One of the strengths of this study lies in the subgroup analysis, which reported OR values for any stimulant use as well as for methamphetamine use alone. The authors acknowledged limitations such as incomplete drug use histories and the effect of chronic disease on drug use.

Otorhinolaryngological disease

No relevant articles were found addressing associations between diseases of the ear, nose, or throat as a consequence of illicit stimulant, hallucinogen, barbiturate, or benzodiazepine use.

Nervous system disease

Based on our review, LSD and barbiturate use and abuse does not appear to contribute to diseases of the nervous system; however, the association between stimulant use and nervous system pathology has been well studied. Of the studies exploring the effects of methamphetamine and MDMA on the nervous system, a number of these use a variety of imaging techniques to assess drug effects on brain structure, neurotransmitters, and their receptors. One case study of stroke after methamphetamine use is also included. Additionally, three articles were found that discuss cognitive dysfunction in relation to long-term benzodiazepine use.

Amphetamines and MDMA

Seeking to explore and explain functional consequences of chronic methamphetamine use, Baicy & London (2007) reviewed several neuroimaging studies comparing chronic

Table 6.6 Methamphetamine use and pulmonary arterial hypertension

Study	Method	Sample	Incidence	Results
Chin et al. (2006)	Retrospective study Relationship between stimulant use and PAH	340 cases of PAH	Methamphetamine use is 7.73 times more common in patients with idiopathic PAH than PAH with known risk factors (95% CI 2.55–23.5; $p < 0.0002$); methamphetamine use is 11.61 times more common in patients with idiopathic PAH than in patients with chronic thrombotic pulmonary hypertension (95% CI 3.34–23.5; $p < 0.0001$)	Stimulant uses, especially methamphetamine use, is more common in patients with idiopathic PAH than patients with other types of PAH

MDMA, 3,4-methylenedioxymethamphetamine; PAH, pulmonary arterial hypertension.

methamphetamine users now abstinent with normal controls. The duration of abstinence varied among the studies. Deficits were observed in markers of both dopaminergic and serotonergic transmission as well as gray and white matter. These deficits appeared to correlate well with observed cognitive deficits. The authors suggested that these deficits may interfere with drug users' ability to remain abstinent.

Volkow et al. (2001a) examined the effect of methamphetamine on brain glucose metabolism using PET to compare glucose metabolism in brains of 15 abstinent methamphetamine users and 21 healthy controls. The duration of abstinence ranged from two weeks to 35 months. Their data showed that abstinent users had increased glucose metabolism (14% higher). The highest rate was observed in the parietal region (20% higher), with lowest rates in thalamus and striatum. Given that the parietal region lacks dopaminergic activity, the authors concluded that methamphetamine use affects circuits lacking dopamine-dependent neurotransmission as well as dopamine circuits.

Ernst et al. (2000) used proton magnetic resonance spectroscopy (MRS) to detect long-term metabolic derangements in the brains of 26 abstinent methamphetamine users compared with 24 normal, healthy controls. Abstinence was defined as no drug use for at least two weeks prior to the start of the study. N-Acetyl aspartate, a neuronal marker, was significantly decreased (5–6%) in brains of abstinent users. In this same group, myo-inositol, a marker of inflammation, was increased (11%) when compared with controls. The authors proposed that abnormal concentrations of these markers imply long-term neuronal damage despite abstinence from methamphetamine.

Noting the presence of ischemic brain lesions in methamphetamine abusers and gender differences in methamphetamine-related neurotoxicity in animal studies, Bae et al. (2006) used T_2-weighted MRI to assess white matter hyperintensities among male and female methamphetamine users. When compared with non-using controls, white matter hyperintensities were more prevalent in methamphetamine users (OR, 7.06), with male users showing a greater number of lesions than female users (OR, 10.00) (CI values not given). The investigators hypothesized that estrogen plays a protective role in the brains of female drug users.

Chang et al. (2005) observed parallels between the cognitive deficits of individuals with HIV-associated dementia and methamphetamine users. Questioning whether HIV and concurrent methamphetamine use had an additive effect on brain injury, the authors employed proton MRS to assess neuronal and glial markers among 24 HIV-positive chronic methamphetamine users, 44 HIV-positive non-users, 36 HIV-negative methamphetamine users, and 39 HIV-negative non-users. The HIV-infected methamphetamine users had the greatest decrease in the concentration of the neuronal marker N-acetyl aspartate in the frontal white matter (6.1%; $p = 0.02$), frontal gray matter (5.7%; $p = 0.03$), and basal ganglia (9%; $p = 0.0001$). Among this same group, myo-inositol, a marker of inflammation or glial activation, was increased in the frontal white matter (12.2%; $p = 0.02$). These results suggest that HIV infection and chronic methamphetamine use injure the brain in an additive manner.

Rothrock $et\ al.$ (1988) documented three cases of young men presenting with stroke after inhaling methamphetamine. The patients ranged in age from 22 to 35 years and denied use of other drugs. Duration of drug use ranged from single use to multiple times weekly over a one-year period. Development of symptoms occurred between 12 hours and two weeks after last use. Head CT showed acute frontal (two patients) and frontoparietal stroke (one patient). Arteriography showed occlusion of the internal carotid artery and/or its branches (two patients) and beading of branches (one patient). All patients had some degree of residual unilateral weakness (two), hemiparesis (one), or aphasia (one) at one year of follow-up. The authors proposed that the delay between drug use and the development of symptoms could represent the growth of a thrombus as well as a progressive vasculitis.

Given that methamphetamine was previously shown to be neurotoxic to dopamine terminals in animal models, Volkow $et\ al.$ (2001b) investigated whether similar toxicity occurs in humans. Using PET imaging and neuropsychological testing, 15 abstinent methamphetamine users were compared with 18 healthy controls. Abstinence was defined as no drug use for at least two weeks prior to the study. Among abstinent drug users, dopamine transporters were reduced in the striatum and caudate by 27.8% and 21.1%, respectively. This reduction was associated with poorer performance on motor and memory tests when compared with controls. Further, the reduction in transporters remained after 11 months of abstinence. The authors proposed that these findings can be used to drive therapies that improve dopamine neurotransmission in abstinent methamphetamine users.

McCann $et\ al.$ (2008) hypothesized that, despite abstinence, methamphetamine users would have deficits in domains involving dopaminergic neurotransmission. Using psychometric testing and PET imaging, the brain function of 22 abstinent methamphetamine users were compared with 17 controls. Abstinence was defined as no drug use for at least two weeks prior to the study. While some deficits in short-term memory, executive function, and manual dexterity were observed among drug users, only short-term memory deficits were associated with aberrant dopamine neurotransmission. The authors suggested that these data support existing work demonstrating that methamphetamine use has lasting effects on central dopaminergic function.

Chana $et\ al.$ (2006) sought to determine the relationship between damage to neuronal circuits and cognitive impairment in HIV-positive methamphetamine users. They correlated neuropathological data from autopsy studies with premortem neurobehavioral assessment. Their data showed that eight HIV-positive methamphetamine users had greater loss of interneurons in frontal cortex compared with 12 non-users. In these patients, decreased density of interneurons was associated with decreased global neurocognitive impairment score and memory score (both $p < 0.05$). The authors propose that the cognitive deficits in HIV-positive methamphetamine users may result from the additive neurotoxic effect of HIV proteins and methamphetamine use.

These studies on methamphetamine users are summarized in Table 6.7.

In one of two studies examining the effects of MDMA on the CNS, Reneman *et al.* (2001c) used diffusion and perfusion magnetic resonance to assess structural differences between eight abstinent MDMA users and six controls. Abstinence was defined as no drug use for three weeks prior to the study. The globus pallidus of MDMA users showed higher mean apparent diffusion coefficients ($p < 0.025$) and higher cerebral volume ratios ($p < 0.025$) compared with the control group. There was a positive correlation between length of exposure to MDMA and increased cerebral volume ratio in the globus pallidus. The authors attributed the difference in the apparent diffusion coefficient values to axonal loss while the increase in cerebral volume was thought to be secondary to MDMA-induced removal of serotonin-induced vasoconstriction.

In a second study, Reneman *et al.* (2001a) sought to examine the consequence of MDMA dose, long-term abstinence, and gender on the density of brain serotonergic neurons. Long-term abstinence was defined as no MDMA use for at least one year prior to the study. The authors used single-photon emission CT and radioligands specific for serotonin transporters. The data showed that serotonin-binding ratios were lower in female heavy MDMA users when compared with controls ($p < 0.01$). Binding ratios were increased among abstinent female users when compared with heavy female users ($p = 0.004$). The authors concluded that men and women differ in vulnerability to MDMA-induced neurotoxicity. This neurotoxicity may be reversible in women.

Four studies examine the relationship between MDMA use and cognition with a focus on memory. In the first of these, Zakzanis & Young (2001) performed neuropsychological testing on a small group ($n = 15$) of self-reported MDMA users. Users were tested at the start of the study and again at one year. At one year, large declines were observed in total Rivermead Behavioral Memory Test (RBMT) scores ($p < 0.001$). Delayed and immediate story recall were preferentially affected ($p < 0.01$). The authors concluded that continued use of MDMA correlates with different facets of memory decline.

Zakzanis & Campbell (2006) retested this same study group ($n = 15$) at two years of follow-up. Since the one-year testing, seven subjects continued to use MDMA; eight subjects reported abstinence from MDMA. On intragroup comparison, former users demonstrated improved scores on vocabulary ($p < 0.01$), block design ($p < 0.05$), and total RBMT ($p < 0.01$) scores. Current users showed significant decline in vocabulary and total RBMT score, decreasing from 17.4 (one year) to 9.1 (two years) ($p < 0.001$). Considering that now-abstinent MDMA users showed improvement or no further decline, the authors concluded that MDMA-induced cognitive deficits may persist after abstinence but these deficits are not progressive.

MDMA has been shown to harm serotonin neural circuits in animal models. Reneman *et al.* (2001b) examined the effect of MDMA on serotonin circuits and memory function in 22 recent (mean time since last dose of 2.4 ± 2.4 months) and 16 abstinent (mean time since last dose of 29.0 ± 20.4 months) MDMA users compared with 13 healthy controls. The recent MDMA users had decreased serotonin transporter density as identified by PET only when compared with controls (1.17 vs. 1.28; a decrease of 9%). Verbal memory testing showed recent and abstinent users recalled fewer words than controls (47.0, 48.0, and 60.0, respectively; $p = 0.001$). There was a correlation between increasing MDMA dose and increasing impairment. The authors proposed that MDMA effects on serotonergic neurons

Table 6.7 Methamphetamine and the nervous system

Study	Method	Sample	Incidence	Results
Baicy & London (2007)	Review Markers of dopamine and serotonin in chronic methamphetamine users Neuroimaging	Abstinent methamphetamine users, healthy controls	Brains of chronic methamphetamine users showed derangements, deficits of markers of various neurotransmitters, white and gray matter deficits; deficits accompanied cognitive impairments	Success in maintaining abstinence may be impaired by cortical deficits resulting from chronic drug use
Volkow et al. (2001a)	Case–control Effect of methamphetamine on brain glucose metabolism	15 detoxified methamphetamine users, 21 healthy controls	Brain glucose metabolism increased in abstinent users (14% higher) with highest rates in parietal region (20% higher); lowest rates in thalamus, striatum	Methamphetamine use affects circuits lacking dopamine-dependent neurotransmission (parietal lobe) as well as dopamine circuits
Ernst et al. (2000)	Case–control study Cerebral metabolite concentrations Proton magnetic resonance spectroscopy	26 abstinent methamphetamine users, 24 healthy controls	Abstinent methamphetamine users compared with controls: significant decrease (5–6%) in N-acetyl aspartate (specific neuronal marker indicating inflammation) in frontal white matter; myo-inositol (glial marker) increased (11%)	Despite abstinence, methamphetamine may induce long-term neuronal damage
Bae et al. (2006)	Case–control study White matter hyperintensities in methamphetamine users T_2-weighted MRI	33 methamphetamine users (22 males, 11 females), 32 healthy controls	White matter hyperintensities increased among methamphetamine users (OR 7.06 for all lesions); severity of lesions correlated with use ($p = 0.027$; lesions more severe in male users than male controls (OR 18.86)	Lesions in the white matter are increased in users of methamphetamine, with the greatest increase observed among male users; estrogen may have a protective effect, ameliorating the drug effect in women
Chang et al. (2005)	Case–control study Neuronal and glial markers in HIV infection and in methamphetamine users Proton magnetic resonance spectroscopy	68 HIV-positive patients (24 methamphetamine users, 44 non-users, 75 HIV-negative patients (36 methamphetamine users, 39 non-users).	Greatest difference in metabolite concentration (lower neuronal markers, higher glial markers) was observed in HIV-positive methamphetamine users	Brain imaging of patients with HIV who are chronic methamphetamine users shows additional neuronal injury and glial activation
Rothrock et al. (1988)	Case study Stroke and methamphetamine inhalation Head CT and arteriography	3 patients, aged 22–35 years	Duration of methamphetamine use ranging from single occasion to several times weekly for 1 year; symptoms occurred 12 h to 2 weeks after last use Head CT and arteriography showed acute stroke with occlusion or "beading" of intracranial arteries and/or major vessels; residual unilateral weakness (2), hemiparesis (1), aphasia (1)	Internal carotid stenosis or occlusion as well as ischemic stroke are potential complications of methamphetamine inhalation

Table 6.7 Cont.

Study	Method	Sample	Incidence	Results
Volkow (2001b)	Case–control study Dopamine transporters in methamphetamine users PET imaging and psychomotor testing	15 abstinent (> 2 weeks) methamphetamine users, 18 healthy controls	Methamphetamine users compared with controls: dopamine transporters reduced in striatum (27.8%) and caudate (21.1%); reduction associated with poor performance on motor and memory tests	The reduction in dopamine transporter levels seen in methamphetamine users correlates with poorer performance on tests of motor function and memory; decreased transporter function persisted for at least 11 months after commencing abstinence
McCann et al. (2008)	Case–control study Dopamine transporter binding potential and psychomotor deficits PET and psychometric testing	22 abstinent (> 2 weeks) methamphetamine users, 17 healthy controls	Methamphetamine users compared with controls: mild deficits in short-term memory, executive function, manual dexterity; only memory loss correlated with decreases in the binding potential of striatal dopamine transporters	There may be a relationship between dopamine transporter binding potential and memory deficits in abstinent methamphetamine users; methamphetamine use produces lasting effects on brain function
Chana et al. (2006)	Case–control study Patterns of neuronal degeneration and cognitive impairment in HIV-positive methamphetamine users Neurocognitive and memory scores and subsequent structural analysis	20 HIV-seropositive autopsy cases (8 methamphetamine users, 12 non-users) with previous neurocognitive and memory scores	Methamphetamine users compared with non-users: greater loss of interneurons in frontal cortex; decreased density of interneurons associated with decreased global neurocognitive impairment score and memory score (both $p < 0.05$)	The reduction in frontal cortex interneurons observed in HIV-positive methamphetamine users is associated with neurocognitive deficits, especially in memory performance

CT, computed tomography; HIV, human immunodeficiency virus; MRI, magnetic resonance imaging; OR, odds ratio; PET, positron emission tomography.

may be reversible with abstinence but MDMA effects on memory function persist despite abstinence.

Schilt *et al.* (2007) investigated the effect of initial, low-dose MDMA use on performance on a battery of neurocognitive tests. Testing of 118 MDMA-naive subjects was repeated at follow-up after 58 subjects reported initial MDMA use. Initially no differences in testing were observed. On follow-up, subjects reporting MDMA use showed deficits in verbal recognition and delayed verbal recall (both $p = 0.03$). The authors concluded that even in low dose, incident MDMA use adversely affects verbal memory.

Rusyniak & Sprague (2005) reviewed three hyperthermic syndromes: serotonin syndrome, malignant hyperthermia, and neuroleptic malignant syndrome. Of interest is the key role that stimulant use plays in the pathogenesis of serotonin syndrome: MDMA acts centrally to deregulate thermogenesis and increased motor activity compounds the toxicity of stimulants on thermoregulatory mechanisms. These findings have important implications for MDMA users who may use drugs while dancing in crowded areas with high ambient temperatures. Treatment for serotonin syndrome includes central serotonin antagonists or benzodiazepines.

Table 6.8 summarizes these studies on MDMA.

Comments

The 16 studies presented above for amphetamines and MDMA describe numerous facets of the relationship between neurological pathology and cognitive impairments and stimulant use. The first eight studies compared abstinent drug users with healthy, non-using controls. The definition of abstinence varied widely between studies. Drug use was commonly ascertained by self-report. The authors acknowledged the difficulty inherent in determining amount of previous drug use and the ability to correlate use with findings. Only two studies used DMV-IV criteria to define methamphetamine dependence. History of polydrug use was the most common confounder. Seven of the studies described above document the relationship between stimulant use and neurocognitive deficits. These studies include small case–control studies (four/seven) as well as a two-part longitudinal study and a prospective study. The strength of these studies lies in the thoroughness of the neuropsychological battery used to test subjects. In four of the studies, this battery was correlated with brain imaging or immunohistochemical analysis of brain tissue. Limitations of the studies include self-report of drug use and self-report of polydrug use. Finally, the last article reviewed above describes the role of stimulants in the pathogenesis of serotonin syndrome. In particular, MDMA use appears to promote this hyperthermic syndrome by its induction of serotonin release as well through the environmental situations and activities that often occur with its use.

Benzodiazepines

In a review article, Stewart (2005) discussed the risk of cognitive impairment as a result of long-term benzodiazepine use. A meta-analysis was done that incorporated literature up to and including 2004. In the studies reviewed, reported dysfunctions associated with long-term use include deficits in concentration, verbal learning, decreased IQ, and impaired visuospatial abilities. However, other investigators failed to associate deficits in psychomotor speed, attention, and verbal memory with long-term. Whatever deficits did exist in long-term users, they appeared to recover some cognitive capabilities after withdrawal, according to some observations. Stewart concluded that any study of the subject was

Table 6.8 Nervous system disorders and MDMA use

Study	Method	Sample	Incidence	Results
Reneman et al. (2001c)	Case–control study Effects of MDMA on brain structure	8 abstinent (3 weeks) MDMA users, 6 healthy non-users	MDMA users versus controls: globus pallidus showed higher mean apparent diffusion coefficients ($p < 0.025$) and higher cerebral volume ratios ($p < 0.025$); positive correlation between length of exposure to MDMA and cerebral volume ratio in globus pallidus	MDMA use appears to induce structural changes in the globus pallidus
Reneman et al. (2001a)	Case–control study Effects of MDMA dose, use patterns, and gender on brain serotonergic neurons SPECT	54 MDMA users (15 moderate, 23 heavy, 16 abstinent 1 year), 15 healthy controls	Serotonin binding ratios were decreased in female, heavy MDMA users ($p < 0.01$); binding ratios were increased among abstinent female users compared with females with heavy use ($p = 0.004$)	Men and women differ in vulnerability to MDMA-induced neurotoxicity in serotonergic neurons; this neurotoxicity may be reversible in women
Zakzanis & Young (2001)	Longitudinal study, investigation of long-term functional consequences of continued MDMA use	15 MDMA users Neuropsychiatric testing at baseline and again at 1 year	Large decline in total RBMT score (everyday functional memory) at 1 year ($p < 0.001$); immediate and delayed story recall affected ($p < 0.01$)	Continued use of MDMA correlates with different facets of memory decline
Zakzanis & Campbell (2006)	Longitudinal study Long-term functional consequences of continued MDMA use Neuropsychiatry testing	15 MDMA users testing at baseline, 1 year and 2 years	Intragroup comparison showed former users with improved scores on vocabulary ($p < 0.01$), block design ($p < 0.05$), total RBMT ($p < 0.01$) scores; current users showed significant decline in vocabulary and total RBMT score, decreasing from 17.4 (1 year) to 9.1 (2 years) ($p < 0.001$)	MDMA-induced cognitive deficits may persist after abstinence but they do not continue to progress
Reneman et al. (2001b)	Case–control study MDMA-induced changes in serotonin transporter density and memory function	22 recent MDMA users (average use 2.4 ± 24 months), 16 abstinent MDMA users (29.0 ± 20.4 months), 13 healthy controls	Recent MDMA users had decreased serotonin transporter density compared with controls (1.17 vs. 1.28 [9%]); recent and abstinent users recall fewer words than controls on verbal memory testing	MDMA effects on serotonergic neurons may be reversible with abstinence; MDMA effects on memory function appear to persist despite abstinence

| Schilt et al. (2007) | Prospective cohort study Relationship between MDMA and subsequent cognitive performance | 118 MDMA-naive subjects: 58 with subsequent MDMA use, 60 remaining MDMA naive | Incident MDMA users showed deficits in verbal recognition and delayed verbal recall (both $p = 0.03$) | Low cumulative dose of MDMA is associated with decline in verbal memory |
| Rusyniak & Sprague (2005) | Review of research Stimulants and their role in serotonin syndrome; malignant hyperthermia, neuroleptic malignant syndrome also reviewed | Case reports and research using human and animal studies | MDMA can deregulate thermogenesis | MDMA acts centrally to precipitate serotonin syndrome in some drug users; higher ambient temperatures and increased muscle activity increase toxicity |

MDMA, 3,4-methylenedioxymethamphetamine; RBMT, Rivermead Behavioral Memory Test; SPECT, single-photon emission computed tomography.

301

Table 6.9 Benzodiazepines and the nervous system

Study	Method	Sample	Incidence	Results
Stewart (2005)	Meta-analysis	Literature up to 2004		Long-term treatment with benzodiazepines is associated with cognitive performance impairment; observable changes in brain activity only temporary; impairment lessened once patients stopped use
Barker et al. (2004)	Meta-analysis	13 studies meeting criteria, including neuropsychological tests categorized into 12 cognitive domains	Mean number of users 33.5 (SD, 28.9); mean number of controls 27.9 (SD, 19.6); mean duration of use 9.9 years Across all cognitive categories examined: long-term users consistently impaired (effect sizes ranging in magnitude from −1.30 to −0.42; mean −0.74 [SD, 0.25]); no effect size had 95% confidence interval that spanned zero	Data suggest that long-term benzodiazepine users are significantly impaired; study size was limited
Busto et al. (2000)	Case–control study CT	20 long-term benzodiazepine users, 36 age- and sex-matched controls	CT measuring atrophy and size of ventricles: V1–V3, sulci, fissures, cisterns and folia: no atrophy differences between users and controls; V1 measurements (mean ± SD) higher in users (12.1 ± 1.3 vs. 11.1 ± 2.0; $p = 0.02$); 3rd and 4th largest sulci higher in controls	CT scans did not indicate any significant differences in long-term users

CT, computed tomography; SD, standard deviation.

possibly confounded by the nature of the subject population, since target ailments, such as anxiety, have been shown to cause deficits in concentration.

Another meta-analysis was performed by Barker et al. (2004), in which 13 studies were included. Each study utilized neuropsychological testing. Results were categorized into 12 specific cognitive domains (e.g., sensory processing, verbal/non-verbal memory, problem solving). Throughout the studies, the mean age of long-terms users was 33.5 years (SD, 28.9); the mean number of controls was 27.9 (SD, 19.6); and the mean duration of use was 9.9 years (range, 1–34). Across all 12 cognitive categories, long-term users were consistently and demonstrably impaired, with effect sizes ranging in magnitude from −1.30 to −0.42, with a mean of −0.74 (SD, 0.25). Findings were significant and different from zero because no effect size had a 95% CI that spanned zero. The authors conceded that this study was very limited, particularly in its sample size.

These analyses are summarized in Table 6.9.

Comments

Both studies described above agree that evidence of cognitive dysfunction is demonstrated through the literature. However, they also agree that these results are not definitive. A major point of concern is the need for careful methodization of future sample populations. In the meta-analysis of Barker *et al.* (2004), it is stated that only 13 studies could be included in accordance with the study criteria, but even then, results may be confounded because of the nature of the subject pool, as discussed by Stewart (2005). Furthermore, it is also noted by Stewart (2005) that no long-term physical abnormalities have been documented as a result of long-term benzodiazepine use. This is confirmed by a CT study (Busto *et al.* (2000) in which no brain abnormalities could be found in long-term users. Therefore, if cognitive dysfunction is evident, confounding variables need to be removed from a larger pool of data in order to better treat and inform the general population.

Ocular disease

A single case report describes the relationship between stimulant use and ocular nerve pathology. Two cases studies are also presented linking LSD to ocular disorders.

MDMA

Schroeder & Brieden (2000) described a case of bilateral sixth nerve palsy. A 17-year-old male with a history of once weekly MDMA use over a two month period presented with bilateral sixth nerve palsy and mild bilateral upper and lower extremity paresthesias, which developed after MDMA use. An extensive work-up was performed including serology, imaging, and electroencephalography – all of which returned negative. These deficits resolved within five days without treatment. The authors concluded that report of recent MDMA use should be considered as a possible cause of transient sixth nerve palsy (Table 6.10).

Comments

This is a single case report describing transient neurological deficits developing in a young man after two months of chronic MDMA use. The patient reported last drug use 24 hours prior to the onset of symptoms. Urine toxicology was not performed. It is not known whether the patient was using other illicit drugs concurrently.

LSD

In an article that reviewed evidence from 1955 to 2001, Halpern & Pope (2003) presented what was known at that time about HPPD or "flashbacks" and stated that information was somewhat limited. Cases are most commonly connected to illicit LSD use. The disorder may persist for months or years after drug use and is associated with substantial morbidity. It is less commonly observed with other hallucinogens and in research and treatment settings. They concluded that HPPD appears to be a genuine but uncommon disorder.

Kawasaki & Purvin (1996) presented three cases of persistent palinopsia. During LSD intoxication, each individual experienced prolonged images and continued to be symptomatic for up to three years after use. No abnormalities were found in neuro-ophthalmological and neurological examinations or in neuroimaging and electrophysiological studies.

Gaillard & Borruat (2003) presented a series of cases, one of which described a patient who had a history of multiple drug abuse, including six years of LSD use. Following heavy intake of alcohol, the patient experienced hallucinations and afterimages (palinopsia) even

Table 6.10 Ocular disease in MDMA use

Study	Method	Sample	Incidence	Results
Schroeder & Brieden (2000)	Case report	17-year-old male with bilateral sixth nerve palsy: 2 month history of once-weekly MDMA use	Bilateral sixth nerve palsy developed after MDMA use and resolved within 5 days without treatment	MDMA use may cause sixth nerve palsy

MDMA, 3,4-methylenedioxymethamphetamine.

Table 6.11 Ocular disorders with LSD

Study	Method	Sample	Incidence	Results
Halpern & Pope (2003)	Literature review 1955–2001	Hallucinogen persisting perception disorder (flashbacks)	Most common in LSD users, can persist for months, years after use	Flashbacks are genuine, but uncommon disorder; current cases are difficult to categorize
Kawasaki & Purvin (1996)	Case report	3 with painopsia at a neuro-ophthalmology center	Persistent palinopsia following LSD use; normal results were found in neuro-ophthalmological and neurological examinations as well as neuroimaging and electrophysiological studies	LSD history should be considered in patients presenting with palinopsia
Gaillard & Borruat (2003)	Case report	1 patient with history of multiple drug abuse, including LSD (6 years use, 20 years abstinence)	Following heavy intake of ethanol, the patient experienced hallucinations and palinopsia even though drug use had ceased 20 years previously; examination showed abnormal visual fields with preserved visual acuity; electroencephalography was also abnormal, suggesting an underlying toxic encephalopathy	Flashbacks may recur years after LSD use; precipitated by ethanol, other medication, anesthesia

LSD, ᴅ-lysergic acid diethylamide.

though drug use had ceased 20 years previously. The patient was examined and was found to have abnormal visual fields with preserved visual acuity. Electroencephalography was also abnormal, suggesting an underlying toxic encephalopathy. The authors noted that it is rare for flashbacks to recur so long after drug use, but when they do so, they are precipitated by factors such as alcohol, medication, or anesthesia. Such phenomena demonstrate the cortical dysfunctions that can be induced by LSD.

These studies are summarized in Table 6.11.

Comments

Although HPPD is rare, even in hallucinogen users, it is recognized as a legitimate disorder. As demonstrated in the case studies above, the disorder has multiple manifestations. Visual images that occur while intoxicated may persist long after LSD use. Those with substantial histories of use may suffer from unwanted hallucinations many years after the last ingestion. The disorder may or may not be associated with measurable physiological abnormalities. In some cases, flashbacks are associated with mental and physical precipitates such as anxiety, fatigue, neuroleptics, alcohol, and marijuana intoxication. The rarity and singularity of each case makes HPPD difficult to identify and analyze. Study is further confounded by the fact that the term "flashback" is almost valueless because it is somewhat subjective. Most studies provide too little information to determine how many patients meet DSM-IV criteria.

Male urological disease

No relevant articles were recovered that described an association between urological disease and illicit stimulant, hallucinogen, barbiturate, or benzodiazepine use.

Female genital and neonatal/congenital disease

The literature review retrieved 16 studies describing the teratogenic effects of stimulants, benzodiazepines, and barbiturates. No articles were found linking use of hallucinogens to gynecological or obstetric pathology. The typical method of investigation was to observe and analyze groups of neonates and their development after antenatal maternal exposure to the drug of interest. Literature reviews as well as analysis of birth registries were included.

Amphetamines and MDMA

McElhatton *et al.* (1999) collected follow-up data on 136 pregnancies with reported maternal exposure to MDMA (74 pregnant women) or MDMA and other drugs of abuse including alcohol. The vast majority (127) of these exposures occurred in the first trimester. Of the 78 live births (59 pregnancies were either terminated or ended in miscarriage), 12 infants had congenital anomalies (15.4%; 95% CI 8.2–25.4). Of these, there was an increased rate of musculoskeletal defects (38/1000; 95% CI 8–109) especially among mothers reporting MDMA use only. Among mothers reporting exposure to MDMA and other drugs, cardiovascular defects (26/1000; 95% CI 3.0–90.0) predominated. The authors noted that the sample size was too small to establish causality in fetal effect (Table 6.12).

Little *et al.* (1988) were one of the first groups to investigate the relationship between methamphetamine use throughout pregnancy and congenital anomalies. They compared two cohorts: 52 pregnant self-reported methamphetamine abusers and 52 pregnant non-users of methamphetamine. Women who injected methamphetamine were more likely than their counterparts to use other drugs of abuse, as well as alcohol and tobacco. Pregnancy complications as well as congenital abnormalities were not significantly different between the two groups (OR 0.72; $p < 0.39$). However, infants born to methamphetamine users showed reductions in weight, length, and head circumference that were not attributable to concurrent tobacco use.

With the specific intention of exploring the relationship between methamphetamine use during pregnancy and fetal growth, Smith *et al.* (2006) performed a large multicenter prospective cohort study of 1618 women; 82 were self-reported methamphetamine users

Table 6.12 Congenital defects and maternal exposure to MDMA

Study	Method	Sample	Incidence	Results
McElhatton et al. (1999)	Prospective, follow-up study Pregnancies with maternal exposure to MDMA	136 pregnancies: 74 women took MDMA only, 62 women took MDMA plus other drugs of abuse; 127 exposed in first trimester	78 live-born infants: 66 normal, 12 with congenital abnormalities (15.4%; 95% CI 8.2–25.4]; increased musculoskeletal defects (38/1000; 95% CI 8–109), especially in MDMA users; increased cardiovascular defects in users of MDMA and other drugs (26/1000; 95% CI 3.0–90.0)	There appears to be a relationship between maternal use of MDMA alone and in combination with other drugs of abuse and increased risk of congenital defects, especially cardiovascular and musculoskeletal defects

CI, confidence interval; MDMA, 3,4-methylenedioxymethamphetamine.

and two were identified when fetal meconium tested positive for methamphetamine. Growth parameters included fetal birthweight and gestational age. Their data showed that infants born to methamphetamine-exposed mothers had significantly lower birthweights ($p < 0.05$). These infants were also more likely to be small for gestational age than infants born to mothers not exposed to methamphetamine (19% vs. 8.5%; OR 3.48; $p < 0.001$). Additionally, infants born to methamphetamine-exposed mothers were born earlier than infants born to mothers in the control group, but this was not statistically significant (38.7 ± 2.4 weeks [range, 25–44]; vs. 39.2 ± 1.9 weeks [range, 25–44]; $p = 0.36$).

Dixon & Bejar (1989) compared three groups of term neonates in order to determine whether antenatal stimulant use was associated with increased incidence of brain abnormalities. These groups included 74 neonates exposed to stimulants in utero, 87 drug-free infants at risk for hypoxic ischemia, and 19 healthy controls; 26 (35.1%) of the stimulant-exposed neonates had abnormal echoencephalography (ECHO) compared with 24 (27.6%) of the at-risk group and 1 (5.3%) of the healthy control group. Within the stimulant-exposed group, subgroup analysis showed that of the methamphetamine exposed infants (24/74), nine (37.5%) had abnormal ECHO. Abnormalities (some of which were not apparent on ECHO) included white matter cavities (1), white matter hyperdensities (3), hemorrhage (11), and ventricular enlargement (3). Of all these types of abnormality, there was only one infant with subependymal hemorrhage in the healthy control group. The authors concluded that there is an increased incidence of ECHO abnormalities in neonates exposed antenatally to stimulants and lacking other risk factors for cerebral injury.

These studies on methamphetamine are summarized in Table 6.13.

Comments

The effects of prenatal methamphetamine exposure on the developing fetus have yet to be well described. Reported above are two studies examining the relationship between exposure and fetal anomalies and one study with a specific focus on examining the effect of exposure on fetal growth parameters. Drug use was by self-report and was not quantified. Tobacco use and polydrug use was more common in methamphetamine-positive pregnant women than controls.

Table 6.13 Congenital defects and maternal exposure to methamphetamine

Study	Method	Sample	Incidence	Results
Little *et al.* (1988)	Case–control study Pregnancy/outcome in women who used methamphetamine throughout pregnancy	52 pregnant intravenous methamphetamine users, 52 pregnant women who reported no methamphetamine use	Methamphetamine users were likely to abuse other drugs; infant size decreased among mothers using methamphetamine; no significant difference in congenital anomalies (OR 0.72; $p < 0.39$)	Methamphetamine use during pregnancy significantly delays fetal growth; use does not appear to increase risk of congenital anomalies
Smith *et al.* (2006)	Prospective large cohort, multicenter study Methamphetamine use during pregnancy and fetal growth	84 methamphetamine-exposed pregnant women, 1534 unexposed controls	Infants born to methamphetamine-exposed mothers were more likely to be small for gestational age (OR 3.48; $p < 0.001$)	Methamphetamine exposure during pregnancy is associated with decreased growth parameters in the neonate
Dixon & Bejar (1989)	Case–control study Antenatal stimulant use and incidence of structural brain abnormalities in neonates Echoencephalography	Three groups: 74 term neonates with prenatal stimulant exposure, 87 drug-free neonates at risk for hypoxic–ischemic encephalopathy, 19 healthy controls	26 (35.1%) of stimulant-exposed neonates with abnormal echoencephalography vs. 24 (27.6%) of at-risk group and 1 (5.3%) of healthy control group; of methamphetamine-exposed infants (24/74), 9 (37.5%) had abnormal echoencephalography	There is an increased incidence of echoencephalography abnormalities in neonates exposed antenatally to stimulants and lacking other risk factors for cerebral injury

OR, odds ratio.

A single study compared ECHO findings among three groups of neonates: stimulant-exposed, "ill" with risk of cerebral pathology, and healthy. Infants were identified by toxicology screen. The strength of this study is the subgroup analysis, which divided the stimulant group into cocaine exposed, methamphetamine exposed and stimulant-narcotic exposed. The types of abnormality for each subgroup are listed.

Benzodiazepines

A report by Laegreid *et al.* (1989) described eight children exposed to benzodiazepines in utero. Five mothers were regular benzodiazepine users, while blood tests confirmed use in the remaining three mothers during their pregnancies. All of the children suffered from a combination of CNS and physical malformations somewhat reminiscent of fetal alcohol syndrome, including growth and facial abnormalities. The authors concluded that this may indicate that benzodiazepines are teratogenic.

In a case–control study, Laegreid *et al.* (1990) compared the serum of mothers who gave birth to children with similar dysmorphic features (embryopathy and fetopathy, unspecified; unspecified congenital malformations of the nervous system; cleft palate and cleft lip; congenital malformations of the urinary tract), with a control group of 60 mothers. These selected abnormalities were noted in 25 out of 10 646 live-born infants observed, 18 of whom had available maternal plasma for analysis. While 8 mothers of the 18 with infants with abnormalities (44%) used benzodiazepines, only 2 of 60 (3.3%) control group mothers were users. The authors concluded that this disparity may demonstrate a teratogenic effect of benzodiazepines.

In a longitudinal study, Laegreid *et al.* (1992) compared the development of 17 children born to mothers who used therapeutic benzodiazepines during pregnancy with that of 29 children born to non-users. Development was assessed at 6, 10, and 18 months. Of the 17 benzodiazepine-exposed children, five displayed craniofacial abnormalities. The exposed children had a comparatively low mean birthweight but quickly reached parity with the control group. However, the exposed children retained a slightly smaller cranial circumference size. The exposed children also demonstrated delays in neuromotor development, but development approached normal levels at 18 months.

Bergman *et al.* (1992) reviewed data for 104 000 women and their deliveries from the US Medicaid system database for the period 1980–1983. Fetal outcomes were analyzed through medical claim profiles up to six to nine years after delivery. Of 80 records showing maternal benzodiazepine use, 64 records were found in medical claims profiles six to nine years after delivery. There were three fetal intrauterine deaths, two cases of congenital abnormalities, and six diagnoses consistent with teratogenic abnormalities. However, the findings are confounded by the fact that these sample mothers' records show multiple substance abuse and disorder histories.

Dolovich *et al.* (1998) reviewed the available literature, including Medline, Embase, Reprotox, as well as texts, in order to examine the risk of neonate facial malformations after benzodiazepine exposure. Of the over 1400 studies reviewed, 23 studies spanning the years 1966 to 1998 were included. No association was demonstrated between benzodiazepine use during pregnancy and fetal malformations in the cohort studies: major malformations (OR 0.90; 95% CI 0.61–1.35) or oral cleft (OR 1.19; 95% CI 0.34–4.15). However, an association appeared to exist in case–control studies: major malformations (OR 3.01; 95% CI 1.32–6.84) or oral cleft alone (OR 1.79; 95% CI 1.13–2.82).

A longitudinal study carried out by Czeizel *et al.* (1999) monitored the somatic, neurological, mental, and behavioral development of children at birth, 8, 15, and 24 months. The children were divided into groups based on in utero exposure: 126 diazepam, 127 promethazine, 256 unexposed negative control, and 102 unexposed positive control. The positive control group consisted of mothers with pregnancy complications similar to those in the drug-exposed group. At birth, only the diazepam-exposed group had a lower birthweight, but at eight months, no major differences were recorded between the groups.

A series of Medline searches were performed by Iqbal *et al.* (2002) to collect all available literature regarding benzodiazepine use and pregnancy, fetuses, and neonates between 1966 and 2000. Based on results, the authors concluded that diazepam is safe to take during pregnancy, though it should be avoided during lactation because of possible effects on the infant. According to the authors' observations, the use of chlordiazepoxide consistently appeared to be safe, and alprazolam use was associated with a higher risk. There was no evidence entirely precluding the medical use of benzodiazepines during pregnancy. However, there is reason for caution, especially if benzodiazepines are taken in concert with other substances.

Wikner *et al.* (2007) used data from the Swedish Medical Birth Register to analyze the relationship between fetal malformations, morbidity, and maternal exposure to benzodiazepines or hypnotic benzodiazepine receptor agonists (HBRA). The study group consisted of 1944 mothers who used benzodiazepines/HBRA during pregnancy and 390 mothers who were prescribed these drugs late in their pregnancy. Their neonatal outcomes were compared with the general registered population (n = 873 879). Neonates who had been exposed to benzodiazepines/HBRA tended to have lower birthweights and more preterm births were also observed in this group. Those who were exposed early also had a moderately increased risk of serious congenital malformations, including pylorostenosis or alimentary tract atresia (AOR 1.24; 95% CI 1.00–1.55). No increased risk for orofacial clefts was apparent. The authors concluded that while the teratogenic potential of benzodiazepines/HBRA may not be particularly strong, it exists.

Table 6.14 summarizes these studies on benzodiazepines.

Comments
The studies described above demonstrate that there is no clear relationship between benzodiazepines and developmental disorders. There does appear to be a common observation that initial development is delayed in neonates born to benzodiazepine users. However, fetuses that have been exposed to benzodiazepines demonstrate little or no difference from unexposed neonates after about a year. Although there appears to be no long-term effects on the exposed neonates, the influence that benzodiazepines exert on fetal development is unknown. There are limited case studies that indicate maternal benzodiazepine use may precipitate physical abnormalities, including facial clefts. The risk of maternal benzodiazepine use does not appear to outweigh the medical benefit. In an article by McElhatton (1994), it is argued that evidence for benzodiazepine-related neonatal disease is flawed and limited. Although some earlier research suggests a connection to multiple malformations, most of the sample populations in subsequent studies consisted of pregnancies in women who suffered from different illnesses and used multiple drugs, making analysis difficult and no direct causality can be linked between benzodiazepines and these neonatal complications.

Barbiturates
In a multiple cohort study, Lindhout *et al.* (1992) examined the proportion of congenital abnormalities appearing in two consecutive groups of infants (cohort A, 1972–1979; cohort B, 1980–1985) who had been exposed to antiepileptic drugs. Cohort A consisted of 151 infants exposed to polytherapies consisting of either carbamazepine, phenobarbital, and valproate with or without phenytoin, or phenobarbital, phenytoin, and primidone. In cohort B, prescriptions of polytherapeutic antiepileptic treatments including phenobarbital, phenytoin, and primidone were significantly reduced. Fifteen (10%) of the infants in cohort A demonstrated congenital anomalies including facial clefts, congenital heart defects, and retardation. Of the 172 exposed infants in cohort B, 13 (7.6%) developed abnormalities that were slightly different, including spinal defects, glandular hypospadias, and inguinal hernia. The difference between the two cohorts in rate of abnormal birth was not significant.

In order to investigate congenital malformations as a result of antiepileptic drug use, Kaneko *et al.* (1999) carried out a prospective study of 983 cases in Japan, Italy, and Canada. The incidence of malformation was found to be 9% in exposed infants and only 3.1% in those who were not exposed to antiepileptic treatments (primidone, valproate, phenytoin, carbamazepine, and phenobarbital). Regarding those infants who were exposed to a single drug, phenobarbital had the lowest incidence (5.1%), and primidone had the highest (14.3%). It was observed that increasing the number of antiepileptic drugs used increased the incidence of malformation. Additionally, specific combinations of drugs (e.g., valproate and carbamazepine) produced

Table 6.14 Congenital defects and maternal exposure to benzodiazepines

Study	Method	Sample	Incidence	Results
Laegreid et al. (1989)	Case report	Eight children exposed to benzodiazepines in utero	Each of the children presented with characteristic dysmorphic features, growth aberrations, and CNS abnormalities at birth	Observations indicate a positive correlation between maternal benzodiazepine use and developmental abnormalities
Laegreid et al. (1990)	Case–control study Characteristic dysmorphic features in children Maternal plasma analysis	10 646 live born infants: 25 with embryopathy, fetopathy, unspecified nervous system malformation, cleft palate and lip, urinary tract malformations; 60 maternal–infant dyads as controls	Plasma analyzed for 18 mothers of infants with dysmorphic features; 8 (44%) tested positive for benzodiazepines; 2/60 (3.3%) positive for benzodiazepines in control group	An association exists between maternal benzodiazepine use and characteristic dysmorphic features selected by investigators
Laegreid et al. (1992)	Longitudinal study Growth and neurodevelopment of benzodiazepine-exposed infants at 6, 10 and 18 months	17 children with antenatal benzodiazepine exposure, 29 infants born to mothers with no known psychotropic drug use	Benzodiazepine-exposed children compared with those with no exposure had lower mean birth-rate and smaller cranial circumference; neuromotor development was typically delayed at 6 and 10 months but normal at 18 months; 5 exposed infants had craniofacial anomalies	Antenatal benzodiazepine use appears to negatively affect neonatal growth parameters, neuromotor development, and craniofacial development; deficits in weight and neuromotor development at normal levels at 18 months
Bergman et al. (1992)	Review of US Medicaid records 1980–1983 Fetal outcomes	104 000 pregnancies: 80 with benzodiazepine use; 64 records reviewed up to 6 to 9 years after delivery	Three fetal intrauterine deaths, 2 cases of congenital abnormality, and 6 (9.4%) diagnoses consistent with teratogenic abnormalities	Benzodiazepine use was simultaneous with various drugs and alcohol, thus confounding results
McElhatton (1994)	1994 article	Review of the evidence regarding maternal benzodiazepine use and effects on pregnancy and lactation		Evidence up to that date is found to be inconclusive; benzodiazepine exposure may delay growth temporarily
Dolovich et al. (1998)	Literature review Medline, Embase, Reprotox, research texts Risk for facial malformations secondary to benzodiazepine exposure	>1400 studies 1996–1998, 23 studies analyzed	Cohort studies indicated no association between benzodiazepines and malformations (OR 0.90; 95% CI 0.61–1.35) and oral clefts (OR 1.19; 95% CI 0.34–4.15); case–control studies did indicate an association for major malformations (OR 3.01; 95% CI 1.32–6.84) or oral cleft alone (OR 1.79; 95% CI 1.13–2.82)	A discrepancy exists between cohort studies and case–control studies regarding benzodiazepine use and fetal malformations

Study	Description	Sample	Results	Comment
Czeizel et al. (1999)	Longitudinal observational study Postnatal development and exposure to benzodiazepine	126 exposed to diazepam, 127 exposed to promethazine, 256 unexposed negative controls, 102 (unexposed positive controls)	Assessment at 8, 15, 24 months: at birth, those exposed to diazepam had a lower weight, but reached parity with the other groups after 8 months	Evidence suggests that benzodiazepines may have delayed intrauterine growth, but effect is negligable after 8 months
Iqbal et al. (2002)	Literature review. Medline Safety of benzodiazepines during pregnancy	Fetuses, and neonates between 1966 and 2000 with maternal benzodiazepine use during pregnancy	Alprazolam may cause complications during pregnancy and lactation; diazepam may cause issues during lactation; Chlordiazepoxide was safe	No evidence reviewed suggested that benzodiazepines are generally harmful enough to preclude their use in most circumstances
Wikner et al. (2007)	Review of Swedish Medical Birth Register Risk of malformations and morbidity in fetuses exposed by their mothers to benzodiazepines or HBRA	1944 mothers who used benzodiazepines /HBRA during pregnancy; 390 mothers who were prescribed such drugs late in their pregnancy; control group the general registered population ($n = 873\ 879$)	Those exposed to benzodiazepines/HBRA tended to have lower birthweights and preterm births; those exposed early in the pregnancy had an increased risk of serious congenital malformations (AOR 1.24; 95% CI 1.00–1.55)	A teratogenic potential exists, but to a small degree in these substances

AOR, adjusted odds ratio; CI, confidence interval; HBRA, hypnotic benzodiazepine receptor agonists; OR, odds ratio.

higher incidence. The only background factor associated with increased incidence was malformation in siblings. This study suggests that polytherapies and individual antiepileptic drugs, to a lesser extent, are responsible for an increase in malformations in exposed infants.

In order to analyze the rate of teratogenicity in infants exposed to antiepileptic drugs, Dravet *et al.* (1992) observed 299 patients between 1984 and 1988 in southeastern France. The authors found a higher percentage of infants were born with malformations to mothers with epilepsy (16/229) than those born within the general population (1640/117 183) as listed within the local Birth Defects Registry. No significant correlation existed between the rate of malformation and severity or type of epilepsy. Fourteen epileptic mothers went without antiepileptic drugs and their infants demonstrated no abnormalities. Eight infants with congenital heart defects were noted from the group of 146 mothers exposed to phenobarbital and no such defects in the infants of the 69 mothers not exposed to it ($p = 0.0424$). Phenobarbital in combination with phenytoin was found to be especially teratogenic.

In a case–control study, van der Pol *et al.* (1991) described the detrimental effects of antenatal exposure to anticonvulsant drugs on CNS development. The sample observed consisted of children aged 6–13 years born to epileptic mothers who were treated with phenobarbital ($n = 13$), carbamazepine ($n = 12$), phenobarbital plus carbamazepine ($n = 12$), or no medication ($n = 24$) during pregnancy. A control group ($n = 61$) consisting of non-epileptic mothers was included to minimize confounding variables. The results showed little correlation between a particular antiepileptic medication and congenital anomalies. However, antenatal exposure to phenobarbital appeared to be associated with smaller head circumference and appeared to have a negative effect on cognitive development.

These studies are summarized in Table 6.15.

Comments

The articles described above document concerns regarding antenatal maternal barbiturate use. Each study examined barbiturate use related to antiepileptic treatment and did not address complications arising from illicit use. An association between barbiturate anticonvulsant treatment and developmental complications was documented, including reduced head circumference, reduced cognition, congenital heart and spinal defects. Although barbiturate anticonvulsants correlated with developmental defects, such results were by no means exclusive to them. Further investigation is needed to determine what risks exists for recreational barbiturate users.

Cardiovascular disease

The review of the literature located several studies that describe the detrimental effects of stimulants on the cardiovascular system. No literature was retrieved describing the relationship between hallucinogens, barbiturates, or benzodiazepines and cardiovascular disease.

Amphetamine and MDMA

Two studies, both conducted at the University of Hawaii, examined the association between methamphetamine use and cardiomyopathy. Wijetunga *et al.* (2003) examined four years of hospital discharge data to obtain a group of 21 patients with a diagnosis of cardiomyopathy and a history of methamphetamine use. The duration of drug use ranged from 2 to 20 years. Echocardiography performed on 19 patients showing left ventricular dilatation in 16 (84%), right ventricular dilatation in 16 (84%), and global hypokinesis in 18 (95%). The

Table 6.15 Congenital defects and maternal exposure to barbiturates

Study	Method	Sample	Incidence	Results
Lindhout et al. (1992)	Multiple cohort study	Two groups of infants: cohort A (1972–1979), exposed to polytherapies consisting of carbamazepine plus phenobarbital plus valproate, with or without phenytoin, or phenobarbital plus phenytoin plus primidone, (n = 151); cohort B (1980–1985) exposed to polytherapeutic antiepileptic treatments including phenobarbital, phenytoin, and primidone were reduced (n = 172)	Cohort A had increased incidence of abnormalities (10%) compared with cohort B (7.6%)	Barbiturate-containing antiepileptic medication used by mothers may contribute to increased risk of various congenital abnormalities in their infants
Kaneko et al. (1999)	Prospective cohort study	983 infants born in Japan, Italy, and Canada	Incidence of congenital malformations: exposed, 9.0%; non-exposed, 3.1% Incidence of those exposed to a single drug were primidone (14.3%), valproate (11.1%), phenytoin (9.1%), carbamazepine (5.7%), phenobarbital (5.1%) Specific combinations led to higher incidence of congenital malformations	Results indicate that antiepileptic treatments may have contributed to congenital malformation incidence; use of multiple drugs increases risk
Dravet et al. (1992)	Prospective cohort study (1984–1988)	Malformation rates of neonates born to a population of pregnant antiepileptic drug users in southeastern France were compared with the rates found in birth defects registry	Significantly higher percentage of infants were born with malformations to mothers with epilepsy (16/229; 7%) than those born within the general population (1640/117 183; 1.36%)	Phenobarbital was found to be teratogenic but more so when in combination with phenytoin
van der Pol et al. (1991)	Case–control study Antenatal exposure to anticonvulsant drugs and CNS development	Children aged 6–13 years born to mothers who treated their epilepsy with phenobarbital (n = 13), carbamazepine (n = 12), phenobarbital plus carbamazepine (n = 12), or no medication (n = 24); control group (n = 61)	Children exposed to phenobarbital appeared to have smaller head circumference; a possible negative effect on cognitive development	Minimal effect on development was observed

authors concluded that chronic methamphetamine use may result in dilated cardiomyopathy and CHF.

In the second study, Yeo *et al.* (2007) investigated the association between methamphetamine use and cardiomyopathy using data extracted from hospital records. The study group comprised 107 patients who were aged 45 years or younger and who had been hospitalized with a primary discharge diagnosis of cardiomyopathy or heart failure; the control group comprised 114 patients with discharge diagnoses other than cardiomyopathy or heart failure and with ejection fractions of $\geq$ 55%. The data showed that history of methamphetamine use was more common in the study group than controls (42% vs. 20%; OR 3.0; 95% CI 1.6–5.7). Within the study group, the methamphetamine-positive subgroup had a lower mean left ventricular ejection fraction than the methamphetamine-negative group (35% vs. 26%; $p = 0.009$). From these data, the authors concluded that methamphetamine use is associated with cardiomyopathy in patients aged 45 years or younger. The authors proposed that methamphetamine may induce cardiomyopathy through mechanisms secondary to a high catecholamine state.

Seeking to investigate the relationship between MDMA use and valvular heart disease, Droogmans *et al.* (2007) compared echocardiographic data from 29 MDMA users and 29 healthy controls matched for age and gender. Based on the US Food and Drug Administration's criteria for appetite suppressant-induced valvular disease, eight MDMA users (28%) had abnormal echocardiographic results. No abnormal results were found among controls. Mitral insufficiency was observed in four MDMA users. Aortic insufficiency was also observed in four MDMA users. Tricuspid regurgitation was observed in 13 MDMA users. These valvular defects were not observed in controls. The authors concluded that MDMA use appears to be associated with the development of valvular heart disease in young people.

These studies of stimulants are summarized in Table 6.16.

Comments

Described are two studies examining the relationship between methamphetamine and cardiomypathy and one study exploring the relationship between MDMA use and valvular heart disease. These are small studies conducted at a single center or within a single geographical region. Drug use was self-reported and extracted from medical records (two studies) or obtained through an interview with a psychiatrist (one study). No information regarding the duration or severity of drug use was obtained.

Dermatological disease

The literature search yielded no studies describing an association between stimulant, hallucinogen, barbiturate, or benzodiazepine use and skin disease.

Nutritional and metabolic disease

No epidemiological literature was found regarding nutritional deficits or metabolic derangements and hallucinogens, barbiturates, or benzodiazepine use.

MDMA

Rosenson *et al.* (2007) reviewed data from the California Poison Control Center to explore gender differences in patients presenting with MDMA-associated hyponatremia. During

Table 6.16 Stimulants and cardiovascular disease

Study	Method	Sample	Incidence	Results
Wijetunga et al. (2003)	Retrospective case series Methamphetamine use and cardiomyopathy	21 patients with discharge diagnosis of cardiomyopathy and methamphetamine use (for 2 to 20 years)	19 with echocardiography: 16 (84%) with dilated left ventricle, 16 (84%) with dilated right ventricle; 18 (95%) with global hypokinesis	Chronic methamphetamine use may result in dilated cardiomyopathy and CHF
Yeo et al. (2007)	Case–control study and chart review Methamphetamine use and cardiomyopathy	107 patients < 45 years with cardiomyopathy or heart failure, 114 controls with ejection fraction > 55%	Those with cardiomyopathy or heart failure compared with controls: history of methamphetamine use more common (42% vs. 20%; OR 3.0; 95% CI 1.6–5.7); lower left ventricular ejection fraction (35% vs. 26%; $p = 0.009$)	Unexplained cardiomyopathy in patients younger than 45 years of age may be associated with methamphetamine use
Droogmans et al. (2007)	Case–control study MDMA use and valvular heart disease	29 MDMA users, 29 healthy controls	MDMA users compared with controls: pathological echocardiography in 8 patients (28%), 0 controls; valvular insufficiencies of mitral, aortic, and tricuspid valves more common in MDMA group	MDMA use appears to be associated with valvulopathy

AOR, adjusted odds ratio; CHF, congestive heart failure; CI, confidence interval; MDMA, 3,4-methylenedioxy-methamphetamine; OR, odds ratio.

the five-year study period, 545 cases of MDMA toxicity were reported; 296 (54.3%) women and 249 (45.7%) men. Seventy-three subjects had a serum sodium level of < 130 mmol/L; women composed just over 75% of these cases. Female sex was associated with increased odds of hyponatremia (OR 4.0; 95% CI 2.1–7.6). Women with hyponatremia showed increased odds of hyponatremia-associated coma (OR 3.9; 95% CI 1.2–12.9). Odds of coma were not increased among men. The authors suggested that estrogen may play a role as it enhances antidiuretic hormone release (Table 6.17).

Comments

A number of case studies describe hyponatremia among MDMA users. This retrospective review summarizes data for a five-year period from the California Poison Control System. The authors acknowledged that the general public and healthcare professionals report cases and the data are, therefore, subject to reporting bias. Spectrum bias may also exist as not all cases of toxicity are reported. Drug exposure was determined whether by self-report or positive urine toxicology.

Table 6.17 Stimulants and metabolism

Study	Method	Sample	Incidence	Results
Rosenson et al. (2007)	Retrospective review of data in the California Poison Control Center MDMA-associated hyponatremia	545 with MDMA toxicity (296 (54.3%) female, 249 (45.7%) male); 73 with serum sodium < 130 mmol/L	55/73 (75.3%) with low serum sodium were women; female sex associated with increased odds of hyponatremia (OR 4.0; 95% CI 2.1–7.6); women with hyponatremia showed increased odds of coma (OR 3.9; 95% CI 1.2–12.9)	Among patients presenting with MDMA-associated hyponatremia, female sex is associated with increased odds of hyponatremia and hyponatremia-associated coma

MDMA, 3,4-methylenedioxymethamphetamine.

Endocrine system disease

The literature search yielded no associations between stimulant, hallucinogen, barbiturate, or benzodiazepine use and endocrine disorders.

Immune system disease

One study was reviewed that positively associated the use of LSD with the onset of lymphoma.

LSD

Nelson et al. (1997) conducted a case–control study of 378 subjects who had been diagnosed with high- or intermediate-grade NHL, but who had not contracted HIV. The purpose of the study was to determine if a correlation existed between NHL and a history of tobacco, alcohol, or recreational drugs, including cocaine, amphetamines, methaqualone (Quaalude), and LSD. Subjects were matched with controls for age, race, and sex with respect to specific substance use. When drug use included multiple substances, risk for NHL tended to increase (trend $p = 0.005$), and when drug use included five or more different substances risk was greatest (OR 5.8; 95% CI 1.2–28.4). Multivariable analyses demonstrated that cocaine use accounted for much of the risk (Table 6.18).

Comments

Although a positive association between LSD usage and increased risk of NHL was demonstrated, the relationship between LSD and the risk of developing NHL is confounded by the other substances studied.

Environmental disease

The literature review yielded 10 articles regarding trauma, amphetamines, and benzodiazepines. No relevant information was found regarding MDMA, barbiturates, or LSD.

Trauma and amphetamines

Burchell et al. (2000) assessed the effect of methamphetamine use on vital signs, laboratory data, and treatment course for 120 patients presenting to the emergency department with a

Table 6.18 The immune system and LSD

Study	Method	Sample	Incidence	Results
Nelson *et al.* (1997)	Case–control study LSD and the onset of NHL	378 diagnosed with high- or intermediate-grade NHL, but HIV negative	A significant increase in risk for NHL in men was found to exist for those who used cocaine, amphetamines, Quaaludes, and LSD, with greater risk for those who used in greater frequency; when drug use included multiple substances, risk for NHL tended to increase (trend p = 0.005); when drug use included five or more different substances risk was greatest (OR 5.8, 95% CI 1.2–28.4)	Multivariable analysis results demonstrated that cocaine probably accounts for much of the risk, but confounding factors could not be removed from some of the findings

CI, confidence interval; LSD, D-lysergic acid diethylamide; NHL, non-Hodgkin's lymphoma; OR, odds ratio.

methamphetamine-positive urine screen and compared these with 240 controls (methamphetamine-negative urine screen). In both groups, 75% were male and 88% presented with blunt force injury. No differences were found in vital signs, other laboratory values, procedures, treatment, or outcome between groups. Blood alcohol level of patients with methamphetamine-positive urine was significantly lower than that of controls. The authors proposed that the lack of difference may reflect a number of factors, including remote exposure, time lag between peak drug effect and presentation to the emergency department, lack of control for other drugs of abuse, and masking of drug effect in victims of severe trauma. The authors also presented a case of severe metabolic acidosis in a trauma victim who had recently smoked crystal methamphetamine.

Tominaga *et al.* (2004) examined the relationship between methamphetamine use, severity of injury, and resource utilization of patients presenting to the emergency department. Urine toxicology was performed on 212 adult patients with injuries graded as 5 or less on the Injury Severity Score; 57 specimens returned positive for methamphetamine. No difference was observed between this group and controls in terms of Injury Severity Score. However, methamphetamine-positive patients were more likely to have a self-inflicted injury/intentional assault (37% vs. 22%; p = 0.04), be admitted to the hospital (91% vs. 70%; p = 0.001), have longer hospitalization (2.7 vs. 1.7; p = 0.003), or have higher hospital charges ($15 617 ± 1866 vs. $11 600 ± 648; p = 0.01).

Two retrospective studies were conducted at a large level I trauma center in Sacramento, California, a region of increased methamphetamine use and production. Over a six-month period, Richards *et al.* (1999b) examined the demographics of 461 methamphetamine users, their medical problems, and their use of hospital resources. The data showed that users were more likely to be male (64%; OR 1.6; 95% CI 1.4–2.0), white (74%; OR 2.7; 95% CI 2.2–3.4), and uninsured (81%; OR 3.6; 95% CI 2.8–4.5). These patients more commonly arrived at the emergency department by ambulance transport and they were more likely to be admitted to the hospital. Injuries secondary to trauma (especially blunt trauma) were more common in this population when compared with methamphetamine-negative patients (37% vs. 21%; p < 0.001).

In the second California trauma center study, Schermer & Wisner (1999) studied methamphetamine prevalence, demographics, injury mechanisms, and use of hospital resources over a five-year period. Their data showed that the rate of urine toxicology positive for methamphetamine almost doubled (7.4% in 1989, 13.4% in 1994) while the rate of cocaine-positive urine (approximately 6% of patients) remained stable over the study time and the rate of blood testing positive for alcohol decreased (43% in 1989, 35% in 1994). Of all the ethnic groups studied, whites (11.8%) and Hispanics (10.7%) tested positive for methamphetamine more frequently than for cocaine. Methamphetamine-positive patients were more frequently injured in motor vehicle collisions and motorcycle accidents than cocaine-positive patients ($p < 0.0001$). Methamphetamine use did not predict the need for emergency surgery or admission to intensive care.

In one of the largest registry-based reviews to date, Swanson et al. (2007) reviewed data from 4932 consecutive trauma patients undergoing urine toxicology screening. At their center, methamphetamine use rose 70% between the years 2003 and 2005. Methamphetamine-positive patients were more likely than non-users to present with violent interpersonal injuries (47.3% vs. 26.3%; $p < 0.001$) and higher mean Injury Severity Scores (11.2 vs. 10.0; $p < 0.01$). They were 113% more likely to die from their injuries (6.3% vs. 3.0%; $p < 0.001$). Average cost of care for these patients was increased. These patients were also more likely to lack insurance or other funding (47.6% vs. 23.1%; $p < 0.001$). The authors concluded that methamphetamine use increased greatly among patients presenting to the emergency department during the period 2003 to 2005. Their data describe a clear relationship between use and adverse outcome in every variable examined.

These studies on amphetamines and trauma are summarized in Table 6.19.

Comments

With one exception, for patients presenting to the emergency department, methamphetamine use adversely affects numerous factors ranging from cause of injury and course of treatment to patient outcome and resource consumption. All studies described were conducted in areas of the western USA and Hawaii – areas well known for a high prevalence of methamphetamine use. Given the setting (emergency department) of these studies, all subjects were identified by urine toxicology. However, not all patients presenting to the emergency department were screened for illicit drugs; therefore, a screening bias existed. This was acknowledged by several of the authors. While not common, false positives do occur and these may have influenced the data. The studies were not able to control for polydrug use or concomitant use of alcohol, which could further degrade coordination and judgement and negatively impact outcome. The duration of methamphetamine use and when the drug was taken relative to admission to healthcare setting was not known.

Trauma and benzodiazepines

One source of concern regarding benzodiazepine use is the increased risk of accidental trauma while under their influence. In a case–control study, Pariente et al. (2008) investigated the association between benzodiazepines and traumatic falls using follow-up data accessed from the French PAQUID (Personnes Agées QUID) community-based cohort for a 10-year period. The outcome measure observed was whether a fall resulting in injury or death was preceded by a report of exposure to benzodiazepines over the previous two weeks. Such patients were compared with frequency-matched controls (3:1). It was found that age was a relevant factor in the results. Among those subjects ≥80 years,

Study	Method	Sample	Incidence	Results
Burchell et al. (2000)	Retrospective case–control study, including one case report. Methamphetamine and trauma	120 trauma patients with urine toxicology positive for methamphetamine, 240 controls. One case of metabolic acidosis after trauma and smoking crystal methamphetamine	Patients with methamphetamine-positive urine had significantly lower blood alcohol levels; no difference in vital signs, laboratory values, procedures, treatment or outcome	Methamphetamine use does not appear to alter vital signs, treatment, or outcome for patients presenting to the ED, but authors acknowledge confounding factors
Tominaga et al. (2004)	Case series. Methamphetamine use and length of hospital stay given minimal injuries	544 adults with Injury Severity Score of 1–5; 212 urine toxicology screens with 57 methamphetamine positive, 155 methamphetamine negative	No difference was observed between groups in Injury Severity Scores; methamphetamine-positive patients were more likely to have self-inflicted injury/intentional assault ($p = 0.04$), be admitted to the hospital ($p = 0.001$), have longer stays ($p = 0.003$), and higher hospital charges ($p = 0.01$)	Methamphetamine-related injuries consume trauma center resources disproportionate to severity
Richards et al. (1999b)	Retrospective population-based review. Methamphetamine use in patients presenting to ED	32 156 total ED visits in 6-month period: 3102 urine toxicology screens with 461 methamphetamine-positive specimens	Methamphetamine-positive patients were more likely to be male (64% [OR 1.6; 95% CI 1.4–2.0]), Caucasian (74% [OR 2.7; 95% CI 2.2–3.4]), and uninsured (81% [OR 3.6; 95% CI 2.8–4.5]); more trauma-related injuries were seen in this group than in methamphetamine-negative patients in ED (37% vs. 21%; $p < 0.001$)	The methamphetamine-positive patient population presenting to the ED is largely composed of young, white males lacking health insurance; trauma-related injuries are more common in this group
Schermer & Wisner (1999)	Retrospective population-based review. Prevalence of methamphetamine use, demographics, injuries and use of hospital resources in trauma patients	18 004 trauma patients, 5-year period: 12 473 (69%) underwent drug testing, 10 298 (57%) underwent blood alcohol testing	Trauma patients positive for methamphetamine: 7.4% in 1989, 13.4% in 1994; methamphetamine-positive patients more likely to be victims of motor vehicle or motorcycle accident than patients testing positive for cocaine ($p < 0.0001$); methamphetamine use did not predict need for emergency surgery or admission to intensive care	Methamphetamine use is nearly doubled in trauma patients between 1989 and 1994; rates of motor vehicle injuries between methamphetamine are similar to those seen in patients using alcohol
Swanson et al. (2007)	Retrospective registry-based review. Impact of methamphetamine use in trauma patients on variables related to injury and hospital resources	4932 consecutive trauma patients undergoing toxicology screening	12.3% methamphetamine positive; among other results, the methamphetamine-positive group was more likely to have violent mechanisms of injury ($p < 0.001$); 113% more likely to die of their injuries ($p < 0.001$); more likely to have higher costs of care; more frequently unfunded ($p < 0.001$)	Specific types of violent injuries are increased among methamphetamine-positive trauma patients; these patients are more likely to have adverse outcomes; cost of care is increased among this group

CI, confidence interval; ED, emergency department; OR, odds ratio.

benzodiazepines were associated with injurious falls (AOR 2.2; 95% CI 1.4–3.4). The attributable risk in this group for falls after benzodiazepine exposure was 28.1% (95% CI 16.7–43.2). The younger members of the cohort experienced the same association between use and injury, but with an AOR of 1.3 (95% CI 0.9–1.9). The authors concluded that the significant risk demonstrated in these cases warrant a re-evaluation of benzodiazepine use, particularly in the elderly.

In another case–control study, Herings *et al.* (1995) used a Dutch medical record database (PHARMO; $n = 300\,000$) to analyze benzodiazepine use and accidental leg trauma. The patients were compared (1:3) with age-, sex-, and pharmacy-matched controls. Information on dosing, timing, elimination half-life, and type of benzodiazepine used by those who suffered femur fractures was included. Between 1986 and 1992, there were 493 cases of patients aged ≥ 5 years who were hospitalized for such accidental injuries. It was found that there was a significant association between femur fractures and current benzodiazepine use (OR 1.6; 95% CI 1.2–2.1). Specific significant associations with such traumas included short half-life benzodiazepines (OR 1.5; 95% CI 1.1–2.0), sudden dosage increases (OR 3.4; 95% CI 1.0–11.5), and concurrent use of multiple benzodiazepines (OR 2.5; 95% CI 1.3–4.9). Results demonstrated a dose–response relationship ($p < 0.0001$) that indicated dosage as the most significant characteristic involving these patients. The information presented suggests that benzodiazepine use is an independent risk factor for these accidental falls and leg trauma.

The risks associated with benzodiazepine use and motor vehicle accidents are also an issue of concern. In a 1998 article, Thomas performed a meta-analysis of the literature available between 1980 and 1997. The data reviewed included case–control studies, police and emergency reports, and driving tests that included subjects who currently used benzodiazepines. Outcomes of interest included impaired driving, accidents, mortality, postaccident medical attention, emergency ward care, and hospitalization. In the reviewed case–control studies, an association between accidents and time of use and quantity of drug taken was found (OR 1.45–2.40). In police and emergency studies, use was typically a factor in 5–10% of the cases (range, 1–66). Thomas concluded that the available data suggest an increased risk of motor vehicle accidents when driving under the influence of benzodiazepines.

In order to assess the risk of impaired driving, Bramness *et al.* (2002) analyzed the records of Norwegian drivers apprehended for driving under the influence. It is standard practice in Norway for physicians to draw and examine blood samples of such suspected drivers. The study population comprised two groups: 818 drivers with samples containing only a single benzodiazepine and 10 759 drivers with samples containing only alcohol. Of the 818 positive for benzodiazepines, 659 (81%) were classified by the physician as impaired. The investigators determined that background factors, such as gender, age, and time of apprehension, were not significant in the physicians' conclusion. Risk of being assessed as impaired did increase with benzodiazepine levels (OR 1.61, 3.65, and 4.11 for three increasing supratherapeutic drug levels). The corresponding OR values for increasing blood alcohol levels were 1.49, 2.94 and 10.49. Those drivers classified as impaired had significantly higher levels of diazepam ($n = 411$; $p < 0.001$), oxazepam ($n = 73$; $p < 0.05$), and flunitrazepam ($n = 211$; $p < 0.05$). These results suggested to the authors that benzodiazepines were a serious risk factor of impaired driving.

In 2007, Engeland *et al.* (2007) carried out another study of users and driving with population-based registries. It included information on drug prescriptions, traffic accidents, and deaths. Incidence of traffic accidents in exposed and unexposed person-time cases were accessed using standardized incidence ratio. A total of 13 000 incidents were registered involving personal injuries. For users, the risk of being involved in an incident increased in the first seven days after the dispensing of their prescriptions (standardized incidence ratio for both sexes combined 1.4; 95% CI 1.3–1.5). The use of both tranquillizing (standardized incidence ratio 2.9; 95% CI 2.5–3.5) and hypnotic (standardized incidence ratio 3.3; 95% CI 2.1–4.7) benzodiazepines increased the risk of accident. The authors concluded that these results support previous studies, which associate benzodiazepine use with traffic accidents.

These studies on benzodiazepines and trauma are summarized in Table 6.20.

Comments

Generally, two forms of trauma were found in the literature regarding benzodiazepine use: accidental falls and impaired driving. The literature that addressed traumatic falls was typically focused on older populations who were prescribed benzodiazepines as part of their medical regimen. Although the risk of trauma from older patients falling is a serious medical issue, it has limited implications for the risks involved with illicit use and abuse. However, these cases of traumatic falls do demonstrate that benzodiazepines have the capacity to influence motor performance and possibly lead to accidental trauma in users. The literature regarding impairment and motor vehicle accidents has greater relevance to the illicit use and abuse of substances. The studies presented above agree that benzodiazepine use impairs driving capability. Since benzodiazepines are so widely prescribed and available, this is an issue that warrants further study and perhaps as much public awareness as alcohol and driving have today.

Other pathological conditions

The literature search yielded no associations regarding stimulant, hallucinogen, barbiturate, or benzodiazepine use and pathological conditions.

Amphetamines and MDMA: summary and overview

As described in the research cited, the use of stimulants, in particular methamphetamine and MDMA, places the user at risk for a number of health problems. These health problems affect many different organ systems including cardiovascular, nervous, musculoskeletal and hepatic systems. Additionally, stimulant use by pregnant women appears to adversely affect fetal growth, and studies have identified a number of congenital anomalies that have been posited to be related to maternal drug use. What follows is a summary of the primary areas in which our research revealed a correlation between stimulant use and health problems. The strength of the research as well as possible explanations for the relationship will be briefly discussed.

Infections

Bacterial infections

Overall association: supported by some evidence

Historically, most MRSA infections occur in hospitals and other healthcare settings; however, the recent rise in community-acquired MRSA infections has been headline news across the country. While the association between MRSA and injection drug use has been

Table 6.20 Benzodiazepine use and trauma

Study	Method	Sample	Incidence	Results
Pariente et al. (2008)	Case–control study using data from the French PAQUID cohort	10 years of follow-up data with frequency-matched controls (3:1)	Outcome measure of interest included falls resulting in hospitalization, fracture, head injury or death Injurious falls as a result of exposure: subjects aged ≥ 80 years, AOR 2.2 (95% CI 1.4–3.4), subjects aged < 80 years, AOR 1.3 (95% CI 0.9–1.9); for subjects aged 80 years or more, attributable risk for injurious falls after exposure was 28.1% (95% CI 16.7–43.2)	Benzodiazepines contribute to a significant risk of injurious falls in the elderly
Herings et al. (1995)	Case–control study	300 000 subjects from Dutch records: 493 aged ≥ 55 years with femur fracture resulting from accidental fall; age-, sex-, and pharmacy-matched controls (1:3)	Falls significantly associated with current benzodiazepine use (OR, 1.6; 95% CI 1.2–2.1); with sudden dose increases (OR, 3.4; 95% CI 1.0–11.5); with a strong dose–response relationship (p < 0.0001)	Benzodiazepines are a major independent risk of falls resulting in femur fracture
Thomas (1998)	Meta-analysis Benzodiazepines and motor vehicle accidents	Medline review (1980–1997) of case–control studies involving benzodiazepines and motor vehicle accidents; police or emergency studies involving benzodiazepine use; driving tests with subjects currently using benzodiazepines	Case–control studies: mortality and emergency medical treatment, OR 1.45–2.4 in relation to time of use and dose; police and emergency studies, use was a factor in 1–66% of accidents	Benzodiazepine use approximately doubles the risk of motor vehicle accidents in the case-control studies
Bramness et al. (2002)	Multiple cohort study, Norway Benzodiazepine use and driving impairment Blood analysis for benzodiazepines and alcohol	Blood samples from suspected impaired drivers: 818 samples with a single benzodiazepine; 10 759 drivers with samples containing only alcohol (reference group)	659 (81%) benzodiazepine users were considered impaired; those impaired had significantly higher diazepam (n = 411; p < 0.001), oxazepam (n = 73; p < 0.05), and flunitrazepam (n = 211; p < 0.05) levels than those not impaired; risk of impairment rose with blood benzodiazepine level (OR 1.61; 95% CI 3.65–4.11) for the three supratherapeutic levels; corresponding risk of impairment with increasing alcohol levels, OR values of 1.49, 2.94, 10.49	Data suggests that benzodiazepine use is a characteristic associated with driving impairment
Engeland et al. (2007)	Case–control study, Norwegian population-based registry Prescription drugs and traffic accidents Standardized incidence ratio	13 000 traffic accidents with personal injuries registered: Information on prescriptions, personal injuries/deaths in exposed and unexposed person-time cases of accidents	Risk of being involved in an accident 7 days after dispensing of prescribed drug increased (standardized incidence ratio both sexes combined, 1.4; 95% CI 1.3–1.5); risk of accidents increased in groups using benzodiazepine tranquillizers (2.9; 95% CI 2.5–3.5) and hypnotics (3.3; 95% CI 2.1–4.7)	The use of prescription benzodiazepines by a driver increases the incidence of traffic accidents

CI, confidence interval; ED, emergency department; OR, odds ratio.

documented since the 1980s (Levine *et al.* 1982), one study (Cohen *et al.* (2007) described the novel relationship between the presence of MRSA skin and soft tissue infections and use of methamphetamine by non-injecting users in a rural community. The data from this study are strong enough to support the relationship; however, causality is not established. Likewise, a second study (Cooper *et al.* 2007) reported a somewhat weak correlation between increased treatment admissions for methamphetamine and increased number of cases of infective endocarditis. These relationships may reflect immunosuppressive effects, including inhibition of antigen processing and presentation and phagocytosis, which have been well described in animal models (Talloczy *et al.* 2008).

Musculoskeletal system disease
Rhabdomyolysis
Overall association: supported by strong evidence
Stimulants exert effects on the musculoskeletal system either by direct toxic effect on myocytes or by predisposing myocytes to injury. Rhabdomyolysis is the most common musculoskeletal injury occurring in stimulant users, and numerous case reports have documented rhabdomyolysis in MDMA users. The environment in which MDMA is commonly used – a "rave party" where users engage in increased physical activity in high ambient temperatures – increases the risk of hyperthermia and this further compounds the toxicity of the drug on skeletal muscle. One study (Richards *et al.* 1999a) determined that over 40% of patients presenting to the emergency department who were found to have rhabdomyolysis tested positive for methamphetamine. While no difference in renal pathology was observed between users and non-users in this study, the clinical relevance of this work is its establishment of a fairly strong correlation between rhabdomyolysis and methamphetamine use. For these patients, the mechanism of myocyte injury is likely to be quite similar to that observed with MDMA use. Emergency department physicians are advised to screen for illicit drug use when rhabdomyolysis is suspected.

Digestive system disease
Hepatoxicity
Overall association: supported by some evidence
While the literature contains many single case reports of MDMA-induced hepatic pathology, two larger case studies were included (Dykhuizen *et al.* 1995; Ellis *et al.* 1996) that document well the clinical presentation and course of MDMA-induced hepatic damage. The review article by Jones & Simpson (1999) reported on studies examining the mechanisms responsible for MDMA-induced hepatotoxicity. Three primary mechanisms were discussed. First, increased susceptibility to toxicity may result from an inherited defect in the hepatic enzyme CYP2D6, the isoenzyme primarily responsible for MDMA metabolism. Second, the observation that liver damage increased with continued use of MDMA supports the hypothesis that immune-mediated mechanisms play a role. Finally, the hyperthermia preceding or resulting from hepatic dysfunction appears to cause lipid peroxidation resulting in liver damage.

Stomatognathic disease

Increased tooth wear

Overall association: supported by some evidence

Several studies have documented numerous alterations in oral sensations, xerostomia, and increased tooth wear among stimulant users. Xerostomia is universally present among users of stimulants and may be secondary to drug-induced catecholamine release. Bruxism is another well-known side effect of amphetamines and amphetamine derivatives. One study (Redfearn *et al.* 1998) found that MDMA use increased the likelihood of back tooth wear. Animal studies (Arrue *et al.* 2004) have determined that MDMA partially inhibits the jaw-opening reflex, although the mechanism of this is still under active investigation. This animal work runs in parallel with the jaw clenching and tooth grinding that is observed in human users of MDMA. A single study (Richards & Brofeldt 2000) correlated methamphetamine use with increased anterior tooth wear, which the authors posited was caused by stimulant-induced vasoconstriction of the anterior of the mouth. Overall, methamphetamine has pronounced effects on the oral cavity, which led to the development of the term "meth mouth." This term refers to the severe decay often present in the mouths of methamphetamine users, resulting from a combination of xerostomia, tooth wear, poor oral hygiene and creation of an acidic environment in the mouth by consumption of carbonated beverages (Brand *et al.* 2008).

Respiratory system disease

Pulmonary artery hypertension

Overall association: supported by some evidence

Although idiopathic PAH is extremely rare, it appears to be increasing among methamphetamine users. One study (Chin *et al.* 2006) showed that patients with idiopathic PAH were 8 to 10 times more likely to have used stimulants than patients with other forms of pulmonary hypertension. The specific link between stimulant use and development of idiopathic PAH is not completely known; however, methamphetamine-induced release of serotonin may play a role. Serotonin is a potent pulmonary vasoconstrictor and stimulates the mitotic activity of pulmonary artery smooth muscle cells (Eddahibi *et al.* 1999; Marcos *et al.* 2004).

Nervous system disease

Neuronal damage and disruption of neurotransmission

Overall association: supported by strong evidence

Stimulant use appears to induce several patterns of neurological impairments that can be traced to drug-induced disturbances in neurotransmission. MDMA causes a profound release of serotonin, with smaller releases of dopamine and norepinephrine. It also inhibits serotonin reuptake, leading to increased intrasynaptic serotonin concentrations followed by serotonin depletion. Animal studies have demonstrated the toxic effect of MDMA on serotonic neurons and variable rates of recovery after drug discontinuation, with change most pronounced in the striatum, hippocampus, and prefrontal cortex (Morton 2005). In line with this, one of the studies described here (Reneman *et al.* 2001c) observed a correlation with MDMA use and axonal loss in the globus pallidus.

It is well established that the serotonergic system plays a significant role in learning and memory. We report several studies that specifically examined the relationship between MDMA use and cognition with a focus on memory. Two of these studies (Zakanis & Young 2001; Zakanis & Campbell 2006) correlated deficits in delayed and immediate recall with MDMA use and later showed that with abstinence the deficits remained stable or improved. One study (Reneman *et al.* 2001b) showed no difference in memory deficits despite reported abstinence. The authors acknowledged the difficulties in proving the correlation, which include the unreliability of drug use self-report, polydrug use, and variability of street drug concentration.

In contrast to MDMA, methamphetamine causes a massive release of dopamine, with a less intense release of serotonin. Numerous animal studies have shown that methamphetamine is toxic to both serotonin and dopaminergic neurons. Various studies were reported that describe the relationship between disturbances in neurotransmission and cognitive impairments. In their review, Baicy & London (2007) surveyed neuroimaging studies and determined that methamphetamine use correlated with impairments in numerous cognitive functions including verbal memory, working memory, psychomotor speed, attention, and inhibitory control. Additional studies reported other examples of methamphetamine-induced neuronal damage, such as increased white matter hyperintensities (Bae *et al.* 2006) and increased cerebral inflammation (Ernst *et al.* 2000). Three case reports of stroke (Rothrock *et al.* 1988) linked methamphetamine use with subsequent stroke and propose that the mechanism may involve drug-induced vasculitis or the creation of a thrombus.

Of interest is that in terms of both MDMA and methamphetamine neurotoxicity, women seem to fare better (Bae *et al.* 2006; Reneman *et al.* 2001a). It is hypothesized that estrogen plays a role, although the specific mechanism is not known. Two studies (Chana *et al.* 2006; Chang *et al.* 2005) have shown that methamphetamine use and concurrent HIV infection appear to have an additive effect on brain injury and neuronal loss. Finally, the massive serotonergic surge associated with MDMA is a well-known pharmacological trigger of serotonin syndrome. Amphetamines have also been known to cause this syndrome.

Ocular disease

Bilateral sixth nerve palsy

Overall association: supported by some evidence

A single case report (Schroeder & Brieden 2000) of transient sixth nerve palsy was found involving a 17-year-old MDMA user. Onset occurred 24 hours after last MDMA use and deficits resolved within five days without treatment. No other literature regarding MDMA and ocular disease was found.

Female genital and neonatal/congenital disease

Fetal anomalies and growth deficiencies

Overall association: supported by some evidence

Unfortunately, studies of congenital anomalies in neonates of stimulant users often yield results that are difficult to interpret in light of the high prevalence of alcohol and tobacco use among these women, as well as other lifestyle habits. As one would expect given the similar vasoactive properties of both cocaine and methamphetamine, some of the same obstetric complications observed in pregnant cocaine users are also observed in pregnant women using methamphetamine. These include premature labor, placental hemorrhage, and maternal stroke. One study (Dixon & Bejar 1989) describing the increased incidence of abnormal ECHO findings in neonates who had been exposed to stimulants in utero hypothesized that these vasoactive effects may have been partly responsible for these findings. Other studies (Little et al. 1988; Smith et al. 2006) included here reported conflicting results regarding the relationship between methamphetamine use and fetal growth parameters, although the larger of the two studies (Smith et al. 2006) found clear evidence of disturbed fetal growth in neonates of methamphetamine-using women. Nevertheless, causality was unable to be determined in this study because of the confounders described above.

Cardiovascular disease

Cardiomyopathy and valvular heart disease

Overall association: supported by some evidence

Stimulant use results in massive increases in catecholamine activity in the branch of the peripheral nervous system dedicated to regulation of both heart rate and blood pressure. The primary mechanism responsible for the cardiotoxic effects of stimulants, particularly methamphetamine, is thought to be excessive catecholamine activity. These high catecholamine levels cause narrowing and spasm of the blood vessels, tachycardia, and hypertension, and they may also be directly toxic to cardiomyocytes. Two of the studies included (Wijetunga et al. 2003; Yeo et al. 2007) illustrate these cardiotoxic effects as they describe the relationship between patients with a history of methamphetamine use and the increased incidence of cardiomyopathy or CHF among this group.

The association of valvular heart disease with both MDMA and various diet drugs has been well documented. Described here is one study (Droogmans et al. 2007) that demonstrated a solid correlation between MDMA use and the development of valvulopathy in young people. Data from previous studies investigating the mechanism of phentermine- and fenfluramine-induced valvular pathology indicate that activation of 5-HT$_{2B}$ receptors by the serotonergic drugs is primarily responsible for this side effect (Rothman et al. 2000). Interestingly, it is well known that MDMA also activates this particular subtype of serotonin receptor; therefore, this activation may be responsible for the valvular disease observed in MDMA users.

Nutritional and metabolic disease

Hyponatremia

Overall association: supported by some evidence

Numerous case studies have documented the occurrence of hyponatremia after high levels of MDMA ingestion. We report here a single large survey (Rosenson et al. 2007) of cases of hyponatremia associated with MDMA toxicity. Many factors play a role in hyponatremia occurring after MDMA use. These include increased water or carbonated beverage intake, excessive motor activity resulting in significant sweating, and antidiuretic hormone release, resulting in the syndrome of inappropriate antidiuretic hormone secretion (Hall & Henry 2006).

Environmental disease

Trauma

Overall association: supported by some evidence

Since the early 1980s, the prevalence of methamphetamine use has increased at an alarming rate. Given the rapid onset of action when methamphetamine is smoked and the concurrent catecholamine surge, users are frequently violent, behave bizarrely, and exhibit excessive anxiety. Given the effects on dopamine and serotonin neurotransmission, psychotic features including paranoia, hallucinations, mood disturbances, homicidal and suicidal thoughts, and out of control rages are common as well. All of these effects increase the probability that the user will be either the victim or the perpetrator of traumatic bodily injury. Several studies (Richards *et al.* 1999b; Schermer & Wisner 1999; Swanson *et al.* 2007) reported here examined the relationship between methamphetamine use and various factors associated with presentation to an emergency department. As would be expected, in almost every variable assessed – from type of injury to cost of care – use of methamphetamine portended a worse outcome.

Overview

Table 6.21 below gives an overview of the effect on body systems of amphetamines and MDMA, together with those of barbiturates, benzodiazepines, and LSD.

Benzodiazepines, barbiturates, and lysergic acid diethylamide: summary and overview

As cited above, the use and abuse of illicit substances including benzodiazepines, barbiturates, and LSD may result in a variety of physical illnesses. However, this grouping of substances is associated with a relatively small number of adverse effects when compared with other, more prevalent recreational drugs. This may be the result of the substances themselves but also because of the nature and frequency of their use. The barbiturates and benzodiazepines are both available to the public through medical prescription, but barbiturates are being progressively replaced by the safer benzodiazepines, which lessens chance of dependency. Additionally, it is rare for recreational drug users to abuse either barbiturates or benzodiazepines exclusively. Rather, they are used to supplement other drugs of choice, including alcohol and cocaine. Therefore, much of the literature found in our review regarding benzodiazepine and barbiturates comes from within a medical context.

Musculoskeletal system disease

Connective tissue disorders

Overall association: supported by some evidence

Barbiturates, such as phenobarbital, are prescribed for epileptics because of their anticonvulsant capabilities. In some cases, such treatment has been shown to be accompanied by various connective tissue disorders. The prospective study by Mattson *et al.* (1989) found

Table 6.21 Stimulants, hallucinogens, barbiturates, and benzodiazepines: summary table

Body system	Topic and evidence of association
Infection	Bacterial methicillin-resistant *Staphylococcus aureus*, pertussis, and infective endocarditis (methamphetamine, some)
Neoplastic	None identified
Musculoskeletal	Rhabdomyolysis (methamphetamine, strong); connective tissue disorders (barbiturates, some)
Digestive	Hepatoxicity (MDMA, some)
Stomatognathic	Increased tooth wear (methamphetamine, some; MDMA, some)
Respiratory	Pulmonary artery hypertension (methamphetamine, some)
Otorhinolaryngological	None identified
Nervous	Brain damage, neurotransmission disruption (methamphetamine, strong); brain damage, neurotransmission disruption (MDMA, some); cognitive dysfunction (benzodiazepines, some)
Ocular	Bilateral sixth nerve palsy (MDMA, some); hallucinogen persisting perception disorder (LSD, some)
Urologic	None identified
Female genital and neonatal/congenital	Cardiovascular and musculoskeletal defects (methamphetamine, some); decrease in fetal growth (MDMA, some; benzodiazepines, some); cardiovascular abnormalities (MDMA, some); multiple malformations (barbiturates, some)
Cardiovascular	Cardiomyopathy (methamphetamine, some); valvular heart disease (MDMA, some)
Dermatological	None identified
Nutritional and metabolic	Hyponatremia (MDMA, some)
Endocrine	None identified
Immune system	Increased risk of non-Hodgkin's lymphoma (LSD, some)
Environmental	Increased rate and severity of trauma cases (methamphetamine, some); increased risk of injurious fall and impaired driving (benzodiazepines, some)
Other pathologies	None

LSD, D-lysergic acid diethylamide; MDMA, 3,4-methylenedioxymethamphetamine.

a correlation between specific barbiturate treatments and a wide variety of musculoskeletal disorders. This is further supported in the literature by multiple case reports (Saviola *et al.* 1996, 2003; Strzelczyk *et al.* 2008) that correlate rheumatism and fibromatosis. These disorders are a rare but significant side effect to barbiturate use in this treatment context.

Nervous system disease

Cognitive dysfunction

Overall association: supported by some evidence

Three articles were found which reviewed and discussed the implications of long-term benzodiazepine use and cognitive function. Two meta-analyses (Barker *et al.* 2004; Stewart

2005) discussed evidence and documented cases in which cognitive dysfunction is manifested in long-term users. Deficits in motor function, memory, and concentration are found. It is noted that contradictory evidence also exists, including a lack of evidence of permanent CNS changes or abnormalities as a result of long-term use. Evidence of cognitive dysfunction is also confounded by the nature of sample populations. Long-term users of benzodiazepines, in a medical context, tend to suffer from conditions that might already impair cognitive performance.

Ocular disease

Hallucinogen persisting perception disorder

Overall association: supported by some evidence

Although more popular in previous decades, LSD is not heavily used in today's recreational drug culture. The risk of dependence is low and frequent abuse of LSD is rare even for typical users. However, the phenomenon known as "flashbacks" or HPPD has been shown to occur in some users. Halpern & Pope (2003) reviewed the available literature from 1955 to 2001 and found that HPPD does exist as a persistent physical disorder, but in somewhat rare cases. This is supported by case studies presented by Kawasaki & Purvin (1996) and Gaillard & Borruat (2003). In some cases, there is physical evidence of an abnormality, such as abnormal electroencephalography. Other cases involve only the reports given by the patients. More investigation is necessary to better understand the causes of HPPD and the varying manifestations it takes.

Female genital and neonatal/congenital disease

Decrease in fetal growth

Overall association: supported by some evidence

The benzodiazepines are so commonly utilized today precisely because they seem to offer very little risk compared with the medical benefits they provide. However, there is some speculation in the literature regarding whether or not maternal benzodiazepine use is harmful to fetal development. Over four years, Laegreid et al. published three studies (1989, 1990, 1992) to address this question. Initially, multiple cases of CNS and physical abnormalities reminiscent of fetal alcohol syndrome were observed; the authors followed this by reporting a case–control study and longitudinal study. In these, a possible risk of cleft palate and other malformations was discussed, but the longitudinal study demonstrated only delayed growth and neuromotor development. These reached normal levels after 18 months. Czeizel et al. (1999) found similar results in a longitudinal study. Both Bergman et al. (1992) and Wikner et al. (2007) reviewed medical records, through Medicaid and a birth registry, respectively. Bergman et al. (1992) found cases of abnormalities, but most of the evidence was confounded by the fact that the population studied was exposed to multiple substances. Wikner et al. (2007) found results similar to those of the Laegreid group in that benzodiazepine exposure resulted in LBW and moderately increased risk of congenital malformations. Dolovich et al. (1998) and Iqbal et al. (2002) both conducted reviews of literature. Dolovich et al. (1998) found a positive association between exposure and malformations in case–control studies but not in cohort studies. Iqbal et al. (2002)

found that alprazolam should be avoided and that benzodiazepine use during lactation may exert effects on the neonate. Maternal benzodiazepine use appears to exert a weak effect on the developing infant.

Multiple malformations

Overall association: supported by some evidence

There is evidence supporting possible congenital defects as a result of barbiturate treatment. The literature reviewed consisted of small case–control studies as well as larger population reviews. As described above, there is an increased risk of congenital disorders such as facial and heart defects, spinal complications, and disrupted CNS development. This danger is not specifically associated with barbiturates in these studies, but with all antiepileptic medications. The danger in maternal use of barbiturates is increased when used in concert with other drugs.

Immune system disease

Increased risk of non-Hodgkin's lymphoma

Overall association: supported by some evidence

One study (Nelson *et al.* 1997) indicated a possible connection between LSD use and the onset of NHL. This connection is somewhat tenuous because NHL was most strongly associated with multiple drug use, not specifically LSD. No other studies were found associating LSD with immunity disorders.

Environmental disease

Trauma: injurious falls

Overall association: supported by some evidence

Two studies analyzed cases of traumatic accidental falls and found that benzodiazepine use increased the risk of injury and hospitalization. However, both studies used sample populations that were older in age ($\geq$ 55 years) and did not address illicit use.

Trauma: impaired driving

Overall association: supported by some evidence

The second form of trauma addressed in the literature was the association of benzodiazepine use and motor vehicle accidents. Three studies were found, including one meta-analysis. All of the authors concluded that benzodiazepine use was a risk factor for driving impairment and possible injury in their sample populations.

Overview

Table 6.21 summarizes the association of the hallucinogens, stimulants, and barbiturates with research covering various body systems described in this chapter. The "Topic" column indicates the condition described, followed by the rating for the evidence of association in parentheses. The term "strong" suggests there is a significant body of knowledge supporting a direct or indirect association between hallucinogens, stimulants, and barbiturates and the condition (e.g., a significant number of studies, cohort or case–controlled studies, clinical laboratory studies, or a single seminal study). "Strong" suggests that the clinician may find this condition in a hallucinogen, stimulant, or barbiturate user. "Some" suggests that there are some studies supporting a direct or indirect association between hallucinogens, stimulants, and barbiturates and the condition (e. g., a smaller number of studies, case–control or case reports, or a study reporting a rare or under-reported condition). In many cases, "some" suggests more evidence is needed to support a strong association with a condition.

Physical illness does co-occur with use of illicit drugs of abuse. A review of the published PubMed literature from 1988 through 2008 revealed that cocaine, marijuana, opioids, and various hallucinogens, stimulants, and barbiturates have associations with physical illnesses. While the literature is vast on the co-occurring or comorbid associations of these illicit substances with mental health disorders, the recent literature is not as expansive for associations with physical health disorders.

Nonetheless, several summary statements regarding illicit substances and physical illnesses are supported through this review. For cocaine, marijuana, and, to a lesser extent, opioids, the review found literature to support incident or prevalent association between several physical diseases and the drug of abuse. It was somewhat surprising that, despite the level of medical harm supposedly attributable to illicit drugs and the public and legal ramifications from illicit drug use, there was not more – and better – evidence of associations, especially considering the volume of literature reviewed. For our reviews on hallucinogens, stimulants, and barbiturates, few categories of physical illness had any convincing evidence of support.

When undertaking a review of the peer-reviewed literature, it is helpful to examine the literature closely regarding the scientific merit of the study and the ability of the study findings to support the authors' conclusion. While not the purpose of this book, in order to conclude that an association of an illicit drug with a specific physical illness has occurred, the conclusion should be supported by facts and not mere conjecture. Furthermore, readers should be cautioned that a large number of studies that investigate or allude to an association do not justify greater support for an association than a small number or even one study. That single study may have been the pre-eminent study regarding the association.

A formal meta-analysis to determine the strength of the support for each illicit drug to each physical illness would be ideal, but many issues limit the usefulness of such analyses. These issues include the heterogeneity of study designs, paucity of description of study methods, and variability in citing specifics about the abuse (e.g., type of drug[s] of abuse, pattern and volume of use, dosage effects) and outcome of disease (e.g., lack of or vagueness in disease definitions, severity of disease).

Alcohol and tobacco smoking are common among patients who use illicit substances. In addition, many patients who use one illicit substance also use others. In this review, many of the studies reviewed did not examine the influence of alcohol, tobacco, or another illicit substance on the association of disease processes to a particular illicit substance. This is especially true with regard to the case series literature. In addition, many of the studies also used self-report regarding drug use. Therefore, any conclusions regarding an association, or the strength of association, for a particular substance of abuse and a physical illness should be made cautiously.

With this in mind, and despite the paucity of good evidence, especially for certain illicit drugs, Table 7.1 (at end of this chapter) indicates the degree to which physical illness occurs with increased incidence or prevalence according to the review of the literature from 1988 through 2008. The table is not comprehensive; the lack of a named association should not prompt the reader to conclude that there is no association with the drug of abuse and a physical illness, rather that the literature from 1988 to 2008 was not helpful in forming an association.

As in the summary tables in each of the four Results chapters, Table 7.1, below, summarizes the association of the drugs with research covering various body systems described in this book. The "Topic" column indicates the condition described, followed by the rating for the evidence of association in parentheses. The term "strong" suggests there is a significant body of knowledge supporting a direct or indirect association between cocaine and the condition (e.g., a significant number of studies, cohort or case–controlled studies, clinical laboratory studies, or a single seminal study). "Strong" suggests that the clinician may find this condition in an illicit drug user. "Some" suggests that there are some studies supporting a direct or indirect association between a drug and the condition (e.g., a smaller number of studies, case–control or case reports, or a study reporting a rare or under-reported condition). In many cases, "some" suggests more evidence is needed to support a strong association with a condition.

In brief, cocaine is strongly associated with perforated ulcer, gastrointestinal ischemia and infarct, exacerbation of asthma, respiratory signs and symptoms, nasal and midline lesions, cerebrovascular vessel reactivity, strokes and SAH, and altered ANS in newborns. Cocaine is also strongly associated with renal dysfunction, some cardiovascular conditions in infants, coronary artery dysfunction, chest pain, rare incidences of AMI and ECG changes, coagulation defects, rhabdomyolysis, excited delirium, and cocaine toxicity. Trauma and body stuffers and packers are also strongly associated with cocaine.

In brief, marijuana use is strongly associated with liver damage and HCV, acute cardiovascular effects, cannabis arteritis, and trauma. Opioid use is strongly associated with rhabdomyolysis, renal disease associated with rhabdomyolysis, NAS, and torsades de pointes and ventricular tachycardia associated with methadone. The hallucinogens, stimulants, and barbiturates are strongly associated with brain damage and neurotransmission disruption (methamphetamine). All other associations have some evidence not determined as strong.

For a clinician, knowing these associations will enhance the ability to consider comorbid physical illnesses based on the type of drug that the patient may be using or abusing and the risks that the drug use has in developing a physical illness. Or a provider may be faced with a patient who is unwilling or unable to provide a history of illicit drug use. Knowing the type (and patterns) of known physical diseases may help the clinician in deducing the illicit drug of abuse.

This review has several limitations to its methods and conclusions. First, this review only examined the recent evidence (from 1988 to 2008) of the associations between drugs of abuse and physical illness. It was not the reviewers' intentions to discount the findings prior to 1988; as mentioned in the Introduction, the lower bound was set partly for the sake of convenience and also to restrict the search to recent findings. In each chapter, there is some mention of findings prior to 1988, and in general, the findings prior to 1988 seem to mirror those in the search time frame.

Table 7.1 Summary of strength of recent evidence regarding drugs of abuse for physical illness.

Body system	Cocaine	Marijuana	Opioids	Benzodiazepines, barbiturates, methamphetamine, MDMA, and LSD
Infections	Bacterial, mycoses, parasitic, viral (all some)	Bacterial (some); viral (liver damage and hepatitis C virus) (strong)	Abscesses and cellulitis (some); pulmonary infection (some); bacterial endocarditis (some); invasive rhinosinusitis (some)	Bacterial: methicillin-resistant *Staphylococcus aureus*, pertussis, and infective endocarditis (methamphetamine, some)
Neoplastic	Non-Hodgkin's lymphoma (some); pancreatic cancer (some)	Respiratory cancer (some); transitional cell bladder cancer (some)	None	None identified
Musculoskeletal	Crack dancing, see nervous system; rhabdomyolysis, see renal system	Spasticity (some)	Rhabdomyolysis (strong)	Rhabdomyolysis (methamphetamine, strong); connective tissue disorders (barbiturates, some)
Digestive	Perforated ulcer, gastrointestinal ischemia and infarct (strong)	None	None	Hepatoxicity (MDMA, some)
Stomatognathic	Included with otorhinolaryngological	Oral health (some)	None	Increased tooth wear (methamphetamine, some; MDMA, some)
Respiratory	Asthma (strong); respiratory changes, signs and symptoms (strong)	Chronic inflammatory change (some); allergen (some)	Asthma (some); non-cardiogenic pulmonary edema (some); respiratory depression (some)	Pulmonary artery hypertension (methamphetamine, some)
Otorhinolaryngological	Oral lesions (some); nasal, including olfaction (strong); midline lesions (strong)	None	None	None identified
Nervous	Cerebrovascular (some); strokes, subarachnoid hemorrhage (strong); autonomic nervous system in newborns (strong); central nervous system atrophy (some); seizures (strong); crack dancing (some); demyelination (some); neuropsychological (some); altered sleep patterns (some)	Atrophy, decreased brain volume (some); cognitive, psychomotor function (some); cerebral ischemia (some); safety, drug use and antiepileptic drugs (some); tardive dyskinesia (some); sleep disturbances (some)	Seizures (some); cerebral/cerebellar dysfunction (some)	Brain damage, neurotransmission disruption (methamphetamine, strong); brain damage and neurotransmission disruption (MDMA, some); cognitive dysfunction (benzodiazepines, some)

Ocular	Corneal (some); retinal (some); iritis (some); altered color vision (some); acute-angle-closure glaucoma (some)	Visual changes (some)	Strabismus (some); ocular candidiasis (some)	Bilateral sixth nerve palsy (MDMA, some); hallucinogen persisting perception disorder (LSD, some)
Urological	Genital ulcer disease in males (some); male sexual dysfunction, priapism (some); renal (strong)	Transitional cell bladder cancer (some)	Renal disease with rhabdomyolysis (strong); other renal pathology (some)	None identified
Female genital and neonatal/ congenital	Genital ulcer disease (some); pelvic inflammatory disease (some); pregnancy complications (some); infant cardiovascular conditions (strong); congenital syphilis (some); congenital anomalies (some)	Genital infections (some); infertility and ovarian dysfunction (some); pregnancy complications (placenta abruptio [some]; altered newborn growth and development [some]; cardiac abnormalities [some]; gastrointestinal abnormalities [some])	Fetal growth restriction (some); placental changes (some); neonatal abstinence syndrome (strong); congenital disease (some); perinatal stroke (some)	Cardiovascular and musculoskeletal defects (methamphetamine, some); decrease in fetal growth (MDMA, some; benzodiazepines, some); cardiovascular abnormalities (MDMA, some); multiple malformations (barbiturates, some)
Cardiovascular	Coronary artery studies (strong); chest pain, acute myocardial infarction, ECG changes (strong); cardiac morphology (some); coagulation defects (strong)	Acute cardiovascular effects (strong); cannabis arteritis (strong); cardiovascular risk (some)	Coronary artery disease (some); infective endocarditis (some); torsades de pointes, ventricular tachycardia (methadone) (strong)	Cardiomyopathy (methamphetamine, some); valvular heart disease (MDMA, some)
Dermatological	Lesions (some)	None	None	None identified
Nutritional and metabolic	Altered plasma cholinesterase (some); body mass index and cocaine-induced psychosis (some); acid–base imbalance (some); hyperthermia (strong); rhabdomyolysis (strong); excited delirium (strong); cocaine toxicity (strong)	Effect on food intake, metabolic syndrome (some)	Calcium inhibition (some); gastrin, decreased release (some); hypercholesterolemia (some); hypo- and hyperthermia (some); hyperkalemia (some)	Hyponatremia (MDMA, some)

Table 7.1 *Cont.*

Body system	Cocaine	Marijuana	Opioids	Benzodiazepines, barbiturates, methamphetamine, MDMA, and LSD
Endocrine	Altered prolactin (some); diabetes mellitus and ketoacidosis (some)	None	Pituitary enlargement, hormone alteration (some)	None identified
Immune	Autoimmune diseases (some); monocyte dysfunction (some)	None	Immunosuppression (some)	Increased risk of non-Hodgkin's lymphoma (LSD, some)
Environment	Trauma (strong); body stuffer/packers (strong)	Trauma (strong)	None	Increased rate and severity of trauma cases (methamphetamine, some); increased risk of injurious fall and impaired driving (benzodiazepines, some)
Other pathologies	Placental pathology (some); brain pathology (some)	None	None	None

LSD, D-lysergic acid diethylamide; MDMA, 3,4-methylenedioxymethamphetamine.

Second, in theory, this review examined about half of the peer-reviewed searchable literature, as MEDLINE was established in 1966. This estimation is likely conservative as the number of journals in the last 20 years, particularly substance abuse journals, has increased. However, an associated limitation is that this review did not examine literature contained outside of MEDLINE or PubMed. However, it is likely that the most evidence-based journals are included in this search, to this review's credit.

Third, it is likely that studies were missed in this review. While every attempt was made to find and describe epidemiological studies that had any potential for associations between drugs of abuse and physical illnesses, the search strategy was conducted in such a way that some studies may have not been identified. This review was conducted by using MeSH terms for drugs of abuse and a very broad search of MeSH terms for physical illnesses. Drugs of abuse go by many names, and diseases are often misidentified or vaguely defined. Furthermore, some associations may have been found in some studies that did not contain MeSH terms that would have been captured in the search strategy. Finally, MeSH terms may have been inaccurate or omitted in the electronic databases for a particular study, which this review then did not evaluate or describe as a result.

A fourth limitation to this review is that it was restricted to studies and papers in the English language. In part, this was done as the medical literature is increasingly related in English, but mainly for convenience of the reviewers.

Fifth, the review concentrated on four main illicit drugs of abuse: cocaine, marijuana, opioids, and the broad category of barbiturates, hallucinogens, and stimulants. The review did not cover every illicit drug of abuse and, therefore, should not be construed as a comprehensive review of all illicit drugs of abuse and physical illness. Nonetheless, for the four main categories, this review is fairly comprehensive of the literature in the search time frame.

A sixth limitation is that the review did not examine illicit drug use associations to mental health disorders, untoward behavioral problems, or adverse public health consequences. The focus of this book was on associations with physical illness. The literature is much more established on the mental health, environmental, legal, and social harms associated with illicit substance use. These associations should not be discounted; mental health influences physical health, and legal and vocational harm associated with use of illicit substances certainly influences the morbidity and incidence of physical illnesses. For example, activities and behavior patterns associated with alcohol and drug use can result in homelessness, which influences the incidence, severity, and treatment of a host of physical health conditions. In this book, the review concentrated on direct associations and not indirect associations of drug use through other illnesses (e.g., mental illness) or social morbidity (e.g., homelessness) to physical illness.

A seventh limitation engendered much discussion among the authors; the review was intended to discusses direct associations of the illicit drug and physical health conditions, not associations made through the route of drug administration (e.g., intravenous drug use). There is a strong association regarding intravenous drug use – particularly heroin use – and infection with HCV and HIV, yet these are scarcely mentioned in this review. There is scant evidence that the drug itself is the causative agent in the increased risk of acquiring these viral infections. Rather, the risk is attributed to the risky behavior (whether intravenous administration or risky sexual practices). Therefore, the review concentrated on direct associations with the agent (the drug) and the disease process.

That being said, the route of administration of the illicit drug was a factor in other aspects of this review. For example, the association of cocaine with pulmonary diseases likely is secondary to its route of administration (inhalation). It is unlikely that pulmonary disease processes would exist (or be as prominent) if cocaine were administered through subdermal routes. Yet when injected subdermally, cocaine has a direct action on restriction of dermal vasculature inciting dermal pathology; therefore, this direct action would be part of the review. Likewise, when cocaine is inhaled (in crack or freebase forms), direct pulmonary vascular constriction is likely behind the pulmonary findings seen in patients with cocaine use. Therefore, as in subdermal administration, cocaine has direct association with pulmonary disease if inhaled, and these associations are described in this review.

Meanwhile, if a patient was intravenously injecting heroin through sterile needles (and did not have other risky behaviors), it is unlikely that infectious disease would occur. Perhaps non-clinical studies, particularly in the pathophysiology literature, could shed more light on the degree of a direct increased risk of heroin to the incidence of an infectious disease. However, for this review, the act of using needles and other risky behaviors associated with drug use was not explicitly examined as a causative agent for physical illness. As above, a direct association with the drug of abuse and the physical illness was examined; indirect associations were not.

An eighth limitation pertains to the opioid and hallucinogen, stimulants, and barbiturate chapters. Some drugs of abuse are also medications for treatment of physical or mental health disorders; therefore, this review did not concentrate on describing the physical consequences of use of opioids (such as for pain) but of illicit use of opioids. Benzodiazipines and opioids are medications that work effectively for a variety of physical ailments. Their side effects are well known. The literature describes the side effect of constipation with opioid use for pain; however, this review concentrated on constipation that occurs with illicit opioid use.

A ninth limitation is that we did not attempt to describe the pathological or pathophysiological mechanism of the association between the illicit substance and a physical health condition. The review was of human studies and the description of these studies only briefly describes potential pathophysiological mechanisms for observed associations. In the future, as the science of addiction encourages more disease-centric approaches to addiction, the mechanisms for the associations of illicit drug use and physical diseases may be more apparent and, thus, more reviewable.

A final limitation is regarding our assessment of the support of the literature for a particular drug of abuse to a particular physical disease. At least two authors agreed on the support of each of the associations, but these were subjective assessments. In the future, greater scientific rating of the literature may be possible, particularly for specific medical illnesses, such as work initiated by the PRISM project, described in the Introduction.

In future editions, these limitations may be confronted. With this background search completed, a foundation for the observed associations has been compiled that will allow for future, more thorough examination of illicit drug use and physical illness associations. Table 7.1 summarizes for all the systems described in this book. This may include describing indirect associations, such as those with mental illness, or different routes of administration of drugs of abuse, non-English literature, and/or stronger grading of the evidence.

Despite these limitations, this book provides a comprehensive review of the associations in the recent, human, English-speaking, searchable literature regarding illicit substance use and physical illness. Overall, future research is needed in many disease associations, and studies regarding mechanisms and causative effects of the potential or realized associations are essential. As addiction is thought as a "brain disease," the agents of the addiction – the drugs themselves – should be examined as factors in physical disease pathology. It may be through these studies that true integrative assessment and care for patients with addictive disorders by mental and physical health providers may be realized.

References

Abs, R., Verhelst, J., Maeyaert, J., *et al.* (2000). Endocrine consequences of long-term intrathecal administration of opioids. *J. Clin. Endocrinol. Metab*, **85**(6), 2215–2222. PM:10852454.

Aggarwal, S. K., Williams, V., Levine, S. R., Cassin, B. J., & Garcia, J. H. (1996). Cocaine-associated intracranial hemorrhage: absence of vasculitis in 14 cases. *Neurology*, **46**(6), 1741–1743. PM:8649582.

Aldington, S., Harwood, M., Cox, B., *et al.* (2008). Cannabis use and risk of lung cancer: a case–control study. *Eur. Respir. J.*, **31**(2), 280–286. PM:18238947.

Alexandrakis, G., Tse, D. T., Rosa, R. H., Jr., & Johnson, T. E. (1999). Nasolacrimal duct obstruction and orbital cellulitis associated with chronic intranasal cocaine abuse. *Arch. Ophthalmol.*, **117**(12), 1617–1622. PM:10604666.

Alldredge, B. K., Lowenstein, D. H., & Simon, R. P. (1989). Seizures associated with recreational drug abuse. *Neurology*, **39**(8), 1037–1039. PM:2788249.

Altman, A. L., Seftel, A. D., Brown, S. L., & Hampel, N. (1999). Cocaine associated priapism. *J. Urol.*, **161**(6), 1817–1818. PM:10332443.

American Psychiatric Association (2000). *Diagnostic and Statistical Manual of Mental Disorders*, 4th edn. Washington, DC: American Psychiatric Press.

Amin, M., Gabelman, G., Karpel, J., & Buttrick, P. (1990). Acute myocardial infarction and chest pain syndromes after cocaine use. *Am. J. Cardiol.*, **66**(20), 1434–1437. PM:2251988.

Angst, J., Gamma, A., Benazzi, F., *et al.* (2003). Diagnostic issues in bipolar disorder. *Eur. Neuropsychopharmacol.*, **13**(Suppl 2), S43–S50. PM:12957719.

Arrue, A., Gomez, F. M., & Giralt, M. T. (2004). Effects of 3,4-methylenedioxymethamphetamine ("ecstasy") on the jaw-opening reflex and on the alpha-adrenoceptors which regulate this reflex in the anesthetized rat. *Eur. J. Oral Sci.*, **112**(2), 127–133. PM:15056109.

Aryana, A. & Williams, M. A. (2007). Marijuana as a trigger of cardiovascular events: speculation or scientific certainty? *Int. J. Cardiol.*, **118**(2), 141–144. PM:17005273.

Arzt, E. & Holsboer, F. (2006). CRF signaling: molecular specificity for drug targeting in the CNS. *Trends Pharmacol. Sci.*, **27**(10), 531–538. PM:16935354.

Attoussi, S., Faulkner, M. L., Oso, A., & Umoru, B. (1998). Cocaine-induced scleroderma and scleroderma renal crisis. *South. Med. J.*, **91**(10), 961–963. PM:9786294.

Bada, H. S., Bauer, C. R., Shankaran, S., *et al.* (2002a). Central and autonomic system signs with in utero drug exposure. *Arch. Dis. Child Fetal Neonatal Ed.*, **87**(2), F106–F112. PM:12193516.

Bada, H. S., Das, A., Bauer, C. R., *et al.* (2002b). Gestational cocaine exposure and intrauterine growth: maternal lifestyle study. *Obstet. Gynecol.*, **100**(5 Pt 1), 916–924. PM:12423853.

Bae, S. C., Lyoo, I. K., Sung, Y. H., *et al.* (2006). Increased white matter hyperintensities in male methamphetamine abusers. *Drug Alcohol Depend.*, **81**(1), 83–88. PM:16005161.

Baicy, K. & London, E. D. (2007). Corticolimbic dysregulation and chronic methamphetamine abuse. *Addiction*, **102**(Suppl 1), 5–15. PM:17493049.

Bailey, D. N. (1993). Serial plasma concentrations of cocaethylene, cocaine, and ethanol in trauma victims. *J. Anal. Toxicol.*, **17**(2), 79–83. PM:8492571.

Baldwin, G. C., Tashkin, D. P., Buckley, D. M., *et al.* (1997). Marijuana and cocaine impair alveolar macrophage function and cytokine production. *Am. J. Respir. Crit Care Med.*, **156**(5), 1606–1613. PM:9372683.

Baldwin, G. C., Choi, R., Roth, M. D., *et al.* (2002). Evidence of chronic damage to the pulmonary microcirculation in habitual users of alkaloidal ("crack") cocaine. *Chest*, **121**(4), 1231–1238. PM:11948058.

Bansal, D., Eigenbrodt, M., Gupta, E., & Mehta, J.L. (2007). Traditional risk factors and acute myocardial infarction in patients hospitalized with cocaine-associated chest pain. *Clin. Cardiol.*, **30**(6), 290–294. PM:17551964.

Barillo, D.J. & Goode, R. (1996). Substance abuse in victims of fire. *J. Burn Care Rehabil.*, **17**(1), 71–76. PM:8808362.

Barker, M.J., Greenwood, K.M., Jackson, M., & Crowe, S.F. (2004). Cognitive effects of long-term benzodiazepine use: a meta-analysis. *CNS Drugs*, **18**(1), 37–48. PM:14731058.

Bateman, D.A., Ng, S.K., Hansen, C.A., & Heagarty, M.C. (1993). The effects of intrauterine cocaine exposure in newborns. *Am. J. Public Health*, **83**(2), 190–193. PM:8427321.

Bauer, C.R., Langer, J.C., Shankaran, S., *et al.* (2005). Acute neonatal effects of cocaine exposure during pregnancy. *Arch. Pediatr. Adolesc. Med.*, **159**(9), 824–834. PM:16143741.

Bauer, L.O. & Mott, A.E. (1996). Differential effects of cocaine, alcohol, and nicotine dependence on olfactory evoked potentials. *Drug Alcohol Depend.*, **42**(1), 21–26. PM:8889400.

Bauwens, J.E., Orlander, H., Gomez, M.P., *et al.* (2002). Epidemic lymphogranuloma venereum during epidemics of crack cocaine use and HIV infection in the Bahamas. *Sex. Transm. Dis.*, **29**(5), 253–259. PM:11984440.

Behnke, M. & Eyler, F.D. (1993). The consequences of prenatal substance use for the developing fetus, newborn, and young child. *Int. J. Addict.*, **28**(13), 1341–1391. PM:7507469.

Behnke, M., Eyler, F.D., Garvan, C.W., *et al.* (1999). Cranial ultrasound abnormalities identified at birth: their relationship to perinatal risk and neurobehavioral outcome. *Pediatrics*, **103**(4), e41. PM:10103333.

Beigi, R.H., Meyn, L.A., Moore, D.M., Krohn, M.A., & Hillier, S.L. (2004). Vaginal yeast colonization in nonpregnant women: a longitudinal study. *Obstet. Gynecol.*, **104**(5 Pt 1), 926–930. PM:15516380.

Bemanian, S., Motallebi, M., & Nosrati, S.M. (2005). Cocaine-induced renal infarction: report of a case and review of the literature. *BMC Nephrol.*, **6**, 10. PM:16176587.

Bergman, U., Rosa, F.W., Baum, C., Wiholm, B. E., & Faich, G.A. (1992). Effects of exposure to benzodiazepine during fetal life. *Lancet*, **340**(8821), 694–696. PM:1355799.

Binder, T. & Vavrinkova, B. (2008). Prospective randomised comparative study of the effect of buprenorphine, methadone and heroin on the course of pregnancy, birthweight of newborns, early postpartum adaptation and course of the neonatal abstinence syndrome (NAS) in women followed up in the outpatient department. *Neuro. Endocrinol. Lett.*, **29**(1), 80–86. PM:18283247.

Blaho, K., Winbery, S., Park, L., *et al.* (2000). Cocaine metabolism in hyperthermic patients with excited delirium. *J. Clin. Forensic Med.*, **7**(2), 71–76. PM:16083654.

Block, R.I., O'Leary, D.S., Ehrhardt, J.C., *et al.* (2000). Effects of frequent marijuana use on brain tissue volume and composition. *Neuroreport*, **11**(3), 491–496. PM:10718301.

Blondell, R.D., Dodds, H.N., Looney, S.W., *et al.* (2005). Toxicology screening results: injury associations among hospitalized trauma patients. *J. Trauma*, **58**(3), 561–570. PM:15761352.

Blows, S., Ivers, R.Q., Connor, J., *et al.* (2005). Marijuana use and car crash injury. *Addiction*, **100**(5), 605–611. PM:15847617.

Boco, T. & Macdonald, R.L. (2004). Absence of acute cerebral vasoconstriction after cocaine-associated subarachnoid hemorrhage. *Neurocrit. Care*, **1**(4), 449–454. PM:16174948.

Bolla, K.I., Lesage, S.R., Gamaldo, C.E., *et al.* (2008). Sleep disturbance in heavy marijuana users. *Sleep*, **31**(6), 901–908. PM:18548836.

Bonkowsky, J.L., Sarco, D., & Pomeroy, S.L. (2005). Ataxia and shaking in a 2-year-old girl: acute marijuana intoxication presenting as seizure. *Pediatr. Emerg. Care*, **21**(8), 527–528. PM:16096599.

Borges, G., Mondragon, L., Medina-Mora, M.E., *et al.* (2005). A case–control study of alcohol and substance use disorders as risk factors for non-fatal injury. *Alcohol Alcohol.*, **40**(4), 257–262. PM:15851400.

Borne, J., Riascos, R., Cuellar, H., Vargas, D., & Rojas, R. (2005). Neuroimaging in drug and substance abuse part II: opioids and solvents. *Top. Magn. Reson. Imaging*, **16**(3), 239–245. PM:16340648.

Boto de los, B.A., Pereira, V.A., Sanchez Ramos, J.L., *et al.* (2002). Bronchial hyperreactivity in patients who inhale heroin mixed with cocaine vaporized on aluminum foil. *Chest*, **121**(4), 1223–1230. PM:11948057.

Boutros, H.H., Pautler, S., & Chakrabarti, S. (1997). Cocaine-induced ischemic colitis with small-vessel thrombosis of colon and gallbladder. *J. Clin. Gastroenterol.*, **24**(1), 49–53. PM:9013352.

Bowley, D.M., Rein, P., Cherry, R., *et al.* (2004). Substance abuse and major trauma in Johannesburg. *S. Afr. J. Surg.*, **42**(1), 7–10. PM:15181707.

Bramness, J.G., Skurtveit, S., & Morland, J. (2002). Clinical impairment of benzodiazepines: relation between benzodiazepine concentrations and impairment in apprehended drivers. *Drug Alcohol Depend.*, **68**(2), 131–141. PM:12234642.

Brand, H.S., Dun, S.N., & Nieuw Amerongen, A.V. (2008). Ecstasy (MDMA) and oral health. *Br. Dent. J.*, **204**(2), 77–81. PM:18268544.

Brecklin, C.S., Gopaniuk-Folga, A., Kravetz, T., *et al.* (1998). Prevalence of hypertension in chronic cocaine users. *Am. J. Hypertens.*, **11**(11 Pt 1), 1279–1283. PM:9832169.

Brewer, J.D., Meves, A., Bostwick, J.M., Hamacher, K.L., & Pittelkow, M.R. (2008). Cocaine abuse: dermatologic manifestations and therapeutic approaches. *J. Am. Acad. Dermatol.*, **59**(3), 483–487. PM:18467002.

Brick, J. (2008). *Handbook of the Medical Consequences of Alcohol and Drug Abuse*, 2nd edn. New York: Haworth Press.

Brickner, M.E., Willard, J.E., Eichhorn, E.J., Black, J., & Grayburn, P.A. (1991). Left ventricular hypertrophy associated with chronic cocaine abuse. *Circulation*, **84**(3), 1130–1135. PM:1832090.

Brogan, W.C., III, Lange, R.A., Glamann, D.B., & Hillis, L.D. (1992). Recurrent coronary vasoconstriction caused by intranasal cocaine: possible role for metabolites. *Ann. Intern. Med.*, **116**(7), 556–561. PM:1543310.

Brookoff, D., Campbell, E.A., & Shaw, L.M. (1993). The underreporting of cocaine-related trauma: drug abuse warning network reports vs hospital toxicology tests. *Am. J. Public Health*, **83**(3), 369–371. PM:8438974.

Buck, G.M., Sever, L.E., Batt, R.E., & Mendola, P. (1997). Life-style factors and female infertility. *Epidemiology*, **8**(4), 435–441. PM:9209860.

Budd, R.D. (1989). Cocaine abuse and violent death. *Am. J. Drug Alcohol Abuse*, **15**(4), 375–382. PM:2596442.

Budde, M.P., De Lange, T.E., Dekker, G.A., Chan, A., & Nguyen, A.M. (2007). Risk factors for placental abruption in a socio-economically disadvantaged region. *J. Matern. Fetal Neonatal Med.*, **20**(9), 687–693. PM:17701669.

Burchell, S.A., Ho, H.C., Yu, M., & Margulies, D.R. (2000). Effects of methamphetamine on trauma patients: a cause of severe metabolic acidosis? *Crit. Care Med.*, **28**(6), 2112–2115. PM:10890674.

Burkett, G., Yasin, S.Y., Palow, D., LaVoie, L., & Martinez, M. (1994). Patterns of cocaine binging: effect on pregnancy. *Am. J. Obstet. Gynecol.*, **171**(2), 372–378. PM:8059815.

Busto, U.E., Bremner, K.E., Knight, K., terBrugge, K., & Sellers, E.M. (2000). Long-term benzodiazepine therapy does not result in brain abnormalities. *J. Clin. Psychopharmacol.*, **20**(1), 2–6. PM:10653201.

Cabral, G.A. (2006). Drugs of abuse, immune modulation, and AIDS. *J. Neuroimmune Pharmacol.*, **1**(3), 280–295. PM:18040805.

Caldicott, D.G., Holmes, J., Roberts-Thomson, K.C., & Mahar, L. (2005). Keep off the grass: marijuana use and acute cardiovascular events. *Eur. J. Emerg. Med.*, **12**(5), 236–244. PM:16175062.

Carriot, F. & Sasco, A.J. (2000). [Cannabis and cancer.] *Rev. Epidemiol. Sante Publique*, **48**(5), 473–483. PM:11084527.

Cassoux, N., Bodaghi, B., Lehoang, P., & Edel, Y. (2002). Presumed ocular candidiasis in drug misusers after intravenous use of oral high dose buprenorphine (Subutex). *Br. J. Ophthalmol.*, **86**(8), 940–941. PM:12140228.

Cejtin, H.E., Young, S.A., Ungaretti, J., *et al.* (1999). Effects of cocaine on the placenta. *Pediatr. Dev. Pathol.*, **2**(2), 143–147. PM:9949220.

Ch'ng, C.W., Fitzgerald, M., Gerostamoulos, J., et al. (2007). Drug use in motor vehicle drivers presenting to an Australian, adult major trauma centre. *Emerg. Med. Australas.*, 19(4), 359–365. PM:17655640.

Chacko, J.A., Heiner, J.G., Siu, W., Macy, M., & Terris, M.K. (2006). Association between marijuana use and transitional cell carcinoma. *Urology*, 67(1), 100–104. PM:16413342.

Chakko, S., Fernandez, A., Mellman, T.A., et al. (1992). Cardiac manifestations of cocaine abuse: a cross-sectional study of asymptomatic men with a history of long-term abuse of "crack" cocaine. *J. Am. Coll. Cardiol.*, 20(5), 1168–1174. PM:1401618.

Chana, G., Everall, I.P., Crews, L., et al. (2006). Cognitive deficits and degeneration of interneurons in HIV+ methamphetamine users. *Neurology*, 67(8), 1486–1489. PM:17060582.

Chang, L., Ernst, T., Speck, O., & Grob, C.S. (2005). Additive effects of HIV and chronic methamphetamine use on brain metabolite abnormalities. *Am. J. Psychiatry*, 162(2), 361–369. PM:15677602.

Chang, C., Grush, A., McClintock, D.E., Nahid, P., & Tang, J.F. (2006a). Unusual finding on bronchoscopy: trauma patient identified as a body stuffer. *J. Clin. Anesth.*, 18(8), 628–630. PM:17175436.

Chang, L., Yakupov, R., Cloak, C., & Ernst, T. (2006b). Marijuana use is associated with a reorganized visual-attention network and cerebellar hypoactivation. *Brain*, 129(Pt 5), 1096–1112. PM:16585053.

Chao, C., Jacobson, L.P., Tashkin, D., et al. (2008). Recreational drug use and T lymphocyte subpopulations in HIV-uninfected and HIV-infected men. *Drug Alcohol Depend.*, 94(1–3), 165–171. PM:18180115.

Chauhan, S.S., Krishnan, J., & Heffner, D.K. (2004). Solitary fibrous tumor of nasal cavity in patient with long-standing history of cocaine inhalation. *Arch. Pathol. Lab Med.*, 128(1), e1–e4. PM:14692833.

Chavez, G.F., Mulinare, J., & Cordero, J.F. (1989). Maternal cocaine use during early pregnancy as a risk factor for congenital urogenital anomalies. *JAMA*, 262(6), 795–798. PM:2746835.

Cherubin, C.E. & Sapira, J.D. (1993). The medical complications of drug addiction and the medical assessment of the intravenous drug user: 25 years later. *Ann. Intern. Med.*, 119(10), 1017–1028. PM:8214979.

Cherukuri, R., Minkoff, H., Feldman, J., Parekh, A., & Glass, L. (1988). A cohort study of alkaloidal cocaine ("crack") in pregnancy. *Obstet. Gynecol.*, 72(2), 147–151. PM:3393357.

Chin, K.M., Channick, R.N., & Rubin, L.J. (2006). Is methamphetamine use associated with idiopathic pulmonary arterial hypertension? *Chest*, 130(6), 1657–1663. PM:17166979.

Chirgwin, K., DeHovitz, J.A., Dillon, S., & McCormack, W.M. (1991). HIV infection, genital ulcer disease, and crack cocaine use among patients attending a clinic for sexually transmitted diseases. *Am. J. Public Health*, 81(12), 1576–1579. PM:1746652.

Cho, C.M., Hirsch, R., & Johnstone, S. (2005). General and oral health implications of cannabis use. *Aust. Dent. J.*, 50(2), 70–74. PM:16050084.

Choy-Kwong, M. & Lipton, R.B. (1989). Seizures in hospitalized cocaine users. *Neurology*, 39(3), 425–427. PM:2927655.

Ciorba, A., Bovo, R., Prosser, S., & Martini, A. (2009). Considerations on the physiopathological mechanism of inner ear damage induced by intravenous cocaine abuse: cues from a case report. *Auris Nasus Larynx*, 36(2), 213–217. PM:18620828.

Ciszowski, K., Hydzik, P., Waldman, W., & Sein, A.J. (2005). [Cocaine smuggling in the gastrointestinal tract – the case report with the review of literature.] *Przegl. Lek.*, 62(6), 492–498. PM:16225104.

Clark, R.F. & Harchelroad, F. (1991). Toxicology screening of the trauma patient: a changing profile. *Ann. Emerg. Med.*, 20(2), 151–153. PM:1996797.

Close, C.E., Roberts, P.L., & Berger, R.E. (1990). Cigarettes, alcohol and marijuana are related to pyospermia in infertile men. *J. Urol.*, 144(4), 900–903. PM:2398564.

Cobaugh, D.J., Schneider, S.M., Benitez, J.G., & Donahoe, M.P. (1997). Cocaine balloon aspiration: successful removal with bronchoscopy. *Am. J. Emerg. Med.*, 15(5), 544–546. PM:9270402.

Cocores, J.A., Miller, N.S., Pottash, A.C., & Gold, M.S. (1988). Sexual dysfunction in abusers of cocaine and alcohol. *Am. J. Drug Alcohol Abuse*, **14**(2), 169–173. PM:2902781.

Cohen, A.L., Shuler, C., McAllister, S., *et al.* (2007). Methamphetamine use and methicillin-resistant Staphylococcus aureus skin infections. *Emerg. Infect. Dis.*, **13**(11), 1707–1713. PM:18217555.

Cohen, D.E., Russell, C.J., Golub, S.A., & Mayer, K.H. (2006). Prevalence of hepatitis C virus infection among men who have sex with men at a Boston community health center and its association with markers of high-risk behavior. *AIDS Patient Care STDs*, **20**(8), 557–564. PM:16893325.

Colatrella, N. & Daniel, T.E. (1999). Crack eye syndrome. *J. Am. Optom. Assoc.*, **70**(3), 193–197. PM:10457695.

Conway, J.E. & Tamargo, R.J. (2001). Cocaine use is an independent risk factor for cerebral vasospasm after aneurysmal subarachnoid hemorrhage. *Stroke*, **32**(10), 2338–2343. PM:11588323.

Cooper, H.L., Brady, J.E., Ciccarone, D., *et al.* (2007). Nationwide increase in the number of hospitalizations for illicit injection drug use-related infective endocarditis. *Clin. Infect. Dis.*, **45**(9), 1200–1203. PM:17918083.

Cordero, D.R., Medina, C., & Helfgott, A. (2006). Cocaine body packing in pregnancy. *Ann. Emerg. Med.*, **48**(3), 323–325. PM:16934653.

Cornelius, M.D., Taylor, P.M., Geva, D., & Day, N.L. (1995). Prenatal tobacco and marijuana use among adolescents: effects on offspring gestational age, growth, and morphology. *Pediatrics*, **95**(5), 738–743. PM:7724314.

Cornelius, M.D., Goldschmidt, L., Day, N.L., & Larkby, C. (2002). Alcohol, tobacco and marijuana use among pregnant teenagers: 6-year follow-up of offspring growth effects. *Neurotoxicol. Teratol.*, **24**(6), 703–710. PM:12460652.

Cota, D. (2008). Role of the endocannabinoid system in energy balance regulation and obesity. *Front. Horm. Res.*, **36**, 135–145. PM:18230900.

Crandall, C.G., Vongpatanasin, W., & Victor, R.G. (2002). Mechanism of cocaine-induced hyperthermia in humans. *Ann. Intern. Med.*, **136**(11), 785–791. PM:12044126.

Crosby, R., Diclemente, R.J., Wingood, G.M., *et al.* (2002). Predictors of infection with Trichomonas vaginalis: a prospective study of low income African-American adolescent females. *Sex. Transm. Infect.*, **78**(5), 360–364. PM:12407241.

Crowe, A.V., Howse, M., Bell, G.M., & Henry, J. A. (2000). Substance abuse and the kidney. *QJM.*, **93**(3), 147–152. PM:10751233.

Cygan, J., Trunsky, M., & Corbridge, T. (2000). Inhaled heroin-induced status asthmaticus: five cases and a review of the literature. *Chest*, **117**(1), 272–275. PM:10631229.

Czeizel, A.E., Szegal, B.A., Joffe, J.M., & Racz, J. (1999). The effect of diazepam and promethazine treatment during pregnancy on the somatic development of human offspring. *Neurotoxicol. Teratol.*, **21**(2), 157–167. PM:10192276.

Czeizel, A.E., Petik, D., & Puho, E. (2004). Smoking and alcohol drinking during pregnancy. The reliability of retrospective maternal self-reported information. *Cent. Eur. J. Public Health*, **12**(4), 179–183. PM:15666453.

Daras, M., Tuchman, A.J., & Marks, S. (1991). Central nervous system infarction related to cocaine abuse. *Stroke*, **22**(10), 1320–1325. PM:1926246.

Daras, M., Koppel, B.S., & tos-Radzion, E. (1994a). Cocaine-induced choreoathetoid movements ("crack dancing"). *Neurology*, **44**(4), 751–752. PM:8164838.

Daras, M., Tuchman, A.J., Koppel, B.S., *et al.* (1994b). Neurovascular complications of cocaine. *Acta Neurol. Scand.*, **90**(2), 124–129. PM:7801738.

Darke, S., Kaye, S., & Duflou, J. (2006). Comparative cardiac pathology among deaths due to cocaine toxicity, opioid toxicity and non-drug-related causes. *Addiction*, **101**(12), 1771–1777. PM:17156176.

Darling, M.R. & Arendorf, T.M. (1992). Review of the effects of cannabis smoking on oral health. *Int. Dent. J.*, **42**(1), 19–22. PM:1563817.

Darling, M.R. & Arendorf, T.M. (1993). Effects of cannabis smoking on oral soft tissues. *Community Dent. Oral Epidemiol.*, **21**(2), 78–81. PM:8485974.

Darling, M.R., Arendorf, T.M., & Coldrey, N.A. (1990). Effect of cannabis use on oral candidal carriage. *J. Oral Pathol. Med.*, **19**(7), 319–321. PM:2231436.

Das, G. (1993). Cocaine abuse in North America: a milestone in history. *J. Clin. Pharmacol.*, **33**(4), 296–310. PM:8473543.

Davis, S.N. & Perkins, J.M. (2007). Role of the endocannabinoid system in management of patients with type 2 diabetes mellitus and cardiovascular risk factors. *Endocr. Pract.*, **13**(7), 790–804. PM:18194939.

Day, N., Sambamoorthi, U., Taylor, P., *et al.* (1991). Prenatal marijuana use and neonatal outcome. *Neurotoxicol. Teratol.*, **13**(3), 329–334. PM:1886543.

Day, N.L. & Richardson, G.A. (1991). Prenatal marijuana use: epidemiology, methodologic issues, and infant outcome. *Clin. Perinatol.*, **18**(1), 77–91. PM:2040119.

Day, N.L., Richardson, G.A., Geva, D., & Robles, N. (1994). Alcohol, marijuana, and tobacco: effects of prenatal exposure on offspring growth and morphology at age six. *Alcohol Clin. Exp. Res.*, **18**(4), 786–794. PM:7526725.

de Beer, S.A., Spiessens, G., Mol, W., & Fa-Si-Oen, P.R. (2008). Surgery for body packing in the Caribbean: a retrospective study of 70 patients. *World J. Surg.*, **32**(2), 281–285. PM:18060451.

de Mendoza, A.D., Rodriguez, J.A., Carvajal, D.A., *et al.* (2004). [Acute renal insufficiency associated to cocaine consumption.] *Rev. Clin. Esp.*, **204**(4), 206–211. PM:15104930.

Decelle, L., Cosyns, J.P., Georges, B., Jadoul, M., & Lefebvre, C. (2007). Acute interstitial nephritis after cocaine sniffing. *Clin. Nephrol.*, **67**(2), 105–108. PM:17338430.

Des Jarlais, J., Hagan, H., Arasteh, K., *et al.* (2007). Herpes simplex virus-2 and HIV among noninjecting drug users in New York city. *Sex. Transm. Dis.*, **34**(11), 923–927. PM:18049425.

Desai, P., Roy, M., Roy, A., Brown, S., & Smelson, D. (1997). Impaired color vision in cocaine-withdrawn patients. *Arch. Gen. Psychiatry*, **54**(8), 696–699. PM:9283503.

Dettmeyer, R., Schlamann, M., & Madea, B. (2004). Cocaine-associated abscesses with lethal sepsis after splenic infarction in an 17-year-old woman. *Forensic Sci. Int.*, **140**(1), 21–23. PM:15013162.

Dettmeyer, R.B., Preuss, J., Wollersen, H., & Madea, B. (2005). Heroin-associated nephropathy. *Expert Opin. Drug Saf.*, **4**(1), 19–28. PM:15709895.

Dhuna, A., Pascual-Leone, A., Langendorf, F., & Anderson, D.C. (1991). Epileptogenic properties of cocaine in humans. *Neurotoxicology*, **12**(3), 621–626. PM:1745445.

Disdier, P., Granel, B., Serratrice, J., *et al.* (2001). Cannabis arteritis revisited: ten new case reports. *Angiology*, **52**(1), 1–5. PM:11205926.

Dixon, S.D. & Bejar, R. (1989). Echoencephalographic findings in neonates associated with maternal cocaine and methamphetamine use: incidence and clinical correlates. *J. Pediatr.*, **115**(5 Pt 1), 770–778. PM:2681639.

Dolovich, L.R., Addis, A., Vaillancourt, J.M., *et al.* (1998). Benzodiazepine use in pregnancy and major malformations or oral cleft: meta-analysis of cohort and case–control studies. *BMJ*, **317**(7162), 839–843. PM:9748174.

Dombrowski, M.P., Wolfe, H.M., Welch, R.A., & Evans, M.I. (1991). Cocaine abuse is associated with abruptio placentae and decreased birth weight, but not shorter labor. *Obstet. Gynecol.*, **77**(1), 139–141. PM:1984213.

Dravet, C., Julian, C., Legras, C., *et al.* (1992). Epilepsy, antiepileptic drugs, and malformations in children of women with epilepsy: a French prospective cohort study. *Neurology*, **42**(4 Suppl 5), 75–82. PM:1574181.

Dressler, F.A. & Roberts, W.C. (1989a). Infective endocarditis in opiate addicts: analysis of 80 cases studied at necropsy. *Am. J. Cardiol.*, **63**(17), 1240–1257. PM:2711995.

Dressler, F.A. & Roberts, W.C. (1989b). Modes of death and types of cardiac disease in opiate addicts: analysis of 168 necropsy cases. *Am. J. Cardiol.*, **64**(14), 909–920. PM:2801561.

Dressler, F.A., Malekzadeh, S., & Roberts, W.C. (1990). Quantitative analysis of amounts of coronary arterial narrowing in cocaine addicts. *Am. J. Cardiol.*, **65**(5), 303–308. PM:2301258.

Droogmans, S., Cosyns, B., D'Haenen, H., *et al.* (2007). Possible association between 3,

4-methylenedioxymethamphetamine abuse and valvular heart disease. *Am. J. Cardiol.*, **100**(9), 1442–1445. PM:17950805.

Duarte, J.G., do Nascimento, A.F., Pantoja, J.G., & Chaves, C.P. (1999). Chronic inhaled cocaine abuse may predispose to the development of pancreatic adenocarcinoma. *Am. J. Surg.*, **178**(5), 426–427. PM:10612544.

Dusick, A.M., Covert, R.F., Schreiber, M.D., *et al.* (1993). Risk of intracranial hemorrhage and other adverse outcomes after cocaine exposure in a cohort of 323 very low birth weight infants. *J. Pediatr.*, **122**(3), 438–445. PM:8441103.

Dykhuizen, R.S., Brunt, P.W., Atkinson, P., Simpson, J.G., & Smith, C.C. (1995). Ecstasy induced hepatitis mimicking viral hepatitis. *Gut*, **36**(6), 939–941. PM:7615289.

Eddahibi, S., Fabre, V., Boni, C., *et al.* (1999). Induction of serotonin transporter by hypoxia in pulmonary vascular smooth muscle cells. Relationship with the mitogenic action of serotonin. *Circ. Res.*, **84**(3), 329–336. PM:10024307.

Eisenberg, M.J., Jue, J., Mendelson, J., Jones, R.T., & Schiller, N.B. (1995). Left ventricular morphologic features and function in nonhospitalized cocaine users: a quantitative two-dimensional echocardiographic study. *Am. Heart J.*, **129**(5), 941–946. PM:7732983.

Eisenstein, T.K., Rahim, R.T., Feng, P., Thingalaya, N.K., & Meissler, J.J. (2006). Effects of opioid tolerance and withdrawal on the immune system. *J. Neuroimmune Pharmacol.*, **1**(3), 237–249. PM:18040801.

Ellis, A.J., Wendon, J.A., Portmann, B., & Williams, R. (1996). Acute liver damage and ecstasy ingestion. *Gut*, **38**(3), 454–458. PM:8675102.

Eng, J.G., Aks, S.E., Waldron, R., Marcus, C., & Issleib, S. (1999). False-negative abdominal CT scan in a cocaine body stuffer. *Am. J. Emerg. Med.*, **17**(7), 702–704. PM:10597096.

Engeland, A., Skurtveit, S., & Morland, J. (2007). Risk of road traffic accidents associated with the prescription of drugs: a registry-based cohort study. *Ann. Epidemiol.*, **17**(8), 597–602. PM:17574863.

Ernst, T., Chang, L., Leonido-Yee, M., & Speck, O. (2000). Evidence for long-term neurotoxicity associated with methamphetamine abuse: a 1H MRS study. *Neurology*, **54**(6), 1344–1349. PM:10746608.

Evans, D.L., Pantanowitz, L., Dezube, B.J., & Aboulafia, D.M. (2002). Breast enlargement in 13 men who were seropositive for human immunodeficiency virus. *Clin. Infect. Dis.*, **35**(9), 1113–1119. PM:12384846.

Fajemirokun-Odudeyi, O., Sinha, C., Tutty, S., *et al.* (2006). Pregnancy outcome in women who use opiates. *Eur. J. Obstet. Gynecol. Reprod. Biol.*, **126**(2), 170–175. PM:16202501.

Feeney, C.M. & Briggs, S. (1992). Crack hands: a dermatologic effect of smoking crack cocaine. *Cutis*, **50**(3), 193–194. PM:1526174.

Fernandez, W.G., Hung, O., Bruno, G.R., Galea, S., & Chiang, W.K. (2005). Factors predictive of acute renal failure and need for hemodialysis among ED patients with rhabdomyolysis. *Am. J. Emerg. Med.*, **23**(1), 1–7. PM:15672329.

Fessler, R.D., Esshaki, C.M., Stankewitz, R.C., Johnson, R.R., & Diaz, F.G. (1997). The neurovascular complications of cocaine. *Surg. Neurol.*, **47**(4), 339–345. PM:9122836.

Finch, P.M., Roberts, L.J., Price, L., Hadlow, N.C., & Pullan, P.T. (2000). Hypogonadism in patients treated with intrathecal morphine. *Clin. J. Pain*, **16**(3), 251–254. PM:11014399.

Fine, D.M., Garg, N., Haas, M., *et al.* (2007). Cocaine use and hypertensive renal changes in HIV-infected individuals. *Clin. J. Am. Soc. Nephrol.*, **2**(6), 1125–1130. PM:17942770.

Fineschi, V., Centini, F., Monciotti, F., & Turillazzi, E. (2002). The cocaine "body stuffer" syndrome: a fatal case. *Forensic Sci. Int.*, **126**(1), 7–10. PM:11955824.

Finn, R., Groves, C., Coe, M., Pass, M., & Harrison, L.H. (2001). Cluster of serogroup C meningococcal disease associated with attendance at a party. *South. Med. J.*, **94**(12), 1192–1194. PM:11811858.

Finsterer, J., Christian, P., & Wolfgang, K. (2004). Occipital stroke shortly after cannabis consumption. *Clin. Neurol. Neurosurg.*, **106**(4), 305–308. PM:15297005.

Flores, E.D., Lange, R.A., Cigarroa, R.G., & Hillis, L.D. (1990). Effect of cocaine on coronary artery dimensions in atherosclerotic coronary artery disease: enhanced vasoconstriction at sites of significant stenoses. *J. Am. Coll. Cardiol.*, **16**(1), 74–79. PM:2358608.

Forrester, M.B. & Merz, R.D. (2006). Comparison of trends in gastroschisis and prenatal illicit drug use rates. *J. Toxicol. Environ. Health A*, **69**(13), 1253–1259. PM:16754539.

Forrester, M.B. & Merz, R.D. (2007). Risk of selected birth defects with prenatal illicit drug use, Hawaii, 1986–2002. *J. Toxicol. Environ. Health A*, **70**(1), 7–18. PM:17162495.

Frances, R.J., Miller, S.I., & Mack, A.H. (2005). *Clinical Textbook of Addictive Disorders*, 3rd edn. New York: Guilford Press.

Frank, D.A., Bauchner, H., Parker, S., *et al.* (1990). Neonatal body proportionality and body composition after in utero exposure to cocaine and marijuana. *J. Pediatr.*, **117**(4), 622–626. PM:2213392.

Frassica, J.J., Orav, E.J., Walsh, E.P., & Lipshultz, S.E. (1994). Arrhythmias in children prenatally exposed to cocaine. *Arch. Pediatr. Adolesc. Med.*, **148**(11), 1163–1169. PM:7921117.

Fried, P.A. (1989). Cigarettes and marijuana: are there measurable long-term neurobehavioral teratogenic effects? *Neurotoxicology*, **10**(3), 577–583. PM:2626219.

Friedman, H., Pross, S., & Klein, T.W. (2006). Addictive drugs and their relationship with infectious diseases. *FEMS Immunol. Med. Microbiol.*, **47**(3), 330–342. PM:16872369.

Fulroth, R., Phillips, B., & Durand, D.J. (1989). Perinatal outcome of infants exposed to cocaine and/or heroin in utero. *Am. J. Dis. Child.*, **143**(8), 905–910. PM:2756964.

Furnari, C., Ottaviano, V., Sacchetti, G., & Mancini, M. (2002). A fatal case of cocaine poisoning in a body packer. *J. Forensic Sci.*, **47**(1), 208–210. PM:12064655.

Gaillard, M.C. & Borruat, F.X. (2003). Persisting visual hallucinations and illusions in previously drug-addicted patients. *Klin. Monatsbl. Augenheilkd.*, **220**(3), 176–178. PM:12664374.

Galea, S., Ahern, J., Tardiff, K., Leon, A.C., & Vlahov, D. (2002). Drugs and firearm deaths in New York City, 1990–1998. *J. Urban Health*, **79**(1), 70–86. PM:11937617.

Galiegue, S., Mary, S., Marchand, J., *et al.* (1995). Expression of central and peripheral cannabinoid receptors in human immune tissues and leukocyte subpopulations. *Eur. J. Biochem.*, **232**(1), 54–61. PM:7556170.

Garfia, A., Valverde, J.L., Borondo, J.C., Candenas, I., & Lucena, J. (1990). Vascular lesions in intestinal ischemia induced by cocaine-alcohol abuse: report of a fatal case due to overdose. *J. Forensic Sci.*, **35**(3), 740–745. PM:2348187.

Geller, T., Loftis, L., & Brink, D.S. (2004). Cerebellar infarction in adolescent males associated with acute marijuana use. *Pediatrics*, **113**(4), e365–e370. PM:15060269.

Ghosheh, F.R., Ehlers, J.P., Ayres, B.D., *et al.* (2007). Corneal ulcers associated with aerosolized crack cocaine use. *Cornea*, **26**(8), 966–969. PM:17721298.

Giese, M.J. (1994). Ocular findings in abused children and infants born to drug abusing mothers. *Optom. Vis. Sci.*, **71**(3), 184–191. PM:8196944.

Gill, A.C., Oei, J., Lewis, N.L., *et al.* (2003). Strabismus in infants of opiate-dependent mothers. *Acta Paediatr.*, **92**(3), 379–385. PM:12725555.

Gill, J.R. & Graham, S.M. (2002). Ten years of "body packers" in New York City: 50 deaths. *J. Forensic Sci.*, **47**(4), 843–846. PM:12136995.

Giovanardi, D., Castellana, C.N., Pisa, S., *et al.* (2005). Prevalence of abuse of alcohol and other drugs among injured drivers presenting to the emergency department of the University Hospital of Modena, Italy. *Drug Alcohol Depend.*, **80**(1), 135–138. PM:15927417.

Gittelman, P.D., Jacobs, J.B., Lebowitz, A.S., & Tierno, P.M., Jr. (1991). *Staphylococcus aureus* nasal carriage in patients with rhinosinusitis. *Laryngoscope*, **101**(7 Pt 1), 733–737. PM:2062153.

Gomez, M.P., Kimball, A.M., Orlander, H., *et al.* (2002). Epidemic crack cocaine use linked with epidemics of genital ulcer disease and heterosexual HIV infection in the Bahamas: evidence of impact of prevention and control measures. *Sex. Transm. Dis.*, **29**(5), 259–264. PM:11984441.

Gonzalez, R. (2007). Acute and non-acute effects of cannabis on brain functioning and neuropsychological performance.

Neuropsychol. Rev., **17**(3), 347–361. PM:17680367.

Gordon, A.J., Sullivan, L.E., Alford, D.P., *et al.* (2007). Update in addiction medicine for the generalist. *J. Gen. Intern. Med.*, **22**(8), 1190–1194. PM:17492327.

Gordon, E. & Devinsky, O. (2001). Alcohol and marijuana: effects on epilepsy and use by patients with epilepsy. *Epilepsia*, **42**(10), 1266–1272. PM:11737161.

Gordon, S., Toepper, W.C., & Blackman, S.C. (1996). Toxicology screening in adolescent trauma. *Pediatr. Emerg. Care*, **12**(1), 36–39. PM:8677177.

Graham, A.W. & Schultz, T.K. (1998). *Principles of Addiction Medicine*, 2nd edn. Chevy Chase, MD: American Society of Addiction Medicine.

Grant, I., Gonzalez, R., Carey, C.L., Natarajan, L., & Wolfson, T. (2003). Non-acute (residual) neurocognitive effects of cannabis use: a meta-analytic study. *J. Int. Neuropsychol. Soc.*, **9**(5), 679–689. PM:12901774.

Greenberg, M.S., Singh, T., Htoo, M., & Schultz, S. (1991). The association between congenital syphilis and cocaine/crack use in New York City: a case–control study. *Am. J. Public Health*, **81**(10), 1316–1318. PM:1928532.

Greenberger, P.A., Miller, T.P., & Lifschultz, B. (1993). Circumstances surrounding deaths from asthma in Cook County (Chicago) Illinois. *Allergy Proc.*, **14**(5), 321–326. PM:8288113.

Gu, X. & Herrera, G.A. (2007). Thrombotic microangiopathy in cocaine abuse-associated malignant hypertension: report of 2 cases with review of the literature. *Arch. Pathol. Lab Med.*, **131**(12), 1817–1820. PM:18081441.

Gunn, R.A., Montes, J.M., Toomey, K.E., *et al.* (1995). Syphilis in San Diego County 1983–1992: crack cocaine, prostitution, and the limitations of partner notification. *Sex. Transm. Dis.*, **22**(1), 60–66. PM:7709327.

Hagel, J., Andrews, G., Vertinsky, T., Heran, M. K., & Keogh, C. (2005). "Chasing the dragon": imaging of heroin inhalation leukoencephalopathy. *Can. Assoc. Radiol. J*, **56**(4), 199–203. PM:16419370.

Hall, A.P. & Henry, J.A. (2006). Acute toxic effects of "ecstasy" (MDMA) and related compounds: overview of pathophysiology and clinical management. *Br. J. Anaesth.*, **96**(6), 678–685. PM:16595612.

Halpern, J.H. & Pope, H.G., Jr. (2003). Hallucinogen persisting perception disorder: what do we know after 50 years? *Drug Alcohol Depend.*, **69**(2), 109–119. PM:12609692.

Handler, A.S., Mason, E.D., Rosenberg, D.L., & Davis, F.G. (1994). The relationship between exposure during pregnancy to cigarette smoking and cocaine use and placenta previa. *Am. J. Obstet. Gynecol.*, **170**(3), 884–889. PM:8141221.

Hari, C.K., Roblin, D.G., Clayton, M.I., & Nair, R.G. (1999). Acute angle closure glaucoma precipitated by intranasal application of cocaine. *J. Laryngol. Otol.*, **113**(3), 250–251. PM:10435135.

Hashibe, M., Straif, K., Tashkin, D.P., *et al.* (2005). Epidemiologic review of marijuana use and cancer risk. *Alcohol*, **35**(3), 265–275. PM:16054989.

Hashibe, M., Ford, D.E., & Zhang, Z.F. (2002). Marijuana smoking and head and neck cancer. *J. Clin. Pharmacol.*, **42**(11 Suppl), 103S–107S. PM:12412843.

Hashibe, M., Morgenstern, H., Cui, Y., *et al.* (2006). Marijuana use and the risk of lung and upper aerodigestive tract cancers: results of a population-based case–control study. *Cancer Epidemiol. Biomarkers Prev.*, **15**(10), 1829–1834. PM:17035389.

Heesch, C.M., Wilhelm, C.R., Ristich, J., *et al.* (2000). Cocaine activates platelets and increases the formation of circulating platelet containing microaggregates in humans. *Heart*, **83**(6), 688–695. PM:10814631.

Herings, R.M., Stricker, B.H., de Boer, A., Bakker, A., & Sturmans, F. (1995). Benzodiazepines and the risk of falling leading to femur fractures. Dosage more important than elimination half-life. *Arch. Intern. Med.*, **155**(16), 1801–1807. PM:7654115.

Herning, R.I., Better, W., Nelson, R., Gorelick, D., & Cadet, J.L. (1999). The regulation of cerebral blood flow during intravenous cocaine administration in cocaine abusers.

Ann. N. Y. Acad. Sci., **890**, 489–494. PM:10668454.

Herning, R.I., Better, W.E., Tate, K., & Cadet, J.L. (2001). Marijuana abusers are at increased risk for stroke. Preliminary evidence from cerebrovascular perfusion data. *Ann. N. Y. Acad. Sci.*, **939**, 413–415. PM:11462796.

Hézode, C., Zafrani, E.S., Roudot-Thoraval, F., *et al.* (2008). Daily cannabis use: a novel risk factor of steatosis severity in patients with chronic hepatitis C. *Gastroenterology*, **134**(2), 432–439. PM:18242211.

Hoang, M.P., Lee, E.L., & Anand, A. (1998). Histologic spectrum of arterial and arteriolar lesions in acute and chronic cocaine-induced mesenteric ischemia: report of three cases and literature review. *Am. J. Surg. Pathol.*, **22**(11), 1404–1410. PM:9808133.

Hofbauer, G.F., Burg, G., & Nestle, F.O. (2000). Cocaine-related Stevens–Johnson syndrome. *Dermatology*, **201**(3), 258–260. PM:11096201.

Hoffman, R.S., Henry, G.C., Howland, M.A., *et al.* (1992). Association between life-threatening cocaine toxicity and plasma cholinesterase activity. *Ann. Emerg. Med.*, **21**(3), 247–253. PM:1536483.

Hoffman, R.S., Thompson, T., Henry, G.C., Hatsukami, D.K., & Pentel, P.R. (1998). Variation in human plasma cholinesterase activity during low-dose cocaine administration. *J. Toxicol. Clin. Toxicol.*, **36**, (1–2) 3–9. PM:9541034.

Hollander, J.E., Hoffman, R.S., Gennis, P., *et al.* (1994). Prospective multicenter evaluation of cocaine-associated chest pain. Cocaine-Associated Chest Pain (COCHPA) Study Group. *Acad. Emerg. Med.*, **1**(4), 330–339. PM:7614278.

Hollander, J.E., Hoffman, R.S., Burstein, J.L., Shih, R.D., & Thode, H.C., Jr. (1995a). Cocaine-associated myocardial infarction. Mortality and complications. Cocaine-Associated Myocardial Infarction Study Group. *Arch. Intern. Med.*, **155**(10), 1081–1086. PM:7748052.

Hollander, J.E., Hoffman, R.S., Gennis, P., *et al.* (1995b). Cocaine-associated chest pain: one-year follow-up. *Acad. Emerg. Med.*, **2**(3), 179–184. PM:7497030.

Hollander, J.E., Todd, K.H., Green, G., *et al.* (1995c). Chest pain associated with cocaine: an assessment of prevalence in suburban and urban emergency departments. *Ann. Emerg. Med.*, **26**(6), 671–676. PM:7492034.

Holland, J.G., Hume, A.S., & Martin, J.N., Jr. (1997). Drug use and physical trauma: risk factors for preterm delivery. *J. Miss. State Med. Assoc.*, **38**(8), 301–305. PM:9260459.

Holly, E.A., Lele, C., Bracci, P.M., & McGrath, M.S. (1999). Case–control study of non-Hodgkin's lymphoma among women and heterosexual men in the San Francisco Bay Area, California. *Am. J. Epidemiol.*, **150**(4), 375–389. PM:10453814.

Holt, V.L., Cushing-Haugen, K.L., & Daling, J.R. (2005). Risk of functional ovarian cyst: effects of smoking and marijuana use according to body mass index. *Am. J. Epidemiol.*, **161**(6), 520–525. PM:15746468.

Horsburgh, C.R., Jr., Anderson, J.R., & Boyko, E.J. (1989). Increased incidence of infections in intravenous drug users. *Infect. Control Hosp. Epidemiol.*, **10**(5), 211–215. PM:2786903.

Hoskins, I.A., Friedman, D.M., Frieden, F.J., Ordorica, S.A., & Young, B.K. (1991). Relationship between antepartum cocaine abuse, abnormal umbilical artery Doppler velocimetry, and placental abruption. *Obstet. Gynecol.*, **78**(2), 279–282. PM:2067775.

Howard, A.A., Arnsten, J.H., & Gourevitch, M.N. (2004). Effect of alcohol consumption on diabetes mellitus: a systematic review. *Ann. Intern. Med.*, **140**(3), 211–219. PM:14757619.

Howington, J.U., Kutz, S.C., Wilding, G.E., & Awasthi, D. (2003). Cocaine use as a predictor of outcome in aneurysmal subarachnoid hemorrhage. *J. Neurosurg.*, **99**(2), 271–275. PM:12924699.

Hsue, P.Y., Salinas, C.L., Bolger, A.F., Benowitz, N.L., & Waters, D.D. (2002). Acute aortic dissection related to crack cocaine. *Circulation*, **105**(13), 1592–1595. PM:11927528.

Hsue, P.Y., McManus, D., Selby, V., *et al.* (2007). Cardiac arrest in patients who smoke crack cocaine. *Am. J. Cardiol.*, **99**(6), 822–824. PM:17350374.

Hubert, G.W., Jones, D.C., Moffett, M.C., Rogge, G., & Kuhar, M.J. (2008). CART peptides as modulators of dopamine and psychostimulants and interactions with the mesolimbic dopaminergic system. *Biochem. Pharmacol.*, **75**(1), 57–62. PM:17854774.

Hughes, S. & Calverley, P.M. (1988). Heroin inhalation and asthma. *BMJ*, **297**(6662), 1511–1512. PM:3147049.

Insel, J.R. & Dhanjal, N. (2004). Pituitary infarction resulting from intranasal cocaine abuse. *Endocr. Pract.*, **10**(6), 478–482. PM:16033719.

Institute of Medicine (2001). *Crossing the Quality Chasm: A New Health System for the 21st Century*. Washington, DC: National Academies Press.

Institute of Medicine (2005). *Improving the Quality of Healthcare for Mental and Substance-Use Conditions: The Quality Chasm Series*. Washington, DC: National Academies Press.

Iqbal, M.M., Sobhan, T., & Ryals, T. (2002). Effects of commonly used benzodiazepines on the fetus, the neonate, and the nursing infant. *Psychiatr. Serv.*, **53**(1), 39–49. PM:11773648.

Irwin, M.R., Olmos, L., Wang, M., *et al.* (2007). Cocaine dependence and acute cocaine induce decreases of monocyte proinflammatory cytokine expression across the diurnal period: autonomic mechanisms. *J. Pharmacol. Exp. Ther.*, **320**(2), 507–515. PM:17068203.

Ishida, J.H., Peters, M.G., Jin, C., *et al.* (2008). Influence of cannabis use on severity of hepatitis C disease. *Clin. Gastroenterol. Hepatol.*, **6**(1), 69–75. PM:18166478.

Jacobsen, L.K., Mencl, W.E., Westerveld, M., & Pugh, K.R. (2004). Impact of cannabis use on brain function in adolescents. *Ann. N. Y. Acad. Sci.*, **1021**, 384–390. PM:15251914.

Jaffe, J.A. & Kimmel, P.L. (2006). Chronic nephropathies of cocaine and heroin abuse: a critical review. *Clin. J. Am. Soc. Nephrol.*, **1**(4), 655–667. PM:17699270.

Jaffey, P.B., Haque, A.K., el-Zaatari, M., Pasarell, L., & McGinnis, M.R. (1990). Disseminated Conidiobolus infection with endocarditis in a cocaine abuser. *Arch. Pathol. Lab Med.*, **114**(12), 1276–1278. PM:2252425.

Jager, G., van Hell, H.H., de Win, M.M., *et al.* (2007). Effects of frequent cannabis use on hippocampal activity during an associative memory task. *Eur. Neuropsychopharmacol.*, **17**(4), 289–297. PM:17137758.

Jain, P.N. & Shah, S.C. (1993). Respiratory depression following combination of epidural buprenorphine and intramuscular ketorolac. *Anaesthesia*, **48**(10), 898–899. PM:8238835.

Jansson, L.M., Dipietro, J.A., Elko, A., & Velez, M. (2007). Maternal vagal tone change in response to methadone is associated with neonatal abstinence syndrome severity in exposed neonates. *J. Matern. Fetal Neonatal Med.*, **20**(9), 677–685. PM:17701668.

Jaworski, J.N. & Jones, D.C. (2006). The role of CART in the reward/reinforcing properties of psychostimulants. *Peptides*, **27**(8), 1993–2004. PM:16766084.

Johanson, C.E., Roehrs, T., Schuh, K., & Warbasse, L. (1999). The effects of cocaine on mood and sleep in cocaine-dependent males. *Exp. Clin. Psychopharmacol.*, **7**(4), 338–346. PM:10609968.

John, V., Dai, H., Talati, A., Charnigo, R.J., Neuman, M., & Bada, H.S. (2007). Autonomic alterations in cocaine-exposed neonates following orthostatic stress. *Pediatr. Res.*, **61**(2), 251–256. PM:17237731.

Johnson, B.A., Dawes, M.A., Roache, J.D., *et al.* (2005). Acute intravenous low- and high-dose cocaine reduces quantitative global and regional cerebral blood flow in recently abstinent subjects with cocaine use disorder. *J. Cereb. Blood Flow Metab.*, **25**(7), 928–936. PM:15758948.

Johnson, S.D., Phelps, D.L., & Cottler, L.B. (2004). The association of sexual dysfunction and substance use among a community epidemiological sample. *Arch. Sex Behav.*, **33**(1), 55–63. PM:14739690.

Jones, A.L. & Simpson, K.J. (1999). Review article: mechanisms and management of hepatotoxicity in ecstasy (MDMA) and amphetamine intoxications. *Aliment. Pharmacol. Ther.*, **13**(2), 129–133. PM:10102941.

Jossens, M.O., Eskenazi, B., Schachter, J., & Sweet, R.L. (1996). Risk factors for pelvic inflammatory disease. A case control study. *Sex. Transm. Dis.*, **23**(3), 239–247. PM:8724516.

Jovanovic-Cupic, V., Martinovic, Z., & Nesic, N. (2006). Seizures associated with intoxication and abuse of tramadol. *Clin. Toxicol.(Phila)*, **44**(2), 143–146. PM:16615669.

Kaku, D.A. & Lowenstein, D.H. (1990).
Emergence of recreational drug abuse as a
major risk factor for stroke in young adults.
Ann. Intern. Med., **113**(11), 821–827.
PM:2240897.

Kamath, S. & Bajaj, N. (2007). Crack dancing in
the United Kingdom: apropos a video case
presentation. *Mov Disord.*, **22**(8), 1190–1191.
PM:17415801.

Kanayama, G., Rogowska, J., Pope, H.G.,
Gruber, S.A., & Yurgelun-Todd, D.A.
(2004). Spatial working memory in heavy
cannabis users: a functional magnetic
resonance imaging study.
Psychopharmacology (Berl), **176**(3–4),
239–247. PM:15205869.

Kaneko, S., Battino, D., Andermann, E., *et al.*
(1999). Congenital malformations due to
antiepileptic drugs. *Epilepsy Res.*, **33**(2–3),
145–158. PM:10094426.

Kapila, Y.L. & Kashani, H. (1997). Cocaine-
associated rapid gingival recession and dental
erosion. A case report. *J. Periodontol.*, **68**(5),
485–488. PM:9182745.

Karch, S.B., Green, G.S., & Young, S. (1995).
Myocardial hypertrophy and coronary artery
disease in male cocaine users. *J. Forensic Sci.*,
40(4), 591–595. PM:7595294.

Kasper, D.L., Baunwald, E., Fauci, A.S., *et al.*
(2005). *Harrison's Principles of Internal
Medicine*, 16th edn. New York: McGraw-Hill.

Kaufman, M.J., Levin, J.M., Maas, L.C., *et al.*
(1998a). Cocaine decreases relative cerebral
blood volume in humans: a dynamic
susceptibility contrast magnetic resonance
imaging study. *Psychopharmacology (Berl)*,
138(1), 76–81. PM:9694529.

Kaufman, M.J., Levin, J.M., Ross, M.H., *et al.*
(1998b). Cocaine-induced cerebral
vasoconstriction detected in humans with
magnetic resonance angiography. *JAMA*,
279(5), 376–380. PM:9459471.

Kawasaki, A. & Purvin, V. (1996). Persistent
palinopsia following ingestion of lysergic
acid diethylamide (LSD). *Arch. Ophthalmol.*,
114(1), 47–50. PM:8540850.

Kennare, R., Heard, A., & Chan, A. (2005).
Substance use during pregnancy: risk factors
and obstetric and perinatal outcomes in
South Australia. *Aust. N. Z. J. Obstet.
Gynaecol.*, **45**(3), 220–225. PM:15904448.

Kibayashi, K., Mastri, A.R., & Hirsch, C.S.
(1995). Cocaine induced intracerebral
hemorrhage: analysis of predisposing factors
and mechanisms causing hemorrhagic
strokes. *Hum. Pathol.*, **26**(6), 659–663.
PM:7774897.

Kistin, N., Handler, A., Davis, F., & Ferre, C.
(1996). Cocaine and cigarettes: a comparison
of risks. *Paediatr. Perinat. Epidemiol.*, **10**(3),
269–278. PM:8822770.

Klein, T.W., Friedman, H., & Specter, S. (1998).
Marijuana, immunity and infection. *J.
Neuroimmunol.*, **83**(1–2), 102–115.
PM:9610678.

Kline, J., Hutzler, M., Levin, B., *et al.* (1991).
Marijuana and spontaneous abortion of
known karyotype. *Paediatr. Perinat.
Epidemiol.*, **5**(3), 320–332. PM:1881842.

Klockgether, T., Weller, M., Haarmeier, T., *et al.*
(1997). Gluteal compartment syndrome due
to rhabdomyolysis after heroin abuse.
Neurology, **48**(1), 275–276. PM:9008535.

Koehler, S.A., Ladham, S., Rozin, L., *et al.* (2005).
The risk of body packing: a case of a fatal
cocaine overdose. *Forensic Sci. Int.*, **151**(1),
81–84. PM:15935945.

Kolodgie, F.D., Virmani, R., Cornhill, J.F.,
Herderick, E.E., & Smialek, J. (1991).
Increase in atherosclerosis and adventitial
mast cells in cocaine abusers: an alternative
mechanism of cocaine-associated
coronary vasospasm and thrombosis. *J. Am.
Coll. Cardiol.*, **17**(7), 1553–1560. PM:2033185.

Kolodgie, F.D., Virmani, R., Cornhill, J.F., *et al.*
(1992). Cocaine: an independent risk factor
for aortic sudanophilia. A preliminary
report. *Atherosclerosis*, **97**(1), 53–62.
PM:1280144.

Kontos, M.C., Jesse, R.L., Tatum, J.L., & Ornato,
J.P. (2003). Coronary angiographic findings
in patients with cocaine-associated chest
pain. *J. Emerg. Med.*, **24**(1), 9–13.
PM:12554033.

Konzen, J.P., Levine, S.R., & Garcia, J.H. (1995).
Vasospasm and thrombus formation as
possible mechanisms of stroke related to
alkaloidal cocaine. *Stroke*, **26**(6), 1114–1118.
PM:7762031.

Koppel, B.S., Samkoff, L., & Daras, M. (1996).
Relation of cocaine use to seizures and epilepsy.
Epilepsia, **37**(9), 875–878. PM:8814101.

Kraines, S.H. (1934). Bell's mania. *Am. J. Psychiatry*, **91**, 29–40.

Kram, H.B., Hardin, E., Clark, S.R., & Shoemaker, W.C. (1992). Perforated ulcers related to smoking "crack" cocaine. *Am. Surg.*, **58**(5), 293–294. PM:1622009.

Krantz, A.J., Hershow, R.C., Prachand, N., *et al.* (2003). Heroin insufflation as a trigger for patients with life-threatening asthma. *Chest*, **123**(2), 510–517. PM:12576374.

Krantz, M.J., Garcia, J.A., & Mehler, P.S. (2005). Effects of buprenorphine on cardiac repolarization in a patient with methadone-related torsade de pointes. *Pharmacotherapy*, **25**(4), 611–614. PM:15977920.

Krantz, M.J., Rowan, S.B., Schmittner, J., & Bucher, B.B. (2007). Physician awareness of the cardiac effects of methadone: results of a national survey. *J. Addict. Dis.*, **26**(4), 79–85. PM:18032235.

Kranzler, H.R. & Wallington, D.J. (1992). Serum prolactin level, craving, and early discharge from treatment in cocaine-dependent patients. *Am. J. Drug Alcohol Abuse*, **18**(2), 187–195. PM:1314018.

Krause, G., Blackmore, C., Wiersma, S., *et al.* (2001). Marijuana use and social networks in a community outbreak of meningococcal disease. *South. Med. J.*, **94**(5), 482–485. PM:11372796.

Kuczkowski, K.M. (2004). Marijuana in pregnancy. *Ann. Acad. Med. Singapore*, **33**(3), 336–339. PM:15175775.

Kuczkowski, K.M. (2007). The effects of drug abuse on pregnancy. *Curr. Opin. Obstet. Gynecol.*, **19**(6), 578–585. PM:18007137.

Laegreid, L., Olegard, R., Walstrom, J., & Conradi, N. (1989). Teratogenic effects of benzodiazepine use during pregnancy. *J. Pediatr.*, **114**(1), 126–131. PM:2562851.

Laegreid, L., Olegard, R., Conradi, N., *et al.* (1990). Congenital malformations and maternal consumption of benzodiazepines: a case-control study. *Dev. Med. Child Neurol.*, **32**(5), 432–441. PM:1972364.

Laegreid, L., Hagberg, G., & Lundberg, A. (1992). Neurodevelopment in late infancy after prenatal exposure to benzodiazepines: a prospective study. *Neuropediatrics*, **23**(2), 60–67. PM:1351263.

Laffi, G.L. & Safran, A.B. (1993). Persistent visual changes following hashish consumption. *Br. J. Ophthalmol.*, **77**(9), 601–602. PM:8218063.

Lam, S.K., To, W.K., Duthie, S.J., & Ma, H.K. (1992). Narcotic addiction in pregnancy with adverse maternal and perinatal outcome. *Aust. N. Z. J. Obstet. Gynaecol.*, **32**(3), 216–221. PM:1445130.

Lange, R.A., Cigarroa, R.G., Yancy, C.W., Jr., *et al.* (1989). Cocaine-induced coronary-artery vasoconstriction. *N. Engl. J. Med.*, **321**(23), 1557–1562. PM:2573838.

Lee, M.J. (1998). Marihuana and tobacco use in pregnancy. *Obstet. Gynecol. Clin. North Am.*, **25**(1), 65–83. PM:9547760.

Leon-Carrion, J. & Vela-Bueno, A. (1991). Cannabis and cerebral hemispheres: a chrononeuropsychological study. *Int. J. Neurosci.*, **57**(3–4), 251–257. PM:1938167.

Leucht, S., Burkard, T., Henderson, J.H., Maj, M., & Sartorius, N. (2007). *Physical Illness and Schizophrenia, A Review of the Evidence.* Cambridge, UK: Cambridge University Press.

Levi, L. & Miller, N.R. (1990). Visual illusions associated with previous drug abuse. *J. Clin. Neuroophthalmol.*, **10**(2), 103–110. PM:2141849.

Levine, D.P., Cushing, R.D., Jui, J., & Brown, W.J. (1982). Community-acquired methicillin-resistant Staphylococcus aureus endocarditis in the Detroit Medical Center. *Ann. Intern. Med.*, **97**(3), 330–338. PM:7114630.

Levine, S.R., Brust, J.C., Futrell, N., Ho, K.L., *et al.* (1990). Cerebrovascular complications of the use of the "crack" form of alkaloidal cocaine. *N. Engl. J. Med.*, **323**(11), 699–704. PM:2388668.

Levinson, D.F. & Simpson, G.M. (1986). Neuroleptic-induced extrapyramidal symptoms with fever. Heterogeneity of the "neuroleptic malignant syndrome." *Arch. Gen. Psychiatry*, **43**(9), 839–848. PM:2875701.

Levy, M. & Koren, G. (1990). Obstetric and neonatal effects of drugs of abuse. *Emerg. Med. Clin. North Am.*, **8**(3), 633–652. PM:2201525.

Levy, R.S., Hebert, C.K., Munn, B.G., & Barrack, R.L. (1996). Drug and alcohol use in orthopedic trauma patients: a prospective study. *J. Orthop. Trauma*, **10**(1), 21–27. PM:8926551.

Li, Y., Wang, X., Tian, S., *et al.* (2002). Methadone enhances human immunodeficiency virus infection of human immune cells. *J. Infect. Dis.*, **185**(1), 118–122. PM:11756991.

Liau, A., Diclemente, R.J., Wingood, G.M., *et al.* (2002). Associations between biologically confirmed marijuana use and laboratory-confirmed sexually transmitted diseases among African American adolescent females. *Sex. Transm. Dis.*, **29**(7), 387–390. PM:12170126.

Lim, K.O., Choi, S.J., Pomara, N., Wolkin, A., & Rotrosen, J.P. (2002). Reduced frontal white matter integrity in cocaine dependence: a controlled diffusion tensor imaging study. *Biol. Psychiatry*, **51**(11), 890–895. PM:12022962.

Lim, K.O., Wozniak, J.R., Mueller, B.A., *et al.* (2008). Brain macrostructural and microstructural abnormalities in cocaine dependence. *Drug Alcohol Depend.*, **92**(1–3), 164–172. PM:17904770.

Lindenbaum, G.A., Carroll, S.F., Daskal, I., & Kapusnick, R. (1989). Patterns of alcohol and drug abuse in an urban trauma center: the increasing role of cocaine abuse. *J. Trauma*, **29**(12), 1654–1658. PM:2593196.

Lindhout, D., Meinardi, H., Meijer, J.W., & Nau, H. (1992). Antiepileptic drugs and teratogenesis in two consecutive cohorts: changes in prescription policy paralleled by changes in pattern of malformations. *Neurology*, **42**(4 Suppl 5), 94–110. PM:1574185.

Lipshultz, S.E., Frassica, J.J., & Orav, E.J. (1991). Cardiovascular abnormalities in infants prenatally exposed to cocaine. *J. Pediatr.*, **118**(1), 44–51. PM:1986097.

Little, B.B., Snell, L.M., & Gilstrap, L.C., III (1988). Methamphetamine abuse during pregnancy: outcome and fetal effects. *Obstet. Gynecol.*, **72**(4), 541–544. PM:3419732.

Little, B.B., Snell, L.M., Klein, V.R., & Gilstrap, L.C., III (1989). Cocaine abuse during pregnancy: maternal and fetal implications. *Obstet. Gynecol.*, **73**(2), 157–160. PM:2911419.

Little, B.B., Snell, L.M., Breckenridge, J.D., *et al.* (1990). Effects of T's and blues abuse on pregnancy outcome and infant health status. *Am. J. Perinatol.*, **7**(4), 359–362. PM:2222629.

Loiselle, J.M., Baker, M.D., Templeton, J.M., Jr., Schwartz, G., & Drott, H. (1993). Substance abuse in adolescent trauma. *Ann. Emerg. Med.*, **22**(10), 1530–1534. PM:8214830.

Lozsadi, D.A., Forster, A., & Fletcher, N.A. (2004). Cannabis-induced propriospinal myoclonus. *Mov. Disord.*, **19**(6), 708–709. PM:15197714.

Lynn, K.L., Pickering, W., Gardner, J., Bailey, R.R., & Robson, R.A. (1998). Intravenous drug use and glomerular deposition of lipid-like material. *Nephron*, **80**(3), 274–276. PM:9807035.

Lyoo, I.K., Streeter, C.C., Ahn, K.H., *et al.* (2004). White matter hyperintensities in subjects with cocaine and opiate dependence and healthy comparison subjects. *Psychiatry Res.*, **131**(2), 135–145. PM:15313520.

Macdonald, S., Anglin-Bodrug, K., Mann, R.E., *et al.* (2003). Injury risk associated with cannabis and cocaine use. *Drug Alcohol Depend.*, **72**(2), 99–115. PM:14636965.

Macones, G.A., Sehdev, H.M., Parry, S., Morgan, M.A., & Berlin, J.A. (1997). The association between maternal cocaine use and placenta previa. *Am. J. Obstet. Gynecol.*, **177**(5), 1097–1100. PM:9396901.

Maher, L., Li, J., Jalaludin, B., Chant, K.G., & Kaldor, J.M. (2007). High hepatitis C incidence in new injecting drug users: a policy failure? *Aust. N. Z. J. Public Health*, **31**(1), 30–35. PM:17333606.

Maj, M. (2008). The WPA Action Plan 2008–2011. *World Psychiatry*, **7**(3), 129–130. PM:18836578.

Majid, P.A., Cheirif, J.B., Rokey, R., *et al.* (1992). Does cocaine cause coronary vasospasm in chronic cocaine abusers? A study of coronary and systemic hemodynamics. *Clin. Cardiol.*, **15**(4), 253–258. PM:1563128.

Makower, R.M., Pennycook, A.G., & Moulton, C. (1992). Intravenous drug abusers attending an inner city accident and emergency department. *Arch. Emerg. Med.*, **9**(1), 32–39. PM:1567526.

Malbrain, M.L., Neels, H., Vissers, K., *et al.* (1994). A massive, near-fatal cocaine intoxication in a body-stuffer. Case report and review of the literature. *Acta Clin. Belg.*, **49**(1), 12–18. PM:8191810.

Maloney, C. (2002). Talc rentinopathy: how history can aid diagnosis. *Optometry Today*, **Dec**, 34–36.

March, J.C., Oviedo-Joekes, E., & Romero, M. (2007). Factors associated with reported hepatitis C and HIV among injecting drug users in ten European cities. *Enferm. Infecc. Microbiol. Clin.*, **25**(2), 91–97. PM:17288906.

Marcos, E., Fadel, E., Sanchez, O., *et al.* (2004). Serotonin-induced smooth muscle hyperplasia in various forms of human pulmonary hypertension. *Circ. Res.*, **94**(9), 1263–1270. PM:15059929.

Marmor, M., Penn, A., Widmer, K., Levin, R.I., & Maslansky, R. (2004). Coronary artery disease and opioid use. *Am. J. Cardiol.*, **93**(10), 1295–1297. PM:15135709.

Martin, D.H. & DiCarlo, R.P. (1994). Recent changes in the epidemiology of genital ulcer disease in the United States. The crack cocaine connection. *Sex. Transm. Dis.*, **21**(2 Suppl), S76–S80. PM:8042123.

Martinez, A., Larrabee, K., & Monga, M. (1996). Cocaine is associated with intrauterine fetal death in women with suspected preterm labor. *Am. J. Perinatol.*, **13**(3), 163–166. PM:8688108.

Marzuk, P.M., Tardiff, K., Leon, A.C., *et al.* (1995). Fatal injuries after cocaine use as a leading cause of death among young adults in New York City. *N. Engl. J. Med.*, **332**(26), 1753–1757. PM:7760893.

Mateo, I., Infante, J., Gomez, B.M., & Garcia-Monco, J.C. (2006). [Cannabis and cerebrovascular disease.] *Neurologia*, **21**(4), 204–208. PM:16832776.

Mateo, I., Pinedo, A., Gomez-Beldarrain, M., Basterretxea, J.M., & Garcia-Monco, J.C. (2005). Recurrent stroke associated with cannabis use. *J. Neurol. Neurosurg. Psychiatry*, **76**(3), 435–437. PM:15716544.

Matias, I. & Di, M., V (2007). Endocannabinoids and the control of energy balance. *Trends Endocrinol. Metab*, **18**(1), 27–37. PM:17141520.

Matochik, J.A., Eldreth, D.A., Cadet, J.L., & Bolla, K.I. (2005). Altered brain tissue composition in heavy marijuana users. *Drug Alcohol Depend.*, **77**(1), 23–30. PM:15607838.

Mattson, R.H., Cramer, J.A., & McCutchen, C.B. (1989). Barbiturate-related connective tissue disorders. *Arch. Intern. Med.*, **149**(4), 911–914. PM:2705840.

Mayo-Smith, M.F. & Spinale, J. (1997). Thermal epiglottitis in adults: a new complication of illicit drug use. *J. Emerg. Med.*, **15**(4), 483–485. PM:9279700.

McCann, U.D., Kuwabara, H., Kumar, A., *et al.* (2008). Persistent cognitive and dopamine transporter deficits in abstinent methamphetamine users. *Synapse*, **62**(2), 91–100. PM:17992686.

McDonald, A., Duncan, N.D., & Mitchell, D.I. (1999). Alcohol, cannabis and cocaine usage in patients with trauma injuries. *West Indian Med. J.*, **48**(4), 200–202. PM:10639839.

McElhatton, P.R. (1994). The effects of benzodiazepine use during pregnancy and lactation. *Reprod. Toxicol.*, **8**(6), 461–475. PM:7881198.

McElhatton, P.R., Bateman, D.N., Evans, C., Pughe, K.R., & Thomas, S.H. (1999). Congenital anomalies after prenatal ecstasy exposure. *Lancet*, **354**(9188), 1441–1442. PM:10543673.

McFadden, C.B., Brensinger, C.M., Berlin, J.A., & Townsend, R.R. (2005). Systematic review of the effect of daily alcohol intake on blood pressure. *Am. J. Hypertens.*, **18**(2 Pt 1), 276–286. PM:15752957.

McGill, V., Kowal-Vern, A., Fisher, S.G., Kahn, S., & Gamelli, R.L. (1995). The impact of substance use on mortality and morbidity from thermal injury. *J. Trauma*, **38**(6), 931–934. PM:7602638.

McGonigal, M.D., Cole, J., Schwab, C.W., *et al.* (1993). Urban firearm deaths: a five-year perspective. *J. Trauma*, **35**(4), 532–536. PM:8411275.

McGrath, C. & Chan, B. (2005). Oral health sensations associated with illicit drug abuse. *Br. Dent. J.*, **198**(3), 159–162. PM:15706386.

McKee, S.A., Applegate, R.J., Hoyle, J.R., *et al.* (2007). Cocaine use is associated with an increased risk of stent thrombosis after percutaneous coronary intervention. *Am. Heart J.*, **154**(1), 159–164. PM:17584570.

McLane, N.J. & Carroll, D.M. (1986). Ocular manifestations of drug abuse. *Surv. Ophthalmol.*, **30**(5), 298–313. PM:2872731.

Medina, K.L., Schweinsburg, A.D., Cohen-Zion, M., Nagel, B.J., & Tapert, S.F. (2007). Effects of alcohol and combined marijuana and alcohol use during adolescence on hippocampal volume and asymmetry. *Neurotoxicol. Teratol.*, **29**(1), 141–152. PM:17169528.

Mehra, R., Moore, B.A., Crothers, K., Tetrault, J., & Fiellin, D.A. (2006). The association between marijuana smoking and lung cancer: a systematic review. *Arch. Intern. Med.*, **166**(13), 1359–1367. PM:16832000.

Mehta, S.K., Finkelhor, R.S., Anderson, R.L., *et al.* (1993). Transient myocardial ischemia in infants prenatally exposed to cocaine. *J. Pediatr.*, **122**(6), 945–949. PM:8501575.

Melandri, R., Re, G., Lanzarini, C., *et al.* (1996). Myocardial damage and rhabdomyolysis associated with prolonged hypoxic coma following opiate overdose. *J. Toxicol. Clin. Toxicol.*, **34**(2), 199–203. PM:8618254.

Meleca, R.J., Burgio, D.L., Carr, R.M., & Lolachi, C.M. (1997). Mucosal injuries of the upper aerodigestive tract after smoking crack or freebase cocaine. *Laryngoscope*, **107**(5), 620–625. PM:9149163.

Menaker, J., Farcy, D.A., Boswell, S.A., *et al.* (2008). Cocaine-induced agitated delirium with associated hyperthermia: a case report. *J. Emerg. Med.*, epub ahead of print. PM:18823733.

Merigian, K.S., Park, L.J., Leeper, K.V., Browning, R.G., & Giometi, R. (1994). Adrenergic crisis from crack cocaine ingestion: report of five cases. *J. Emerg. Med.*, **12**(4), 485–490. PM:7963395.

Mertens, J.R., Lu, Y.W., Parthasarathy, S., Moore, C., & Weisner, C.M. (2003). Medical and psychiatric conditions of alcohol and drug treatment patients in an HMO: comparison with matched controls. *Arch. Intern. Med.*, **163**(20), 2511–2517. PM:14609789.

Mertz, K.J., Weiss, J.B., Webb, R.M., *et al.* (1998). An investigation of genital ulcers in Jackson, Mississippi, with use of a multiplex

polymerase chain reaction assay: high prevalence of chancroid and human immunodeficiency virus infection. *J. Infect. Dis.*, **178**(4), 1060–1066. PM:9806035.

Messinis, L., Kyprianidou, A., Malefaki, S., & Papathanasopoulos, P. (2006). Neuropsychological deficits in long-term frequent cannabis users. *Neurology*, **66**(5), 737–739. PM:16534113.

Michael, W.J., Flegel, R., Atkins, R., *et al.* (2005). Drug and alcohol use among drivers admitted to a level-1 trauma center. *Accid. Anal. Prev.*, **37**(5), 894–901. PM:15927139.

Minkoff, H., Zhong, Y., Strickler, H.D., *et al.* (2008). The relationship between cocaine use and human papillomavirus infections in HIV-seropositive and HIV-seronegative women. *Infect. Dis. Obstet. Gynecol.*, **2008**, 587082. PM:18437233.

Minor, R.L., Jr., Scott, B.D., Brown, D.D., & Winniford, M.D. (1991). Cocaine-induced myocardial infarction in patients with normal coronary arteries. *Ann. Intern. Med.*, **115**(10), 797–806. PM:1929028.

Mitchell, J.D. & Schwartz, A.L. (1996). Acute angle-closure glaucoma associated with intranasal cocaine abuse. *Am. J. Ophthalmol.*, **122**(3), 425–426. PM:8794717.

Mittleman, M.A., Mintzer, D., Maclure, M., *et al.* (1999). Triggering of myocardial infarction by cocaine. *Circulation*, **99**(21), 2737–2741. PM:10351966.

Mittleman, M.A., Lewis, R.A., Maclure, M., Sherwood, J.B., & Muller, J.E. (2001). Triggering myocardial infarction by marijuana. *Circulation*, **103**(23), 2805–2809. PM:11401936.

Mochizuki, Y., Zhang, M., Golestaneh, L., Thananart, S., & Coco, M. (2003). Acute aortic thrombosis and renal infarction in acute cocaine intoxication: a case report and review of literature. *Clin. Nephrol.*, **60**(2), 130–133. PM:12940616.

Moeller, F.G., Hasan, K.M., Steinberg, J.L., *et al.* (2007). Diffusion tensor imaging eigenvalues: preliminary evidence for altered myelin in cocaine dependence. *Psychiatry Res.*, **154**(3), 253–258. PM:17321725.

Mohs, M.E., Watson, R.R., & Leonard-Green, T. (1990). Nutritional effects of marijuana, heroin, cocaine, and nicotine. *J. Am. Diet. Assoc.*, **90**(9), 1261–1267. PM:2204648.

Mokdad, A.H., Marks, J.S., Stroup, D.F., & Gerberding, J.L. (2004). Actual causes of death in the United States, 2000. *JAMA*, **291**(10), 1238–1245. PM:15010446.

Moliterno, D.J., Willard, J.E., Lange, R.A., *et al.* (1994). Coronary-artery vasoconstriction induced by cocaine, cigarette smoking, or both. *N. Engl. J. Med.*, **330**(7), 454–459. PM:8289850.

Mooney, E.E., Boggess, K.A., Herbert, W.N., & Layfield, L.J. (1998). Placental pathology in patients using cocaine: an observational study. *Obstet. Gynecol.*, **91**(6), 925–929. PM:9610997.

Moore, B.A., Augustson, E.M., Moser, R.P., & Budney, A.J. (2005). Respiratory effects of marijuana and tobacco use in a US sample. *J. Gen. Intern. Med.*, **20**(1), 33–37. PM:15693925.

Morgan, P.T. & Malison, R.T. (2007). Cocaine and sleep: early abstinence. *Sci. World J.*, 7, 223–230. PM:17982597.

Morgan, P.T., Pace-Schott, E.F., Sahul, Z.H., *et al.* (2006). Sleep, sleep-dependent procedural learning and vigilance in chronic cocaine users: evidence for occult insomnia. *Drug Alcohol Depend.*, **82**(3), 238–249. PM:16260094.

Morton, J. (2005). Ecstasy: pharmacology and neurotoxicity. *Curr. Opin. Pharmacol.*, **5**(1), 79–86. PM:15661630.

Moussouttas, M. (2004). Cannabis use and cerebrovascular disease. *Neurologist*, **10**(1), 47–53. PM:14720314.

Mueller, B.A., Daling, J.R., Weiss, N.S., & Moore, D.E. (1990). Recreational drug use and the risk of primary infertility. *Epidemiology*, **1**(3), 195–200. PM:2081252.

Mukamal, K.J., Maclure, M., Muller, J.E., & Mittleman, M.A. (2008). An exploratory prospective study of marijuana use and mortality following acute myocardial infarction. *Am. Heart J.*, **155**(3), 465–470. PM:18294478.

Munarriz, R., Hwang, J., Goldstein, I., Traish, A.M., & Kim, N.N. (2003). Cocaine and ephedrine-induced priapism: case reports and investigation of potential adrenergic mechanisms. *Urology*, **62**(1), 187–192. PM:12837464.

Munckhof, W.J., Konstantinos, A., Wamsley, M., Mortlock, M., & Gilpin, C. (2003). A cluster of tuberculosis associated with use of a marijuana water pipe. *Int. J. Tuberc. Lung Dis.*, **7**(9), 860–865. PM:12971670.

Murphy, E.L., DeVita, D., Liu, H., *et al.* (2001). Risk factors for skin and soft-tissue abscesses among injection drug users: a case–control study. *Clin. Infect. Dis.*, **33**(1), 35–40. PM:11389492.

Nademanee, K., Gorelick, D.A., Josephson, M.A., *et al.* (1989). Myocardial ischemia during cocaine withdrawal. *Ann. Intern. Med.*, **111**(11), 876–880. PM:2817640.

Nanda, A., Vannemreddy, P., Willis, B., & Kelley, R. (2006). Stroke in the young: relationship of active cocaine use with stroke mechanism and outcome. *Acta Neurochir. Suppl.*, **96**, 91–96. PM:16671433.

Narongchai, P., Narongchai, S., & Thampituk, S. (2007). The incidence of drug abuse in unnatural deaths in northern Thailand. *J. Med. Assoc. Thai.*, **90**(1), 137–142. PM:17621744.

National Institute on Drug Abuse (2009). *Principles of Drug Treatment: A Research-Based Guide*, 2nd edn. Bethesda, MD: National Institute on Drug Abuse, National Institutes of Health, US Department of Health and Human Services.

Nelson, R.A., Levine, A.M., Marks, G., & Bernstein, L. (1997). Alcohol, tobacco and recreational drug use and the risk of non-Hodgkin's lymphoma. *Br. J. Cancer*, **76**(11), 1532–1537. PM:9400954.

Ness, R.B., Grisso, J.A., Hirschinger, N., *et al.* (1999). Cocaine and tobacco use and the risk of spontaneous abortion. *N. Engl. J. Med.*, **340**(5), 333–339. PM:9929522.

Neumeister, A.S., Pilcher, L.E., Erickson, J.M., *et al.* (2007). Hepatitis-C prevalence in an urban native-American clinic: a prospective screening study. *J. Natl. Med. Assoc.*, **99**(4), 389–392. PM:17444428.

Ney, J.A., Dooley, S.L., Keith, L.G., Chasnoff, I.J., & Socol, M.L. (1990). The prevalence of substance abuse in patients with suspected preterm labor. *Am. J. Obstet. Gynecol.*, **162**(6), 1562–1565. PM:2360589.

Nieder, A.M., Lipke, M.C., & Madjar, S. (2006). Transitional cell carcinoma associated with marijuana: case report and review of the literature. *Urology*, **67**(1), 200. PM:16413373.

Nissen, S.E., Nicholls, S.J., Wolski, K., *et al.* (2008). Effect of rimonabant on progression of atherosclerosis in patients with abdominal obesity and coronary artery disease: the STRADIVARIUS randomized controlled trial. *JAMA*, **299**(13), 1547–1560. PM:18387931.

Noel, B., Ruf, I., & Panizzon, R.G. (2008). Cannabis arteritis. *J. Am. Acad. Dermatol.*, **58**(5 Suppl 1), S65–S67. PM:18489050.

Nolte, K.B., Brass, L.M., & Fletterick, C.F. (1996). Intracranial hemorrhage associated with cocaine abuse: a prospective autopsy study. *Neurology*, **46**(5), 1291–1296. PM:8628469.

Norfolk, G.A. (2007). The fatal case of a cocaine body-stuffer and a literature review: towards evidence based management. *J. Forensic Leg. Med.*, **14**(1), 49–52. PM:16442337.

Norris, K.C., Thornhill-Joynes, M., Robinson, C., *et al.* (2001). Cocaine use, hypertension, and end-stage renal disease. *Am. J. Kidney Dis.*, **38**(3), 523–528. PM:11532684.

Nyenwe, E.A., Loganathan, R.S., Blum, S., *et al.* (2007). Active use of cocaine: an independent risk factor for recurrent diabetic ketoacidosis in a city hospital. *Endocr. Pract.*, **13**(1), 22–29. PM:17360297.

O'Donnell, A.E. & Pappas, L.S. (1988). Pulmonary complications of intravenous drug abuse. Experience at an inner-city hospital. *Chest*, **94**(2), 251–253. PM:3396399.

O'Malley, S., Adamse, M., Heaton, R.K., & Gawin, F.H. (1992). Neuropsychological impairment in chronic cocaine abusers. *Am. J. Drug Alcohol Abuse*, **18**(2), 131–144. PM:1562011.

Oeltmann, J.E., Oren, E., Haddad, M.B., *et al.* (2006). Tuberculosis outbreak in marijuana users, Seattle, Washington, 2004. *Emerg. Infect. Dis.*, **12**(7), 1156–1159. PM:16836841.

Office of National Drug Control Policy (2004). *The Economic Costs of Drug Abuse in the United States, 1992–2002.* [Publication No. 207303] Washington, DC: Executive Office of the President.

Oh, S., Havlen, P.R., & Hussain, N. (2005). A case of polymicrobial endocarditis caused by anaerobic organisms in an injection drug user. *J. Gen. Intern. Med.*, **20**(10), C1–C2. PM:16191149.

Om, A., Warner, M., Sabri, N., Cecich, L., & Vetrovec, G. (1992). Frequency of coronary artery disease and left ventricle dysfunction in cocaine users. *Am. J. Cardiol.*, **69**(19), 1549–1552. PM:1598868.

Orozco-Cabal, L., Liu, J., Pollandt, S., *et al.* (2008). Dopamine and corticotropin-releasing factor synergistically alter basolateral amygdala-to-medial prefrontal cortex synaptic transmission: functional switch after chronic cocaine administration. *J. Neurosci.*, **28**(2), 529–542. PM:18184795.

Osborn, H.H., Tang, M., Bradley, K., & Duncan, B.R. (1997). New-onset bronchospasm or recrudescence of asthma associated with cocaine abuse. *Acad. Emerg. Med.*, **4**(7), 689–692. PM:9223692.

Osorio, J., Farreras, N., Ortiz De, Z.L., & Bachs, E. (2000). Cocaine-induced mesenteric ischaemia. *Dig. Surg.*, **17**(6), 648–651. PM:11155017.

Pace-Schott, E.F., Stickgold, R., Muzur, A., *et al.* (2005). Sleep quality deteriorates over a binge–abstinence cycle in chronic smoked-cocaine users. *Psychopharmacology (Berl)*, **179**(4), 873–883. PM:15672273.

Pachigolla, G., Blomquist, P., & Cavanagh, H.D. (2007). Microbial keratitis pathogens and antibiotic susceptibilities: a 5-year review of cases at an urban county hospital in north Texas. *Eye Contact Lens*, **33**(1), 45–49. PM:17224678.

Papi, C., Candia, S., Masci, P., *et al.* (1999). Acute ischaemic colitis following intravenous cocaine use. *Ital. J. Gastroenterol. Hepatol.*, **31**(4), 305–307. PM:10425576.

Pariente, A., Dartigues, J.F., Benichou, J., *et al.* (2008). Benzodiazepines and injurious falls in community dwelling elders. *Drugs Aging*, **25**(1), 61–70. PM:18184030.

Parry, C.D., Pluddemann, A., Donson, H., *et al.* (2005). Cannabis and other drug use among trauma patients in three South African cities, 1999–2001. *S. Afr. Med. J.*, **95**(6), 429–432. PM:16100892.

Pascual-Leone, A., Dhuna, A., Altafullah, I., & Anderson, D.C. (1990). Cocaine-induced seizures. *Neurology*, **40**(3 Pt 1), 404–407. PM:2107459.

Pascual-Leone, A., Dhuna, A., & Anderson, D.C. (1991). Cerebral atrophy in habitual cocaine abusers: a planimetric CT study. *Neurology*, **41**(1), 34–38. PM:1985292.

Patkar, A.A., Mannelli, P., Certa, K.M., et al. (2004). Relationship of serum prolactin with severity of drug use and treatment outcome in cocaine dependence. *Psychopharmacology (Berl)*, **176**(1), 74–81. PM:15064918.

Peces, R., Navascues, R.A., Baltar, J., Seco, M., & Alvarez, J. (1999). Antiglomerular basement membrane antibody-mediated glomerulonephritis after intranasal cocaine use. *Nephron*, **81**(4), 434–438. PM:10095180.

Peden, M., van der Spuy, J., Smith, P., & Bautz, P. (2000). Substance abuse and trauma in Cape Town. *S. Afr. Med. J.*, **90**(3), 251–255. PM:10853402.

Perneger, T.V., Klag, M.J., & Whelton, P.K. (2001). Recreational drug use: a neglected risk factor for end-stage renal disease. *Am. J. Kidney Dis.*, **38**(1), 49–56. PM:11431181.

Petitti, D.B., Sidney, S., Quesenberry, C., & Bernstein, A. (1998). Stroke and cocaine or amphetamine use. *Epidemiology*, **9**(6), 596–600. PM:9799166.

Petronis, K.R. & Anthony, J.C. (1989). An epidemiologic investigation of marijuana- and cocaine-related palpitations. *Drug Alcohol Depend.*, **23**(3), 219–226. PM:2787738.

Peyrot, I., Garsaud, A.M., Saint-Cyr, I., et al. (2007). Cannabis arteritis: a new case report and a review of literature. *J. Eur. Acad. Dermatol. Venereol.*, **21**(3), 388–391. PM:17309465.

Pillay, S.S., Rogowska, J., Kanayama, G., et al. (2008). Cannabis and motor function: fMRI changes following 28 days of discontinuation. *Exp. Clin. Psychopharmacol.*, **16**(1), 22–32. PM:18266549.

Pilon, A.F. & Scheiffle, J. (2006). Ulcerative keratitis associated with crack-cocaine abuse. *Cont. Lens Anterior Eye*, **29**(5), 263–267. PM:17052948.

Polen, M.R., Sidney, S., Tekawa, I.S., Sadler, M., & Friedman, G.D. (1993). Health care use by frequent marijuana smokers who do not smoke tobacco. *West J. Med.*, **158**(6), 596–601. PM:8337854.

Pope, H.G., Jr., Gruber, A.J., & Yurgelun-Todd, D. (1995). The residual neuropsychological effects of cannabis: the current status of research. *Drug Alcohol Depend.*, **38**(1), 25–34. PM:7648994.

Qureshi, A.I., Akbar, M.S., Czander, E., et al. (1997). Crack cocaine use and stroke in young patients. *Neurology*, **48**(2), 341–345. PM:9040718.

Qureshi, A.I., Suri, M.F., Guterman, L.R., & Hopkins, L.N. (2001). Cocaine use and the likelihood of nonfatal myocardial infarction and stroke: data from the Third National Health and Nutrition Examination Survey. *Circulation*, **103**(4), 502–506. PM:11157713.

Ramaekers, J.G., Kauert, G., van Ruitenbeek, P., et al. (2006). High-potency marijuana impairs executive function and inhibitory motor control. *Neuropsychopharmacology*, **31**(10), 2296–2303. PM:16572123.

Rana, J., Ebert, G.A., & Kappy, K.A. (1995). Adverse perinatal outcome in patients with an abnormal umbilical coiling index. *Obstet. Gynecol.*, **85**(4), 573–577. PM:7898836.

Rao, H., Wang, J., Giannetta, J., et al. (2007). Altered resting cerebral blood flow in adolescents with in utero cocaine exposure revealed by perfusion functional MRI. *Pediatrics*, **120**(5), e1245–e1254. PM:17974718.

Rastegar, D.A. & Fingerhood, M.I. (2005). *Addiction Medicine: An Evidence-Based Handbook*. Philadelphia, PA: Lippincott, Williams & Wilkins.

Rawstron, S.A., Jenkins, S., Blanchard, S., Li, P.W., & Bromberg, K. (1993). Maternal and congenital syphilis in Brooklyn, NY. Epidemiology, transmission, and diagnosis. *Am. J. Dis. Child.*, **147**(7), 727–731. PM:8322741.

Rayman, N., Lam, K.H., van, Leeuwen, J., et al. (2007). The expression of the peripheral cannabinoid receptor on cells of the immune system and non-Hodgkin's lymphomas. *Leuk. Lymphoma*, **48**(7), 1389–1399. PM:17613768.

Redfearn, P.J., Agrawal, N., & Mair, L.H. (1998). An association between the regular use of 3,4-methylenedioxy-methamphetamine (ecstasy) and excessive wear of the teeth. *Addiction*, 93(5), 745–748. PM:9692273.

Regidor, E., Barrio, G., de la, F.L., & Rodriguez, C. (1996). Non-fatal injuries and the use of psychoactive drugs among young adults in Spain. *Drug Alcohol Depend.*, 10(3), 249–259. PM:8861404.

Reimer, J., Lorenzen, J., Baetz, B., et al. (2007). Multiple viral hepatitis in injection drug users and associated risk factors. *J. Gastroenterol. Hepatol.*, 22(1), 80–85. PM:17201886.

Reis, A.D., Figlie, N.B., & Laranjeira, R. (2006). Prevalence of substance use among trauma patients treated in a Brazilian emergency room. *Rev. Bras. Psiquiatr.*, 28(3), 191–195. PM:17063218.

Reneman, L., Booij, J., de Boer, K., et al. (2001a). Effects of dose, sex, and long-term abstention from use on toxic effects of MDMA (ecstasy) on brain serotonin neurons. *Lancet*, 358(9296), 1864–1869. PM:11741626.

Reneman, L., Lavalaye, J., Schmand, B., et al. (2001b). Cortical serotonin transporter density and verbal memory in individuals who stopped using 3,4-methylenedioxymethamphetamine (MDMA or "ecstasy"): preliminary findings. *Arch. Gen. Psychiatry*, 58(10), 901–906. PM:11576026.

Reneman, L., Majoie, C. B., Habraken, J.B., & den Heeten, G.J. (2001c). Effects of ecstasy (MDMA) on the brain in abstinent users: initial observations with diffusion and perfusion MR imaging. *Radiology*, 220(3), 611–617. PM:11526257.

Reynolds, E.W., Riel-Romero, R.M., & Bada, H.S. (2007). Neonatal abstinence syndrome and cerebral infarction following maternal codeine use during pregnancy. *Clin. Pediatr.(Phila)*, 46(7), 639–645. PM:17704497.

Rice, E.K., Isbel, N.M., Becker, G.J., Atkins, R.C., & McMahon, L.P. (2000). Heroin overdose and myoglobinuric acute renal failure. *Clin. Nephrol.*, 54(6), 449–454. PM:11140805.

Richards, J.R. & Brofeldt, B.T. (2000). Patterns of tooth wear associated with methamphetamine use. *J. Periodontol.*, 71(8), 1371–1374. PM:10972655.

Richards, J.R., Johnson, E.B., Stark, R.W., & Derlet, R.W. (1999a). Methamphetamine abuse and rhabdomyolysis in the ED: a 5-year study. *Am. J. Emerg. Med.*, 17(7), 681–685. PM:10597089.

Richards, J.R., Bretz, S.W., Johnson, E.B., et al. (1999b). Methamphetamine abuse and emergency department utilization. *West. J. Med.*, 170(4), 198–202. PM:10344172.

Rivara, F.P., Mueller, B.A., Fligner, C.L., et al. (1989). Drug use in trauma victims. *J. Trauma*, 29(4), 462–470. PM:2565405.

Rivero, M., Karlic, A., Navaneethan, S.D., & Singh, S. (2006). Possible cocaine-induced acute renal failure without rhabdomyolysis. *J. Nephrol.*, 19(1), 108–110. PM:16523435.

Rizzo, M., Lamers, C.T., Sauer, C.G., et al. (2005). Impaired perception of self-motion (heading) in abstinent ecstasy and marijuana users. *Psychopharmacology (Berl)*, 179(3), 559–566. PM:15723231.

Rodondi, N., Pletcher, M.J., Liu, K., Hulley, S.B., & Sidney, S. (2006). Marijuana use, diet, body mass index, and cardiovascular risk factors (from the CARDIA study). *Am. J. Cardiol.*, 98(4), 478–484. PM:16893701.

Rofsky, J.E., Townsend, J.C., Ilsen, P.F., & Bright, D.C. (1995). Retinal nerve fiber layer defects and microtalc retinopathy secondary to free-basing "crack" cocaine. *J. Am. Optom. Assoc.*, 66(11), 712–720. PM:8576537.

Rogge, G., Jones, D., Hubert, G.W., Lin, Y., & Kuhar, M.J. (2008). CART peptides: regulators of body weight, reward and other functions. *Nat. Rev. Neurosci.*, 9(10), 747–758. PM:18802445.

Rome, L.A., Lippmann, M.L., Dalsey, W.C., Taggart, P., & Pomerantz, S. (2000). Prevalence of cocaine use and its impact on asthma exacerbation in an urban population. *Chest*, 117(5), 1324–1329. PM:10807818.

Ropper, A.H. & Blair, R. (2003). Symmetric deep cerebellar lesions after smoking heroin. *Arch. Neurol.*, 60(11), 1605–1606. PM:14623734.

Rosenblatt, K.A., Daling, J.R., Chen, C., Sherman, K.J., & Schwartz, S.M. (2004). Marijuana use and risk of oral squamous cell carcinoma. *Cancer Res.*, **64**(11), 4049–4054. PM:15173020.

Rosenson, J., Smollin, C., Sporer, K.A., Blanc, P., & Olson, K.R. (2007). Patterns of ecstasy-associated hyponatremia in California. *Ann. Emerg. Med.*, **49**(2), 164–171. PM:17084942.

Ross, D.L. (1998). Factors associated with excited delirium deaths in police custody. *Mod. Pathol.*, **11**(11), 1127–1137. PM:9831212.

Ross, M.W., Risser, J., Peters, R.J., & Johnson, R.J. (2006). Cocaine use and syphilis trends: findings from the arrestee drug abuse monitoring (ADAM) program and syphilis epidemiology in Houston. *Am. J. Addict.*, **15**(6), 473–477. PM:17182451.

Rosse, R., Deutsch, S., & Chilton, M. (2005). Cocaine addicts prone to cocaine-induced psychosis have lower body mass index than cocaine addicts resistant to cocaine-induced psychosis: implications for the cocaine model of psychosis proneness. *Isr. J. Psychiatry Relat Sci.*, **42**(1), 45–50. PM:16134406.

Roth, M.D., Arora, A., Barsky, S.H., *et al.* (1998). Airway inflammation in young marijuana and tobacco smokers. *Am. J. Respir. Crit Care Med.*, **157**(3 Pt 1), 928–937. PM:9517614.

Roth, M.D., Whittaker, K., Salehi, K., Tashkin, D.P., & Baldwin, G.C. (2004). Mechanisms for impaired effector function in alveolar macrophages from marijuana and cocaine smokers. *J. Neuroimmunol.*, **147**(1–2), 82–86. PM:14741433.

Roth, T., Roehrs, T., & Pies, R. (2007). Insomnia: pathophysiology and implications for treatment. *Sleep Med. Rev.*, **11**(1), 71–79. PM:17175184.

Rothman, R.B., Baumann, M.H., Savage, J.E., *et al.* (2000). Evidence for possible involvement of 5-HT(2B) receptors in the cardiac valvulopathy associated with fenfluramine and other serotonergic medications. *Circulation*, **102**(23), 2836–2841. PM:11104741.

Rothrock, J.F., Rubenstein, R., & Lyden, P.D. (1988). Ischemic stroke associated with methamphetamine inhalation. *Neurology*, **38**(4), 589–592. PM:3352918.

Roy, E., Alary, M., Morissette, C., *et al.* (2007). High hepatitis C virus prevalence and incidence among Canadian intravenous drug users. *Int. J. STD AIDS*, **18**(1), 23–27. PM:17326858.

Rozhinskaia, I.V., Rott, G.M., & Poverennyi, A.M. (1989). [The content of the chief amount of myoglobin in the blood serum as an immune complex.] *Biull. Eksp. Biol. Med.*, **107**(3), 308–310. PM:2653451.

Rusyniak, D.E. & Sprague, J.E. (2005). Toxin-induced hyperthermic syndromes. *Med. Clin. North Am.*, **89**(6), 1277–1296. PM:16227063.

Ruttenber, A.J., Lawler-Heavner, J., Yin, M., *et al.* (1997). Fatal excited delirium following cocaine use: epidemiologic findings provide new evidence for mechanisms of cocaine toxicity. *J. Forensic Sci.*, **42**(1), 25–31. PM:8988571.

Ruttenber, A.J., McAnally, H.B., & Wetli, C.V. (1999). Cocaine-associated rhabdomyolysis and excited delirium: different stages of the same syndrome. *Am. J. Forensic Med. Pathol.*, **20**(2), 120–127. PM:10414649.

Sacerdote, P. (2008). Opioid-induced immunosuppression. *Curr. Opin. Support. Palliat. Care*, **2**(1), 14–18. PM:18685388.

Sachs, R., Zagelbaum, B.M., & Hersh, P.S. (1993). Corneal complications associated with the use of crack cocaine. *Ophthalmology*, **100**(2), 187–191. PM:8437825.

Santibanez, S.S., Garfein, R.S., Swartzendruber, A., *et al.* (2005). Prevalence and correlates of crack-cocaine injection among young injection drug users in the United States, 1997–1999. *Drug Alcohol Depend.*, **77**(3), 227–233. PM:15734222.

Satran, A., Bart, B.A., Henry, C.R., *et al.* (2005). Increased prevalence of coronary artery aneurysms among cocaine users. *Circulation*, **111**(19), 2424–2429. PM:15883217.

Saviola, G., Taveggia, G., Capodaglio, P., & Grioni, G. (1996). [Rheumatism caused by anticonvulsants: presentation of 2 clinical cases with work reintegration.] *G. Ital. Med. Lav.*, **18**, (1–3) 31–34. PM:9312444.

Saviola, G., Abdi, A.L., Avanzi, S., & Trentanni, C. (2003). [Phenobarbital rheumatism associated with gouty arthritis. Case report with 18-month follow-up.] *Clin. Ter.*, **154**(5), 349–351. PM:14994925.

Schafer, S., Gillette, H., Hedberg, K., & Cieslak, P. (2006). A community-wide pertussis outbreak: an argument for universal booster vaccination. *Arch. Intern. Med.*, **166**(12), 1317–1321. PM:16801516.

Schaper, A., Hofmann, R., Bargain, P., *et al.* (2007). Surgical treatment in cocaine body packers and body pushers. *Int. J. Colorectal Dis.*, **22**(12), 1531–1535. PM:17520265.

Scheenstra, R.J., van Buren, M., & Koopman, J.P. (2007). [A patient with both cocaine-induced nasal septum destruction and antibodies against anti-neutrophil cytoplasmic antibodies (ANCA); potential confusion with Wegener's disease.] *Ned. Tijdschr. Geneeskd.*, **151**(43), 2395–2399. PM:18019218.

Schempf, A.H. (2007). Illicit drug use and neonatal outcomes: a critical review. *Obstet. Gynecol. Surv.*, **62**(11), 749–757. PM:17925048.

Scher, M.S., Richardson, G.A., Coble, P.A., Day, N.L., & Stoffer, D.S. (1988). The effects of prenatal alcohol and marijuana exposure: disturbances in neonatal sleep cycling and arousal. *Pediatr. Res.*, **24**(1), 101–105. PM:3412843.

Schermer, C.R. & Wisner, D.H. (1999). Methamphetamine use in trauma patients: a population-based study. *J. Am. Coll. Surg.*, **189**(5), 442–449. PM:10549732.

Schilt, T., de Win, M.M., Koeter, M., *et al.* (2007). Cognition in novice ecstasy users with minimal exposure to other drugs: a prospective cohort study. *Arch. Gen. Psychiatry*, **64**(6), 728–736. PM:17548754.

Schroeder, B. & Brieden, S. (2000). Bilateral sixth nerve palsy associated with MDMA ("ecstasy") abuse. *Am. J. Ophthalmol.*, **129**(3), 408–409. PM:10704573.

Schuetze, P. & Eiden, R.D. (2006). The association between maternal cocaine use during pregnancy and physiological regulation in 4- to 8-week-old infants: an examination of possible mediators and moderators. *J. Pediatr. Psychol.*, **31**(1), 15–26. PM:15788714.

Schuetze, P., Eiden, R.D., & Coles, C.D. (2007). Prenatal cocaine and other substance exposure: effects on infant autonomic regulation at 7 months of age. *Dev. Psychobiol.*, **49**(3), 276–289. PM:17380506.

Schwartz, R.H., Estroff, T., Fairbanks, D.N., & Hoffmann, N.G. 1989a. Nasal symptoms associated with cocaine abuse during

adolescence. *Arch. Otolaryngol. Head Neck Surg.*, **115**(1), 63–64. PM:2909232.

Schwartz, R.H., Gruenewald, P.J., Klitzner, M., & Fedio, P. 1989b. Short-term memory impairment in cannabis-dependent adolescents. *Am. J. Dis. Child*, **143**(10), 1214–1219. PM:2801665.

Shankaran, S., Das, A., Bauer, C.R., *et al.* (2006). Fetal origin of childhood disease: intrauterine growth restriction in term infants and risk for hypertension at 6 years of age. *Arch. Pediatr. Adolesc. Med.*, **160**(9), 977–981. PM:16953023.

Sharma, R., Organ, C.H., Jr., Hirvela, E.R., & Henderson, V.J. (1997). Clinical observation of the temporal association between crack cocaine and duodenal ulcer perforation. *Am. J. Surg.*, **174**(6), 629–632. PM:9409587.

Shiono, P.H., Klebanoff, M.A., Nugent, R.P., *et al.* (1995). The impact of cocaine and marijuana use on low birth weight and preterm birth: a multicenter study. *Am. J. Obstet. Gynecol.*, **172**(1 Pt 1), 19–27. PM:7847533.

Sidney, S. (2002). Cardiovascular consequences of marijuana use. *J. Clin. Pharmacol.*, **42**(11 Suppl), 64S–70S. PM:12412838.

Siegal, H.A., Falck, R.S., Wang, J., Carlson, R.G., & Massimino, K.P. (2006). Emergency department utilization by crack-cocaine smokers in Dayton, Ohio. *Am. J. Drug Alcohol Abuse*, **32**(1), 55–68. PM:16450643.

Sim, M.E., Lyoo, I.K., Streeter, C.C., *et al.* (2007). Cerebellar gray matter volume correlates with duration of cocaine use in cocaine-dependent subjects. *Neuropsychopharmacology*, **32**(10), 2229–2237. PM:17299505.

Simon, S.L., Domier, C.P., Sim, T., *et al.* (2002). Cognitive performance of current methamphetamine and cocaine abusers. *J. Addict. Dis.*, **21**(1), 61–74. PM:11831501.

Simpson, R.K., Jr., Fischer, D.K., Narayan, R.K., Cech, D.A., & Robertson, C.S. (1990). Intravenous cocaine abuse and subarachnoid haemorrhage: effect on outcome. *Br. J. Neurosurg.*, **4**(1), 27–30. PM:2334523.

Simsek, S., de Vries, X.H., Jol, J.A., *et al.* (2006). Sino-nasal bony and cartilaginous destruction associated with cocaine abuse, S. aureus and antineutrophil cytoplasmic antibodies. *Neth. J. Med.*, **64**(7), 248–251. PM:16929087.

Singer, L., Arendt, R., Song, L.Y., Warshawsky, E., & Kliegman, R. (1994). Direct and indirect interactions of cocaine with childbirth outcomes. *Arch. Pediatr. Adolesc. Med.*, **148**(9), 959–964. PM:8075743.

Sirvent, A.E., Enriquez, R., Andrada, E., *et al.* (2007). Goodpasture's syndrome in a patient using cocaine: a case report and review of the literature. *Clin. Nephrol.*, **68**(3), 182–185. PM:17915623.

Sison, C.G., Ostrea, E.M., Jr., Reyes, M.P., & Salari, V. (1997). The resurgence of congenital syphilis: a cocaine-related problem. *J. Pediatr.*, **130**(2), 289–292. PM:9042134.

Sloan, E.P., Zalenski, R.J., Smith, R.F., *et al.* (1989). Toxicology screening in urban trauma patients: drug prevalence and its relationship to trauma severity and management. *J. Trauma*, **29**(12), 1647–1653. PM:2593195.

Sloan, M.A., Kittner, S.J., Rigamonti, D., & Price, T.R. (1991). Occurrence of stroke associated with use/abuse of drugs. *Neurology*, **41**(9), 1358–1364. PM:1891081.

Smith, L.M., Qureshi, N., Renslo, R., & Sinow, R.M. (2001). Prenatal cocaine exposure and cranial sonographic findings in preterm infants. *J. Clin. Ultrasound*, **29**(2), 72–77. PM:11425091.

Smith, L.M., LaGasse, L.L., Derauf, C., *et al.* (2006). The infant development, environment, and lifestyle study: effects of prenatal methamphetamine exposure, polydrug exposure, and poverty on intrauterine growth. *Pediatrics*, **118**(3), 1149–1156. PM:16951010.

Soderstrom, C.A., Trifillis, A.L., Shankar, B.S., Clark, W.E., & Cowley, R.A. (1988). Marijuana and alcohol use among 1023 trauma patients. A prospective study. *Arch. Surg.*, **123**(6), 733–737. PM:2835941.

Soderstrom, C.A., Dischinger, P.C., Kerns, T.J., & Trifillis, A.L. (1995). Marijuana and other drug use among automobile and motorcycle drivers treated at a trauma center. *Accid. Anal. Prev.*, **27**(1), 131–135. PM:7718074.

Soderstrom, C.A., Dischinger, P.C., Kerns, T.J., *et al.* (2001). Epidemic increases in cocaine

and opiate use by trauma center patients: documentation with a large clinical toxicology database. *J. Trauma*, **51**(3), 557–564. PM:11535910.

Sorvillo, F., Kovacs, A., Kerndt, P., *et al.* (1998). Risk factors for trichomoniasis among women with human immunodeficiency virus (HIV) infection at a public clinic in Los Angeles County, California: implications for HIV prevention. *Am. J. Trop. Med. Hyg.*, **58**(4), 495–500. PM:9574798.

Spence, M.R., Williams, R., DiGregorio, G.J., Kirby-McDonnell, A., & Polansky, M. (1991). The relationship between recent cocaine use and pregnancy outcome. *Obstet. Gynecol.*, **78**, (3 Pt 1) 326–329. PM:1876358.

Sporer, K.A. & Dorn, E. (2001). Heroin-related noncardiogenic pulmonary edema : a case series. *Chest*, **120**(5), 1628–1632. PM:11713145.

Sporer, K.A. & Firestone, J. (1997). Clinical course of crack cocaine body stuffers. *Ann. Emerg. Med.*, **29**(5), 596–601. PM:9140242.

Sprauve, M.E., Lindsay, M.K., Herbert, S., & Graves, W. (1997). Adverse perinatal outcome in parturients who use crack cocaine. *Obstet. Gynecol.*, **89**(5 Pt 1), 674–678. PM:9166299.

Stein, M.D., Herman, D.S., Bishop, S., *et al.* (2004). Sleep disturbances among methadone maintained patients. *J. Subst. Abuse Treat.*, **26**(3), 175–180. PM:15063910.

Steinberger, E.K., Ferencz, C., & Loffredo, C.A. (2002). Infants with single ventricle: a population-based epidemiological study. *Teratology*, **65**(3), 106–115. PM:11877773.

Stevens, D.C., Campbell, J.P., Carter, J.E., & Watson, W.A. (1994). Acid-base abnormalities associated with cocaine toxicity in emergency department patients. *J. Toxicol. Clin. Toxicol.*, **32**(1), 31–39. PM:8308947.

Stewart, S.A. (2005). The effects of benzodiazepines on cognition. *J. Clin. Psychiatry*, **66**(Suppl 2), 9–13. PM:15762814.

Stoduto, G., Vingilis, E., Kapur, B.M., *et al.* (1993). Alcohol and drug use among motor vehicle collision victims admitted to a regional trauma unit: demographic, injury, and crash characteristics. *Accid. Anal. Prev.*, **25**(4), 411–420. PM:8357454.

Stokes, J.R., Hartel, R., Ford, L.B., & Casale, T.B. (2000). Cannabis (hemp) positive skin tests and respiratory symptoms. *Ann. Allergy Asthma Immunol.*, **85**(3), 238–240. PM:11030280.

Stracciari, A., Guarino, M., Crespi, C., & Pazzaglia, P. (1999). Transient amnesia triggered by acute marijuana intoxication. *Eur. J. Neurol.*, **6**(4), 521–523. PM:10362911.

Stratton, S.J., Rogers, C., Brickett, K., & Gruzinski, G. (2001). Factors associated with sudden death of individuals requiring restraint for excited delirium. *Am. J. Emerg. Med.*, **19**(3), 187–191. PM:11326341.

Strzelczyk, A., Vogt, H., Hamer, H.M., & Kramer, G. (2008). Continuous phenobarbital treatment leads to recurrent plantar fibromatosis. *Epilepsia*, **49**(11), 1965–1968. PM:18513351.

Sudhakar, C.B., Al-Hakeem, M., MacArthur, J.D., & Sumpio, B.E. (1997). Mesenteric ischemia secondary to cocaine abuse: case reports and literature review. *Am. J. Gastroenterol.*, **92**(6), 1053–1054. PM:9177533.

Sullivan, L.E., Fiellin, D.A., & O'Connor, P.G. (2005). The prevalence and impact of alcohol problems in major depression: a systematic review. *Am. J. Med.*, **118**(4), 330–341. PM:15808128.

Sundram, S. (2006). Cannabis and neurodevelopment: implications for psychiatric disorders. *Hum. Psychopharmacol.*, **21**(4), 245–254. PM:16783814.

Sutter, F.K. & Landau, K. (2003). Heroin and strabismus. *Swiss Med. Wkly.*, **133**(19–20), 293–294. PM:12844273.

Swaminathan, S., Schoenbaum, E.E., Klein, R.S., *et al.* (2007). Two-step tuberculin skin testing in drug users. *J. Addict. Dis.*, **26**(2), 71–79. PM:17595000.

Swanson, S.M., Sise, C.B., Sise, M.J., *et al.* (2007). The scourge of methamphetamine: impact on a level I trauma center. *J. Trauma*, **63**(3), 531–537. PM:18073597.

Talloczy, Z., Martinez, J., Joset, D., *et al.* (2008). Methamphetamine inhibits antigen processing, presentation, and phagocytosis. *PLoS Pathog.*, **4**(2), e28. PM:18282092.

Tanenbaum, J.H. & Miller, F. (1992). Electrocardiographic evidence of myocardial injury in psychiatrically hospitalized cocaine abusers. *Gen. Hosp. Psychiatry*, **14**(3), 201–203. PM:1601297.

Tanvetyanon, T., Dissin, J., & Selcer, U.M. (2001). Hyperthermia and chronic pancerebellar syndrome after cocaine abuse. *Arch. Intern. Med.*, **161**(4), 608–610. PM:11252123.

Tapert, S.F., Schweinsburg, A.D., Drummond, S.P., *et al.* (2007). Functional MRI of inhibitory processing in abstinent adolescent marijuana users. *Psychopharmacology (Berl)*, **194**(2), 173–183. PM:17558500.

Tashkin, D.P. (1990). Pulmonary complications of smoked substance abuse. *West. J. Med.*, **152**(5), 525–530. PM:2190420.

Tashkin, D.P. (2001). Airway effects of marijuana, cocaine, and other inhaled illicit agents. *Curr. Opin. Pulm. Med.*, **7**(2), 43–61. PM:11224724.

Tashkin, D.P. (2005). Smoked marijuana as a cause of lung injury. *Monaldi Arch. Chest Dis.*, **63**(2), 93–100. PM:16128224.

Tashkin, D.P., Gorelick, D., Khalsa, M.E., Simmons, M., & Chang, P. (1992a). Respiratory effects of cocaine freebasing among habitual cocaine users. *J. Addict. Dis.*, **11**(4), 59–70. PM:1486094.

Tashkin, D.P., Khalsa, M.E., Gorelick, D., *et al.* (1992b). Pulmonary status of habitual cocaine smokers. *Am. Rev. Respir. Dis.*, **145**(1), 92–100. PM:1731605.

Taylor, D.R., Poulton, R., Moffitt, T.E., Ramankutty, P., & Sears, M.R. (2000). The respiratory effects of cannabis dependence in young adults. *Addiction*, **95**(11), 1669–1677. PM:11219370.

Taylor, D.R., Fergusson, D.M., Milne, B.J., *et al.* (2002). A longitudinal study of the effects of tobacco and cannabis exposure on lung function in young adults. *Addiction*, **97**(8), 1055–1061. PM:12144608.

Taylor, F.M., III (1988). Marijuana as a potential respiratory tract carcinogen: a retrospective analysis of a community hospital population. *South. Med. J.*, **81**(10), 1213–1216. PM:3175726.

Teoh, S.K., Mendelson, J.H., Woods, B.T., *et al.* (1993). Pituitary volume in men with concurrent heroin and cocaine dependence. *J. Clin. Endocrinol. Metab*, **76**(6), 1529–1532. PM:8501161.

Tetrault, J.M., Crothers, K., Moore, B.A., *et al.* (2007). Effects of marijuana smoking on pulmonary function and respiratory complications: a systematic review. *Arch. Intern. Med.*, **167**(3), 221–228. PM:17296876.

Thammakumpee, G. & Sumpatanukule, P. (1994). Noncardiogenic pulmonary edema induced by sublingual buprenorphine. *Chest*, **106**(1), 306–308. PM:8020299.

Thomas, R.E. (1998). Benzodiazepine use and motor vehicle accidents. Systematic review of reported association. *Can. Fam. Physician*, **44**(April), 799–808. PM:9585853.

Thompson, S.T. (1993). Preventable causes of male infertility. *World J. Urol.*, **11**(2), 111–119. PM:8343795.

Thomson, W.M., Poulton, R., Broadbent, J.M., *et al.* (2008). Cannabis smoking and periodontal disease among young adults. *JAMA*, **299**(5), 525–531. PM:18252882.

Thorpe, L.E., Ouellet, L.J., Levy, J.R., Williams, I.T., & Monterroso, E.R. (2000). Hepatitis C virus infection: prevalence, risk factors, and prevention opportunities among young injection drug users in Chicago, 1997–1999. *J. Infect. Dis.*, **182**(6), 1588–1594. PM:11069228.

Tobias, J.D. (1997). Seizure after overdose of tramadol. *South. Med. J.*, **90**(8), 826–827. PM:9258310.

Tominaga, G.T., Garcia, G., Dzierba, A., & Wong, J. (2004). Toll of methamphetamine on the trauma system. *Arch. Surg.*, **139**(8), 844–847. PM:15302693.

Torfs, C.P., Velie, E.M., Oechsli, F.W., Bateson, T.F., & Curry, C.J. (1994). A population-based study of gastroschisis: demographic, pregnancy, and lifestyle risk factors. *Teratology*, **50**(1), 44–53. PM:7974254.

Towers, C.V., Pircon, R.A., Nageotte, M.P., Porto, M., & Garite, T.J. (1993). Cocaine intoxication presenting as preeclampsia and eclampsia. *Obstet. Gynecol.*, **81**(4), 545–547. PM:8459963.

Tran, K.H. & Ilsen, P.F. (2007). Peripheral retinal neovascularization in talc retinopathy. *Optometry*, **78**(8), 409–414. PM:17662930.

Trimarchi, M., Nicolai, P., Lombardi, D., *et al.* (2003). Sinonasal osteocartilaginous necrosis in cocaine abusers: experience in 25 patients. *Am. J. Rhinol.*, **17**(1), 33–43. PM:12693654.

Trimarchi, M., Miluzio, A., Nicolai, P., *et al.* (2006). Massive apoptosis erodes nasal mucosa of cocaine abusers. *Am. J. Rhinol.*, **20**(2), 160–164. PM:16686379.

Underdahl, J.P. & Chiou, A.G. (1998). Preseptal cellulitis and orbital wall destruction secondary to nasal cocaine abuse. *Am. J. Ophthalmol.*, **125**(2), 266–268. PM:9467464.

US Substance Abuse and Mental Health Services (2007). *National Survey on Drug Use and Health.* Rockville, MD: US Substance Abuse and Mental Health Services Administration, Office of Applied Studies.

Urey, J.C. (1991). Some ocular manifestations of systemic drug abuse. *J. Am. Optom. Assoc.*, **62**(11), 832–842. PM:1813511.

Uzan, M., Volochine, L., Rondeau, E., *et al.* (1988). [Renal disease associated with heroin abuse.] *Nephrologie*, **9**(5), 217–221. PM:3216943.

Valladares, E.M. & Irwin, M.R. (2007). Polysomnographic sleep dysregulation in cocaine dependence. *Sci. World J.*, **7**, 213–216. PM:17982595.

van der Klooster, J.M. & Grootendorst, A.F. (2001). Severe bullous emphysema associated with cocaine smoking. *Thorax*, **56**(12), 982–983. PM:11758511.

van der Pol, M.C., Hadders-Algra, M., Huisjes, H.J., & Touwen, B.C. (1991). Antiepileptic medication in pregnancy: late effects on the children's central nervous system development. *Am. J. Obstet. Gynecol.*, **164**(1 Pt 1), 121–128. PM:1986598.

van Gorp, W.G., Wilkins, J.N., Hinkin, C.H., *et al.* (1999). Declarative and procedural memory functioning in abstinent cocaine abusers. *Arch. Gen. Psychiatry*, **56**(1), 85–89. PM:9892260.

Van Hoozen, B.E. & Cross, C.E. (1997). Marijuana. Respiratory tract effects. *Clin. Rev. Allergy Immunol.*, **15**(3), 243–269. PM:9358987.

Vemuri, V.K., Janero, D.R., & Makriyannis, A. (2008). Pharmacotherapeutic targeting of the endocannabinoid signaling system: drugs for obesity and the metabolic syndrome. *Physiol Behav.*, **93**(4–5), 671–686. PM:18155257.

Verdejo-Garcia, A.J., Lopez-Torrecillas, F., Aguilar de Arcos, F., & Perez-Garcia, M. (2005). Differential effects of MDMA, cocaine, and cannabis use severity on distinctive components of the executive functions in polysubstance users: a multiple regression analysis. *Addict. Behav.*, **30**(1), 89–101. PM:15561451.

Verdejo-Garcia, A.J. & Perez-Garcia, M. (2007). Profile of executive deficits in cocaine and heroin polysubstance users: common and differential effects on separate executive components. *Psychopharmacology (Berl)*, **190**(4), 517–530. PM:17136401.

Vicentic, A. & Jones, D.C. (2007). The CART (cocaine- and amphetamine-regulated transcript) system in appetite and drug addiction. *J. Pharmacol. Exp. Ther.*, **320**(2), 499–506. PM:16840648.

Vinson, D.C. (2006). Marijuana and other illicit drug use and the risk of injury: a case-control study. *Mo. Med.*, **103**(2), 152–156. PM:16703715.

Vlahov, D., Galea, S., Ahern, J., Resnick, H., & Kilpatrick, D. (2004). Sustained increased consumption of cigarettes, alcohol, and marijuana among Manhattan residents after September 11, 2001. *Am. J. Public Health*, **94**(2), 253–254. PM:14759935.

Voirin, N., Berthiller, J., Haim-Luzon, V., *et al.* (2006). Risk of lung cancer and past use of cannabis in Tunisia. *J. Thorac. Oncol.*, **1**(6), 577–579. PM:17409920.

Volcy, J., Nzerue, C.M., Oderinde, A., & Hewan-Iowe, K. (2000). Cocaine-induced acute renal failure, hemolysis, and thrombocytopenia mimicking thrombotic thrombocytopenic purpura. *Am. J. Kidney Dis.*, **35**(1), E3. PM:10620564.

Volkow, N.D., Chang, L., Wang, G.J., *et al.* (2001a). Higher cortical and lower subcortical metabolism in detoxified methamphetamine abusers. *Am. J. Psychiatry*, **158**(3), 383–389. PM:11229978.

Volkow, N.D., Chang, L., Wang, G.J., *et al.* (2001b). Association of dopamine transporter reduction with psychomotor impairment in methamphetamine abusers. *Am. J. Psychiatry*, **158**(3), 377–382. PM:11229977.

von Mondach, U. (2005). [Drug use in pregnancy.] *Ther. Umsch.*, **62**(1), 29–35. PM:15702704.

Vupputuri, S., Batuman, V., Muntner, P., *et al.* (2004). The risk for mild kidney function decline associated with illicit drug use among hypertensive men. *Am. J. Kidney Dis.*, **43**(4), 629–635. PM:15042540.

Walker, R., Hiller, M., Staton, M., & Leukefeld, C.G. (2003). Head injury among drug abusers: an indicator of co-occurring problems. *J. Psychoactive Drugs*, **35**(3), 343–353. PM:14621132.

Walsh, J.M., Flegel, R., Cangianelli, L.A., *et al.* (2004a). Epidemiology of alcohol and other drug use among motor vehicle crash victims admitted to a trauma center. *Traffic. Inj. Prev.*, **5**(3), 254–260. PM:15276926.

Walsh, J.M., Flegel, R., Cangianelli, L.A., *et al.* (2004b). Epidemiology of alcohol and other drug use among motor vehicle crash victims admitted to a trauma center. *Traffic. Inj. Prev.*, **5**(3), 254–260. PM:15276926.

Wang, E.S. (1991). Cocaine-induced iritis. *Ann. Emerg. Med.*, **20**(2), 192–193. PM:1996804.

Warner, E.A. (1993). Cocaine abuse. *Ann. Intern. Med.*, **119**(3), 226–235. PM:8323092.

Warner, E.A., Greene, G.S., Buchsbaum, M.S., Cooper, D.S., & Robinson, B.E. (1998). Diabetic ketoacidosis associated with cocaine use. *Arch. Intern. Med.*, **158**(16), 1799–1802. PM:9738609.

Warrian, W.G., Halikas, J.A., Crosby, R.D., Carlson, G.A., & Crea, F. (1992). Observations on increased CPK levels in "asymptomatic" cocaine abusers. *J. Addict. Dis.*, **11**(4), 83–95. PM:1486096.

Weathers, W.T., Crane, M.M., Sauvain, K.J., & Blackhurst, D.W. (1993). Cocaine use in women from a defined population: prevalence at delivery and effects on growth in infants. *Pediatrics*, **91**(2), 350–354. PM:8424009.

Webber, M.P. & Hauser, W.A. (1993). Secular trends in New York City hospital discharge diagnoses of congenital syphilis and cocaine dependence, 1982–88. *Public Health Rep.*, **108**(3), 279–284. PM:8497564.

Weber, J.E., Chudnofsky, C.R., Boczar, M., *et al.* (2000). Cocaine-associated chest pain: how common is myocardial infarction? *Acad. Emerg. Med.*, **7**(8), 873–877. PM:10958126.

Weddington, W.W., Brown, B.S., Haertzen, C.A., *et al.* (1990). Changes in mood, craving, and sleep during short-term abstinence reported by male cocaine addicts. A controlled, residential study. *Arch. Gen. Psychiatry,* **47**(9), 861–868. PM:2393345.

Westover, A.N., McBride, S., & Haley, R.W. (2007). Stroke in young adults who abuse amphetamines or cocaine: a population-based study of hospitalized patients. *Arch. Gen. Psychiatry,* **64**(4), 495–502. PM:17404126.

Westreich, R.W. & Lawson, W. (2004). Midline necrotizing nasal lesions: analysis of 18 cases emphasizing radiological and serological findings with algorithms for diagnosis and management. *Am. J. Rhinol.,* **18**(4), 209–219. PM:15490567.

Wetli, C.V. & Fishbain, D.A. (1985). Cocaine-induced psychosis and sudden death in recreational cocaine users. *J. Forensic Sci.,* **30**(3), 873–880. PM:4031813.

Wiesner, O., Russell, K.A., Lee, A.S., et al. (2004). Antineutrophil cytoplasmic antibodies reacting with human neutrophil elastase as a diagnostic marker for cocaine-induced midline destructive lesions but not autoimmune vasculitis. *Arthritis Rheum.,* **50**(9), 2954–2965. PM:15457464.

Wijetunga, M., Seto, T., Lindsay, J., & Schatz, I. (2003). Crystal methamphetamine-associated cardiomyopathy: tip of the iceberg? *J. Toxicol. Clin. Toxicol.,* **41**(7), 981–986. PM:14705845.

Wikner, B.N., Stiller, C.O., Bergman, U., Asker, C., & Kallen, B. (2007). Use of benzodiazepines and benzodiazepine receptor agonists during pregnancy: neonatal outcome and congenital malformations. *Pharmacoepidemiol. Drug Saf,* **16**(11), 1203–1210. PM:17894421.

Williams, J. & Wasserberger, J. (2006). Crack cocaine causing fatal vasoconstriction of the aorta. *J. Emerg. Med.,* **31**(2), 181–184. PM:17044582.

Williams, L.J., Correa, A., & Rasmussen, S. (2004). Maternal lifestyle factors and risk for ventricular septal defects. *Birth Defects Res. A Clin. Mol. Teratol.,* **70**(2), 59–64. PM:14991912.

Williams, M.A., Lieberman, E., Mittendorf, R., Monson, R.R., & Schoenbaum, S.C. (1991). Risk factors for abruptio placentae. *Am. J. Epidemiol.,* **134**(9), 965–972. PM:1951294.

Wilson, P.D., Loffredo, C.A., Correa-Villasenor, A., & Ferencz, C. (1998). Attributable fraction for cardiac malformations. *Am. J. Epidemiol.,* **148**(5), 414–423. PM:9737553.

Wilson, W.H., Ellinwood, E.H., Mathew, R.J., & Johnson, K. (1994). Effects of marijuana on performance of a computerized cognitive-neuromotor test battery. *Psychiatry Res.,* **51**(2), 115–125. PM:8022946.

Witter, F.R. & Niebyl, J.R. (1990). Marijuana use in pregnancy and pregnancy outcome. *Am. J. Perinatol.,* **7**(1), 36–38. PM:2294909.

Woolard, R., Nirenberg, T.D., Becker, B., et al. (2003). Marijuana use and prior injury among injured problem drinkers. *Acad. Emerg. Med.,* **10**(1), 43–51. PM:12511314.

World Health Organization (2002). *World Health Report 2002: Reducing Risks, Promoting Healthy Life.* Geneva: World Health Organization.

Yang, C.C., Yang, G.Y., Ger, J., Tsai, W.J., & Deng, J.F. (1995). Severe rhabdomyolysis mimicking transverse myelitis in a heroin addict. *J. Toxicol. Clin. Toxicol.,* **33**(6), 591–595. PM:8523478.

Yeo, K.K., Wijetunga, M., Ito, H., et al. (2007). The association of methamphetamine use and cardiomyopathy in young patients. *Am. J. Med.,* **120**(2), 165–171. PM:17275458.

Yewell, J., Haydon, R., Archer, S., & Manaligod, J.M. (2002). Complications of intranasal prescription narcotic abuse. *Ann. Otol. Rhinol. Laryngol.,* **111**(2), 174–177. PM:11860072.

Young, M.E., Rintala, D.H., Rossi, C.D., Hart, K.A., & Fuhrer, M.J. (1995). Alcohol and marijuana use in a community-based sample of persons with spinal cord injury. *Arch. Phys. Med. Rehabil.,* **76**(6), 525–532. PM:7763151.

Zachariah, S.B. (1991). Stroke after heavy marijuana smoking. *Stroke,* **22**(3), 406–409. PM:2003312.

Zakzanis, K.K. & Campbell, Z. (2006). Memory impairment in now abstinent MDMA users and continued users: a longitudinal follow-up. *Neurology,* **66**(5), 740–741. PM:16534114.

Zakzanis, K.K. & Young, D.A. (2001). Memory impairment in abstinent MDMA ("ecstasy") users: a longitudinal investigation. *Neurology,* **56**(7), 966–969. PM:11294938.

Zandio, A.B., Erro Aguirre, M.E., Cabada, T., & Ayuso, B.T. (2008). [Cocaine-induced brain stem stroke associated to craneal midline destructive lesions.] *Neurologia*, **23**(1), 55–58. PM:18365781.

Zaretsky, A., Rector, N.A., Seeman, M.V., & Fornazzari, X. (1993). Current cannabis use and tardive dyskinesia. *Schizophr. Res.*, **11**(1), 3–8. PM:7905284.

Zhang, H. & Bracken, M.B. (1996). Tree-based, two-stage risk factor analysis for spontaneous abortion. *Am. J. Epidemiol.*, **144**(10), 989–996. PM:8916510.

Zhang, Z.F., Morgenstern, H., Spitz, M.R., *et al.* (1999). Marijuana use and increased risk of squamous cell carcinoma of the head and neck. *Cancer Epidemiol. Biomarkers Prev.*, **8**(12), 1071–1078. PM:10613339.

Zhou, W., Lin, P.H., Bush, R.L., Nguyen, L., & Lumsden, A.B. (2004). Acute arterial thrombosis associated with cocaine abuse. *J. Vasc. Surg.*, **40**(2), 291–295. PM:15297823.

Zimmerman, J.L., Dellinger, R.P., & Majid, P.A. (1991). Cocaine-associated chest pain. *Ann. Emerg. Med.*, **20**(6), 611–615. PM:2039098.

Ziring, D., Wei, B., Velazquez, P., *et al.* (2006). Formation of B and T cell subsets require the cannabinoid receptor CB2. *Immunogenetics*, **58**(9), 714–725. PM:16924491.

Index

Note: page numbers in *italics* refer to tables

Printed in the United States
by Baker & Taylor Publisher Services